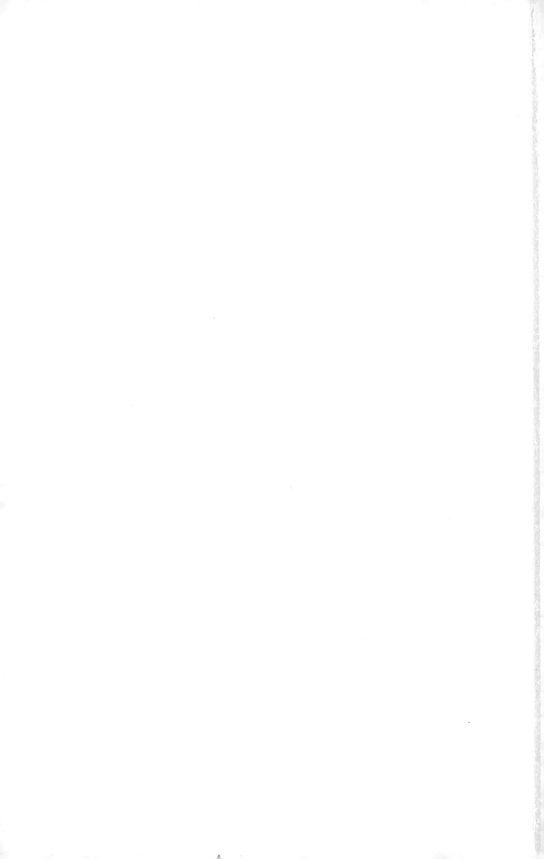

Praise for

EMF*D

"Dr. Mercola's groundbreaking new book on the health effects of EMFs is both a sobering tale and an effective call to action. Dr. Mercola carefully lays out the history and evidence for the deleterious effects of EMF exposure and gives you real time, concrete steps to take to mitigate the damage for you and your family. As a result of reading this important book, I am redoubling my efforts to protect my family and patients from the harmful effects of EMFs, especially in light of the 5G rollout. This is a fight that involves us all, and Dr. Mercola's book can help to light the way in this important struggle."

— **Thomas Cowan, M.D.**, author of *Human Heart, Cosmic Heart*;
Vaccines, Autoimmunity, and the Changing Nature of Childhood Illness;
and *Cancer and the New Biology of Water*

"Ten years ago, my declining health improved overnight after one simple change to my electrical exposures. If I had known about the health effects of wireless and electrical exposures fifteen years ago, it would have saved over a decade of deep personal pain and suffering. Please read this book and share what you have learned to protect yourself and the ones you love."

— **Peter Sullivan**, founder of Clear Light Ventures

"Want to know how EMFs impact your health? This book gives a masterful account of why our lives and our planet are becoming EMF*D up and what we can do about it. Readable and balanced, it's a must-read for anyone truly interested in safeguarding their health."

— **Lloyd Burrell**, author of *EMF Practical Guide* and
founder of ElectricSense.com

"5G technology holds the promise for faster connections, greater bandwidth, low latency, a massive internet-of-things, and smart cities. What's not to like about that? Dr. Mercola has written an easy-to-read and comprehensive book explaining what we know about the potential adverse biological effects of a massive increase in our exposure to EMFs if/when 5G becomes widely available. Even if you don't use the technology, you can't opt out because it will be everywhere. This book is the go-to place if you want to become informed about the dangers of EMFs."

— **Stephanie Seneff, Ph.D.**, senior research scientist,
MIT Computer Science and Artificial Intelligence Laboratory

"Dr. Joseph Mercola's latest book—*EMF*D*—introduces the reader to the concept that electronic and wireless technology emits frequencies in the form of dirty electricity and microwave radiation that can harm and are harming our health. This books comes at an interesting time when governments around the world are racing to roll out 5G, 5th generation, wireless technology, without any testing of the biological and health effects of long-term exposure.
As we are increasingly exposed to more radiation via smart meters, smart appliances, Wi-Fi in schools, and now 5G small cell antennas placed on lamp posts every 100 meters or so, a growing number of people are asking, 'Why the rush to 5G?' and 'Do we really need this technology?' It is no longer enough for us to eat organic, drink purified water, inhale fresh air, exercise, and get plenty of sleep to stay healthy. We must also minimize our exposure to the harmful effects of electromagnetic pollution. Learn how to reduce your exposure and how to repair EMF-related damage by reading Dr. Mercola's book, *EMF*D*. You won't be disappointed!"

— **Dr. Magda Havas, B.Sc., Ph.D.**, Professor Emerita,
Trent University, Canada

"Dr. Joseph Mercola has written the definitive book on electromagnetic fields, with a particular emphasis on how they affect our health. This is an invaluable resource with many practical solutions, especially for those who are EMF-sensitive. For those who don't yet know about EMFs or who refuse to take them seriously, it will be harder to ignore them after reading this book. Everyone needs to know about the dangers of EMFs. This comprehensive manual will help accomplish that."

— **Oram Miller**, certified building biology environmental
consultant and electromagnetic radiation specialist

EMF*D

EMF*D

5G, Wi-Fi & Cell Phones: Hidden Harms and How to Protect Yourself

DR. JOSEPH MERCOLA

HAY HOUSE, INC.

Carlsbad, California • New York City

London • Sydney • New Delhi

Published in the United States by: Hay House, Inc.: www.hayhouse.com®
Published in Australia by: Hay House Australia Pty. Ltd.: www.hayhouse.com.au
Published in the United Kingdom by: Hay House UK, Ltd.: www.hayhouse.co.uk
Published in India by: Hay House Publishers India: www.hayhouse.co.in

Cover design: Jason Gabbert
Interior design: Nick C. Welch
Indexer: J S Editorial, LLC

Image on page 33 reprinted from *The Lancet Planetary Health*, Vol. 2, no. 12, Priyanka Bandara and David O. Carpenter, "Planetary electromagnetic pollution: it is time to assess its impact," pages e512–e514, copyright 2018, with permission from Elsevier.

Illustration on page 153 reprinted from *Ageing Research Reviews*, Vol. 47, Keisuke Yaku, Keisuke Okabe, and Takashi Nakagawa, "NAD metabolism: Implications in aging and longevity," pages 1–17, copyright 2018, with permission from Elsevier.

Cataloging-in-Publication Data is on file at the Library of Congress

Hardcover ISBN: 978-1-4019-5875-6
e-book ISBN: 978-1-4019-5876-3
Audiobook ISBN: 978-1-4019-5877-0

11 10 9 8 7 6 5 4 3 2
1st edition, February 2020

Printed in the United States of America

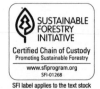

SFI label applies to the text stock

ALSO BY DR. JOSEPH MERCOLA

KetoFast*

KetoFast Cookbook (with Pete Evans)*

Superfuel (with James DiNicolantonio)*

Fat for Fuel*

The Fat for Fuel Ketogenic Cookbook (with Pete Evans)*

Effortless Healing

The No-Grain Diet

Sweet Deception

Dark Deception

The Great Bird Flu Hoax

Freedom at Your Fingertips

Generation XL

Healthy Recipes for Your Nutritional Type

*Available from Hay House
Please visit:

Hay House USA: www.hayhouse.com®
Hay House Australia: www.hayhouse.com.au
Hay House UK: www.hayhouse.co.uk
Hay House India: www.hayhouse.co.in

***

CONTENTS

INTRODUCTION

For many decades in the mid-20th century, cigarette smoking was common practice. People smoked at home, work, and school, while eating at restaurants, driving in cars, and flying on planes. A pack of cigarettes was proudly displayed in most men's shirt pockets and lay nestled in women's purses.

Fast forward to the present. Smoking is outlawed in nearly all public spaces and tobacco use has greatly declined. But cigarettes were such a mainstay of daily life and communal culture throughout the world that it was difficult to imagine things any other way.

We know now that the tobacco industry became aware of the disastrous health effects of smoking in the 1950s, yet it hid the accumulating evidence from the public whom it relied on to buy its products. For decades, the public was blatantly lied to about the safety of cigarettes.

It wasn't until a few brave whistleblowers brought the hidden research and manipulative industry tactics to light that our government began taking steps to reduce dependence on tobacco products. But hundreds of millions of lives worldwide were likely prematurely lost in those intervening years.

As the calendar turned over to the 21st century, something began replacing all of those packs of cigarettes in shirt pockets and purses: cell phones. In the two decades since the turn of the millennium, these communication devices that were once a novelty have become an inescapable part of modern life.

Sadly, smoking and cell phones have more in common than their popularity. They also share the fact that they are each an enormous threat to individual and public health.

The danger of cell phones doesn't come from the cell phones themselves, but from their *electromagnetic fields* (otherwise known as EMFs) that your cell phone—and other electronic devices that communicate wirelessly—use to function.

EMFs are invisible to your eyes and exist in a spectrum of frequencies that include radio and TV waves, microwaves, visible light, ultraviolet light, X-rays, and radioactive elements. Some sources of EMFs are natural, such as sunlight, while others are man-made—such as the energy used to cook foods by micro-wave ovens.

These EMFs have demonstrable negative physiological effects, but very few people fully grasp this. We have been lulled into a false sense of security by an industry that is going to great lengths to keep us in the dark, just like in the early days of smoking.

And our government appears endlessly willing, even eager, to allow technology companies to do pretty much whatever they want—including spending mountains of money to dissuade leg-islators from passing laws that would regulate an industry that is making it harder and harder to understand what the dangers are, much less avoid them.

WHAT YOU CAN'T SEE *CAN* HURT YOU

A conservative estimate is that 3 percent of the population has *electrohypersensitivity*, which means they experience palpable symptoms—headaches, insomnia, fatigue, heart palpitations, sen-sations of skin prickling—when they are exposed to EMFs. The rest of us can't feel EMFs.

But that doesn't mean that the EMFs you are exposed to aren't causing damage.

The wireless industry and the government agencies that are supposed to regulate this industry want you to believe that the science is settled and wireless exposures are safe. Unfortunately, this message is not reality. EMF damage can manifest in myriad ways that include many conditions that are occurring in ever-increasing amounts, such as decreased sperm counts, impaired sleep, anxiety, depression, Alzheimer's disease, and cancer.

I first heard the concerns that cell phones might be harmful more than 20 years ago. At the time, I agreed that it made sense, but I failed to take any action. The truth is, I simply didn't want to believe this to be true. As far as I could tell, the science was ambiguous at best.

And even if it were true, I figured my healthy diet and lifestyle would be more than enough to compensate for these relatively "inconsequential" exposures—sadly, one of the more foolish professional assumptions I have ever made. Hard to believe it, but I fell for the wireless industry's propaganda.

I now see that unless you take serious action to lower your EMF exposure, you will not be able to achieve full health, no matter how carefully you eat or how strategic you are in your lifestyle choices.

I suspect many of you are in the same boat as I was, and you shouldn't feel bad. After all, the wireless industry has far greater resources at its disposal than the tobacco industry ever did.

THE THREAT WILL ONLY CONTINUE TO GROW

I understand that the news I'm delivering may be disheartening. After all, cell phones and Wi-Fi offer incredibly useful conveniences. And they are ubiquitous: Few of us are ever more than a few feet from our cell phones at any given time—even during sleep.

We spend most of our working hours an arm's distance away from a computer that is connected wirelessly to the Internet. We live in homes, neighborhoods, and cities that are in direct and constant contact with these fields through electrical wiring, microwave ovens, cell phone towers, and Wi-Fi.

As society adopts ever more wireless technologies, we are increasingly bathed in high intensities of EMFs. Some EMFs are emitted by devices we own and use ourselves, but even if you refused to ever buy a cell phone or wireless router, you would still be exposed to ever-increasing amounts of EMFs thanks to the growing number of cell towers, wireless hot spots, and satellites that are used to broadcast these signals.

To make matters worse, with the advent of 5G (or the "fifth generation" of cell phone technology) that is rolling out as I write this, your EMF exposures—and the health and environmental ramifications they bring—are about to increase exponentially. By the time this book is in your hands, you will likely have access to 5G if you live in a large urban area.

As you'll learn more about in the chapters ahead, some of the EMFs that 5G will use require new technologies to transmit and receive signals. This means we are about to experience an explosion in new antennas. And all the signals from all of those additional antennas and base stations will be layered on top of the EMF swamp that we are already swimming in.

These new EMFs have never been tested for long-term safety on humans, not to mention microbes, insects, animals, and plants. This means we are all participants in a massive involuntary public health experiment. Once you read this book, however, you won't be an unwitting participant—you'll know what you're being exposed to, as well as what you need to do to protect yourself.

And that's really what this book is about—giving you knowledge so you can minimize health risks for yourself and your family.

After all, if you don't know the risks you're taking every day when you slide your cell phone into your pocket or hold it to your head, buy a smart appliance, or upgrade to a 5G phone, you're essentially gambling with your health, your life span, and even your ability to have children.

Worse yet, you're gambling with your children's health, their life spans, and their ability to have children (which is especially concerning as many children are allowed to start interacting with cell phones—whether to watch a video or just haphazardly press buttons—in an effort to keep them occupied as early as six months old.) [1]

If we don't start taking widespread action to mitigate this ticking time bomb soon, we will be EMF*d.

Am I saying you need to do away with all useful technology? Or even just cell phones and Wi-Fi? Certainly not. But I am saying that you and your family would benefit from educated measures to reduce your exposure to the radiation these technological developments expose you to. I wrote this book to help you do just that.

It is time to take a closer look at the risks of convenient wireless connectivity so that we can mitigate them. After all, you can't correct a problem you don't know you have.

HOW TO USE THIS BOOK

As in all of my work, I want to give you the information you need so that you can understand your options for improving your health and make empowered and informed choices.

To do that, I have organized this book so that by the end of it you will understand:

- Just what EMFs are and how they work
- How the science proves that EMFs are dangerous, as well as how companies and government agencies have conspired—and continue to conspire—to keep this science hidden
- Exactly how EMFs damage your body

- How to repair the damage that has already occurred

- How to curb your EMF exposure and reduce your risk of incurring future damage

Reading this book may be challenging at times: Some of the information is highly technical. I aim to make it as digestible as possible. While some of it may be upsetting, this book will empower you to make choices that will lead to your improved, long-lasting, and radiant health.

It is imperative that you begin making those choices now, because if you wait for the telecommunications industry or the government to protect you, you will be waiting for far too long. There is simply no more time to wait.

CHAPTER 1

UNDERSTANDING EMFS

Think of all the modern electronic conveniences you use throughout the course of your day. The list is practically endless: your dishwasher, oven, washer and dryer, heater, air conditioner, television, computer, and let's not forget your cell phone.

All these devices are powered by an invisible mix of both electric and magnetic energy. In the past few decades, these devices, along with wireless Internet and Wi-Fi, have transformed life as we know it, providing incredible conveniences.

But at what cost?

The enormous time-saving benefits of these amenities make it easy to ignore the harm they may cause. For decades, many well-respected researchers have had serious concerns about the health effects of EMFs. To help you understand the negative impact of wireless EMFs, you need a basic grasp of what EMFs are, how they work, and how they affect things they encounter. That's what you'll find in this chapter.

WHAT ARE EMFS?

Let's keep it simple. There are many different types of EMFs. Each has its own frequency, which is the number of waves that will pass through a fixed point per second. Frequency is measured in units called Hertz, which is named after the 19th century German physicist Heinrich Hertz and abbreviated Hz. One thousand Hz is a kilohertz (KHz), one million Hz is a megahertz, and one billion Hz is a gigahertz (GHz).

As I mentioned in the introduction, EMFs come from both natural sources, such as lightning and sunlight, and man-made sources, such as cell phones, Wi-Fi routers, electrical wiring, and microwaves. They exist in a spectrum, from extremely low frequency (3 Hz to 300 Hz) all the way up to gamma rays, which have a frequency greater than 10^{22} Hz.

You can see the spectrum in the chart below.

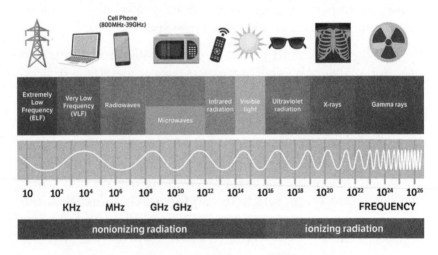

Figure 1.1: The spectrum of EMFs.

As you can also see from this chart, EMFs are typically classified into two major groups: *ionizing* and *nonionizing radiation.*

Ionizing means that that particular EMF has enough energy to disrupt the structure of an atom by knocking off one or more of its tightly bound electrons, transforming that previously neutral atom into an ion with a positive charge.

Ions are a problem because they can produce free radicals. Free radicals are simply molecules that have become ionized and have not found anything to latch on to so as to remove their unbalanced charge. They behave like loose cannons in the ordered and civilized world of your cell's biochemistry.

Free radicals by themselves are not dangerous as your body requires a certain level to stay healthy, but when they are produced in excess quantities they become problematic. They can attack the complex and precisely formed molecules of your cell membranes, proteins, stem cells, and mitochondria and convert them to damaged, and in many cases useless, forms.

Ionizing radiation can also cause DNA damage. This is an undisputed fact, and explains why any time you have ever gotten an X-ray (a form of ionizing radiation) , you have likely been given a protective lead apron to cover your torso and shield your organs from exposure.

The major types of ionizing radiation are: neutrons from radioactive elements like uranium, alpha particles, beta particles, X-rays, and gamma rays. Since alpha and beta particles can be stopped by physical barriers, such as a sheet of paper or an aluminum plate, they are not typically of much concern. But neutrons from radioactive elements and X- and gamma rays are far more penetrating, and exposure to them can cause serious biological damage.[1,2]

Exposure Levels of Different Sources
of Ionizing Radiation

Ionizing radiation exposure	Dose in millirems
Background	0.006
Chest X-ray	10
Flying at 35,000 feet	0.6/hour
CT scan	200–1,000

Data above compiled from the U.S. Nuclear Regulatory Commission.[3]

Nonionizing radiation does not have enough energy to create ions, and thus it has been generally regarded as safe and biologically "harmless" for decades. But we are now learning that there are other mechanisms by which nonionizing radiation can cause damage to living cells.

As you can see in the graphic on page 2, nonionizing radiation is produced by electronics such as cell phones and other wireless devices including baby monitors, cordless phones, and smart appliances.

The classification of nonionizing radiation as universally "safe" in appropriate exposures has been proven to be false, though many still cling to it. (I will explore the science behind this claim further in Chapter 4.)

Not all forms of nonionizing radiation are damaging. The graphic also shows that visible and infrared light are forms of nonionizing radiation; both are important for human health. It is well established that exposure to these forms of light is necessary for optimal health.

And yet, when you review the research and become aware of the efforts made to distort or suppress its findings, you will see compelling proof that nonionizing EMFs have the ability to cause great harm to your health.

Top 6 Sources of EMFs in Your Home

The following devices emit the vast majority of the EMFs you are exposed to in your home. I will cover how to replace these devices, or reduce the level of EMFs they emit, in Chapter 7; for now, put as much distance as you can between yourself and these devices, as proximity increases exposure exponentially.

- Cell phones, laptops, and tablets
- Wi-Fi routers
- Cordless DECT phones (digital enhanced cordless technology)
- Microwave ovens
- Bluetooth devices, such as headphones, AirPods, fitness trackers, keyboards, wireless mice, printers, baby monitors, hearing aids, speakers, gaming consoles and controllers, Amazon Echo and Alexa-enabled devices, any "smart" device including virtually any new TV
- Smart electric, gas, and water meters

BOTH IONIZING AND NONIONIZING RADIATION DAMAGE DNA (JUST VIA DIFFERENT MEANS)

How can nonionizing radiation sometimes be good and sometimes be bad?

To help you understand this seeming contradiction, allow me to drill down a little more deeply on why both ionizing and nonionizing radiation can be so dangerous.

First, I'll explain how ionizing radiation damages your body. As I mentioned earlier, ionizing radiation easily passes through every tissue in your body. It can knock electrons out of the orbit of atoms and turn them into destructive ions that can create damaging free radicals.

One of the most concerning aspects of this process is when the ionizing radiation passes through the nucleus of your cells where most of your DNA is stored. It has enough energy to directly break some of the covalent bonds in your DNA. This is the way that ionizing radiation causes genetic damage, which can then lead to cell death or cancer.

There is also an indirect way that ionizing radiation damages DNA, and that is by converting the water in your nucleus into one of the most dangerous free radicals in your body, the *hydroxyl free radical*. This highly unstable hydroxyl free radical can then go on to cause its own DNA destruction.

This direct and indirect DNA damage by ionizing radiation is illustrated in the graphic below.

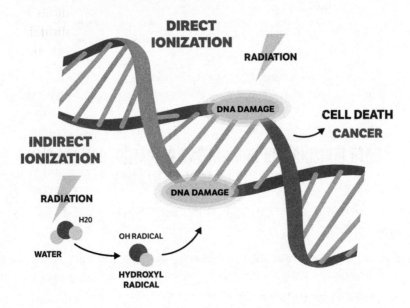

Figure 1.2: How X-rays damage your DNA.

For many years the wireless industry and the federal regulatory agencies have insisted that nonionizing radiation cannot cause DNA damage because it does not have enough energy to directly break DNA bonds.

The concept that nonionizing radiation, the type emitted by your cell phone and Wi-Fi, can cause similar genetic damage as ionizing radiation, is highly controversial. The reason why this issue is so confusing is largely because nonionizing radiation from your wireless devices causes biologic damage by an entirely different mechanism than ionizing radiation.

It's true that nonionizing radiation, by definition, doesn't have enough energy to directly break the covalent bonds in your DNA or produce hydroxyl radicals that do the same. However, wireless radiation results in DNA and biologic damage that is nearly identical to the harm caused by ionizing radiation. It just does it in a different way that very few people are aware of.

Nonionizing radiation from your wireless devices actually creates carbonyl free radicals—instead of the hydroxyl radicals that ionizing radiation gives rise to—that cause virtually identical damage to your nuclear DNA, cell membranes, proteins, mitochondria, and stem cells.

Of course, the full extent of the process is more involved than this simple explanation, which is why I delve deep into the science of how EMFs from nonionizing radiation cause damage in Chapter 4, where you will learn why the nonionizing radiation you are exposed to every day from your wireless devices and Wi-Fi are collectively far more dangerous to you than ionizing radiation.

THE CURRENT WIRELESS SAFETY STANDARDS ARE DANGEROUSLY FLAWED

As a result of the coordinated and costly efforts of the wireless industry, you and your family are left woefully unprotected by the current federal safety guidelines because they are fundamentally flawed.

The Federal Communications Commission (FCC) establishes safety guidelines for the radiation emitted by cell phones by using what's known as a *specific anthropomorphic mannequin* (SAM)—a plastic facsimile of a human head filled with liquid designed to mimic the absorption rate of brain tissue—to determine what's known as *specific absorption rate* (SAR).

The only value of the SAR reading is to measure the short-term thermal effect of the radiation on your body. As I discuss at length in Chapter 4, though, the primary way EMFs damage your body is not through heat but through changes at the cellular level, which the SAR reading does not measure.

There are many additional problems with the SAR:

- SAM is modeled on a six-foot-two-inch man who weighs more than 200 pounds and thus is significantly larger than most of the U.S. population, particularly women and children.

- SAR values are reported to the FCC by phone manufacturers and have been known to vary from the reported number by a factor of two across models of the same phone.

- The SAR value varies with the source of exposure and the person using the phone. For example, if you are in a rural area or in an elevator or a car, where the cell phone uses more power, your brain will get a greater exposure from the higher power required in these instances. Under certain conditions, the SAR value can be 10 to 100 times higher than reported.

- Holding the phone in a slightly different way can actually render the worst SAR value phone less harmful than the best SAR value phone.

Perhaps you might be lulled into purchasing a low SAR phone to ease your mind. But this would be a false sense of security, because the SAR rating has *nothing* to do with the true biological damage done by the EMFs emitted by cell phones. It is merely a gauge of the intensity of the heating effect, which provides only the benefit of being able to compare the SAR of one phone to another.

Even if a low SAR rating did reflect a phone's potential for harm, you would probably still be at risk. All mobile phone manufacturers recommend that you hold your phone at least 5 to 15 millimeters away from your body. Yet very few are aware of this directive. Sadly, your phone company buried it deep within the cell phone manual, which virtually no one ever reads.

Even with all their inaccuracies as an estimate of biological damage, SAR ratings can provide some benefit, as higher ratings are correlated with higher RF radiation and should correspond to greater cellular damage.

Finally, the FCC and other regulatory bodies around the world derive their standards from work done by a private group called the International Commission on Non-Ionizing Radiation Protection (ICNIRP). The ICNIRP even stated in 1998:

> These guidelines are based on short-term, immediate health effects such as stimulation of peripheral nerves and muscles, shocks and burns caused by touching conducting objects, and elevated tissue temperatures resulting from absorption of energy during exposure to EMF.[4]

In other words, they are only intended to "protect" from short-term exposure, and as you'll read more about in Chapter 2, the diseases of EMFs—especially brain cancer—can take decades to develop.

To top it all off, the ICNIRP has also been recently criticized by the group of investigative journalists called Investigate Europe as being part of an industry-controlled cartel of industry-favorable regulatory agencies. [5]

You need to understand that you simply *cannot* determine the safety of your phone from the SAR standards currently set by the FCC.

THE IMPORTANCE OF PULSED VS. NON-PULSED EMFS

In addition to the distinction between ionizing and nonionizing, there is another classification of EMFs that you should be familiar with so you can understand the science I will review in the chapters to come—the difference between alternating current (AC), which is pulsed, and direct current (DC), which is non-pulsed.

An AC charge moves in two different directions, and switches between these directions in regular pulses, similar to your heartbeat. Our electric grid delivers an AC that pulses 60 times per second, known as 60 Hertz (Hz) in the United States and 50 Hz in most countries outside the U.S.

Direct current (DC) electricity, on the other hand, flows only in one direction. DC currents are what you experience in nature. The Earth creates a DC magnetic and electric field. DC electricity is based on the idea of a battery sending the electrons in one direction. All batteries are DC.

Your body's nervous system does the same and uses DC for synapses and signals. The sodium-potassium pump in your cells is essentially a battery that produces DC current. As such, your body is designed to work with DC current.

As I discuss a little later in this chapter, Thomas Edison popularized DC current and that was what people started using when electricity was first distributed to the public. The reason that we use AC electricity over DC electricity is because Nikola Tesla found out that AC can travel greater distances than DC without significant reduction in voltage, which is the pressure of electricity.

This is most unfortunate, because using DC to power the electric grid would have been a far better biological solution—since living organisms have been regularly exposed throughout their biological evolution to the Earth's static electric and magnetic fields, our bodies tolerate DC far better than AC.

In fact, when there are variations of more than 20 percent in the Earth's natural electromagnetic fields during magnetic storms or geomagnetic pulsations that occur approximately every 11 years due to changes in solar activity cycles, there are increased rates of animal and human health incidents, including nervous and psychiatric diseases, hypertensive crises, heart attacks, cerebral accidents, and mortality. [6,7]

Since living organisms do not have defenses against variations of greater than 20 percent of natural EMFs, it is realistic to expect that they do not have defenses against man-made EMFs, which vary unpredictably and at 100 percent or more from average intensity.

To make matters even worse, wireless signals use several different frequencies simultaneously, making the variability even higher. This is likely why living organisms perceive the pulsation of man-made EMFs as an environmental stressor. [8]

For example, it was found that a 2.8 GHz EMF pulsed on 500 Hz was significantly more effective in increasing heart rate in rats than the corresponding continuous wave (unpulsed) 2.8 GHz EMF with the same average intensity and exposure duration.[9]

Also researchers found exposure to 900 MHz radio-frequency (RF) pulses caused changes in human EEGs (diagnostic tests of brain activity), while the corresponding carrier wave signal (same frequency but continuous instead of pulsed) with the same exposure duration did not. [10]

EXTREMELY LOW FREQUENCY EMFS

Most of the EMFs that I cover in this book—primarily those used by cell phones and wireless devices—are classified as very low frequencies and higher. But there is a category of EMFs beneath this group, and that is *extremely low frequencies* (ELFs). ELFs have a frequency between 0 and 300 Hz, and are emitted by power lines, electrical wiring, and electrical appliances, such as hairdryers.

But there are also ELFs associated with regular wireless signals in the form of pulsing and modulation. There is some evidence indicating that the effects of these wireless EMFs on living organisms are due to the included ELFs.[11,12] Moreover, ELFs alone are found independently to be bioactive.[13,14] As you'll read in Chapter 5, there have been many studies on the link between exposure to power lines and breast cancer, impaired sleep, and childhood leukemia.

The potential for ELF exposure to negatively impact health seems to be highest when the ELFs are pulsed. For example, researchers found that a 1.8 GHz RF signal amplitude-modulated by pulsing ELFs caused DNA damage in cultured human cells, while the same signal with an unmodulated continuous wave with the same exposure duration was ineffective.[15]

Common Sources of ELFs

- Power lines
- Electrical wiring
- Electric blankets
- All electrical appliances

MAGNETIC FIELDS VS. ELECTRIC FIELDS

Electromagnetic fields have two components—an electric field and a magnetic field. The Earth has a geomagnetic field, as our planet is essentially one large magnet—its magnetic field is what allows compasses to work and empowers migratory animals to know which way to travel. Your body has a magnetic field too—both these natural magnetic fields are DC, and measured in units of either tesla (T) or gauss (G).

An electric current naturally generates a magnetic field around it. If you've ever played with two magnets, you've already experienced the fact that a magnetic field quickly gets weaker with distance.

However, there is some evidence that magnetic fields have a danger all their own.

THE HEALTH EFFECTS OF MAGNETIC FIELDS

Much of the research into the health effects of magnetic fields has been related to increases in childhood leukemia and brain cancers. A study that scanned a collection of data from 1997 through 2013 examined 11,699 cases and 13,194 controls and concluded that "magnetic field level exposure may be associated with childhood leukemia."[16]

These studies are some of the research that the World Health Organization refers to when admitting that some types of EMFs are indeed related to cancers, are biologically harmful, and should be limited.

Common Indoor Sources of Magnetic Fields

- Faulty wiring and/or grounding issues
- Circuit breaker boxes
- Electric stoves
- Refrigerator motors
- Hair dryers
- Current on metal water pipes (usually found in houses with metal pipes that are on city water)
- Current on other components of the metal grounding system, including TV cable sheathing, indoor metal gas lines, and air ducts
- Point sources, including transformers and motors

Furthermore, in 1979 Nancy Wertheimer and physicist Ed Leeper found that childhood leukemia rates doubled versus controls for children subjected to only 3 milligauss of magnetic field exposure when in the vicinity of neighborhood distribution power lines in Denver.[17] This finding was also repeated in a 1988 study conducted by the New York State Department of Health.[18]

There is also research linking higher levels of exposure to magnetic fields during pregnancy and an increased risk of miscarriage.[19,20]

ANOTHER SOURCE OF RADIATION THAT IS HARMFUL TO YOUR HEALTH: DIRTY ELECTRICITY

This type of EMF is a specific type of electric and magnetic field known by a few different names: the most common one is *dirty electricity* and the most accurate one is *high-frequency voltage transients. Electromagnetic interference* (EMI) is another term frequently used to describe dirty electricity.

Many EMF experts now use the additional term *microsurge electrical pollution,* or MEP, to describe dirty electricity, and define dirty electricity as all electric and magnetic fields from any frequency above 50/60 Hz (which is the fundamental frequency of electricity from electric utilities around the world).

These transients typically occur whenever alternating current (AC) electricity that runs along power lines (with a frequency standardized to 60 Hz in North America and 50 Hz in the rest of the world) is manipulated into other types of electricity (such as direct current, or DC), when it is transformed to another voltage using what's called a *switched mode power supply,* or its flow is interrupted.

Dirty electricity most often ranges from 2,000 Hz (2 kHz) to 100,000 Hz (100 kHz). This is a very special range as it is the frequency in which electric and magnetic fields most easily couple to your body, causing biological damage through a mechanism I will describe later in the book.

The primary way dirty electricity occurs throughout the world is when an electric motor that uses an AC switching power supply is run, such as in your air conditioner, refrigerator, kitchen blender, TV, or computer. The good news about these sources of dirty electricity is that they are locally produced and easily remediated with filters; I will cover exactly how to do that in Chapter 7.

In North America, however, there is another common source of dirty electricity: electric utility substations that deliver power to the community but fail to separate the returning neutral wires from the grounding line from each user back to the utility substation.

Instead, utilities use the cheaper route and allow the actual ground to return a good deal of the current, as the Earth is a conductor of electricity. Since dirty electricity rides along with 60 Hz electricity wherever it goes, this practice contaminates soil with dirty electricity.

Another common source of dirty electricity is compact fluorescent light bulbs. They create dirty electricity because they have a switched mode power supply in their base that converts the 60 Hz AC current first into DC current and then changes the voltage into a higher frequency, typically around 50,000 Hz (50 kHz).

Not only do fluorescent bulbs create dirty electricity, but they also produce digital light with an unhealthy spectrum that is predominately blue, which disrupts your melatonin levels if you view it after sunset. So, an excellent strategy to improve your health is to limit your exposure to fluorescent lights at home and the office.

Newer electronic dimmer switches, which modulate the level of light emitted by bulbs by turning the power source on and off—very quickly for brighter light and more slowly for dimmer light—are also significant sources of dirty electricity. (Older rheostat-based dimmers from decades ago do not cause dirty electricity.)

Computers, monitors, and TVs create dirty electricity because their various components run on DC electricity. They also use switched mode power supplies to convert AC to the various DC voltages, and it is those components that emit the dirty electricity.

Cell phone towers themselves are a substantial source of dirty electricity. When I interviewed Sam Milham, an M.D. and M.P.H. epidemiologist and author of *Dirty Electricity*,[21] on my website, mercola.com, he pointed out:

> Every cell tower in the world makes dirty electricity by the ton. Lots of schools have cell towers on campus. What they're doing is they're bathing the kids [with EMI, or electromagnetic interference—dirty electricity]. It gets back into the wires; the ground wires and power wires that service it. The grid becomes an antenna for all this dirty electricity, which then extends miles downstream.

Solar panels and wind turbines are also major contributors to dirty electricity levels, or rather, their inverters are. Solar panels generate low-voltage DC electricity, which isn't usable by either the wiring in your home or the power grid. So the panels are usually connected to an inverter, which converts the DC into AC and raises the voltage to 120 volts.

Many people who have installed solar panels (photovoltaic panels) on their homes are completely unaware of the fact that their inverters are a source of dirty electricity. Large, commercial solar arrays have a similar problem, as they also use inverters— sometimes thousands of them if they're really big arrays—and they all generate EMI or dirty electricity.

When I had my solar panels installed at my home many years ago, I was unaware of this problem. Once I learned of the issue, I was able to remediate this powerful source of dirty electricity, and I will share how you can do this too later in the book. This is important because it is clear that the country is moving rapidly toward renewable energy, which uses these inverters that produce dirty electricity. So eventually it will be a problem for most of us.

Common Sources of Dirty Electricity

- Compact fluorescent bulbs (CFLs)
- Cordless phones
- Fans with multiple speeds
- Most energy-efficient appliances and furnaces, as they are likely saving energy by turning the current on and off repeatedly
- Many LED lights
- Computers and laptops
- Any electronic appliance with a transformer box at the end of the power cord
- Hair dryers
- Dimmer switches
- Refrigerators
- Printers
- Cell phone chargers
- Televisions
- Wi-Fi routers
- Smart utility meters
- Smart appliances
- Cell towers
- Solar panel inverters

HOW DID WE GET HERE? THE EARLY HISTORY OF EMFS

In my book *Fat for Fuel*, I chronicled how processed vegetable oils, such as cottonseed, soybean, and canola, debuted at the end of the 19th century and then proliferated through the food system at an ever-expanding rate—as did incidences of heart disease.

The relationship between the rise in electrification and chronic diseases follows an eerily similar trajectory and, I believe, presents a compelling reason why this electrification—and the expansion of devices that emit EMFs that came along with it—is one of the primary reasons for the epidemic of chronic diseases that we are now experiencing.

THOMAS EDISON HERALDS INTRODUCTION OF FIRST ELECTRICAL SERVICES

It seems like we've always had instant and widespread access to electrical power, but the reality is that it never really existed prior to 150 years ago. And it took nearly another 75 years before it became widely available in the U.S. outside of urban areas.

The introduction of electrical services all started during the late 1870s, when Thomas Edison was working in his New Jersey lab to develop an incandescent light bulb that used DC power to heat a filament that then glowed. It took him 14 months of testing, but on October 21, 1879, Edison got an incandescent light bulb to glow for 13 ½ hours. He patented his light bulb in 1880.

The first people to enjoy on-demand incandescent light in their homes were well-to-do families in New York City, with small generators used to power each individual home. The question then became, how to get electricity to multiple homes in multiple locations?

MANY STILL DON'T HAVE ELECTRICAL SERVICES

Rural areas remained largely without power, however, and for more than 50 years there were basically two populations in the U.S.: those who lived in urban areas and had access to electricity, and those who lived in rural areas and did not. It wasn't until the

1950s that the electric grid reached most outlying areas, thanks to the Rural Electrification Project.

Of course, there are still vast swaths of the world without electricity—primarily in sub-Saharan Africa and central Asia. In fact, as of 2016 an estimated 13 percent of the world's population didn't have access to electricity.[22]

The number of people worldwide who don't have electricity is still significant, although it does get smaller every year; 2017 was the first year that number fell below 1 billion,[23] and 100 million people throughout the world gain access to electricity every year.[24]

That means we haven't yet achieved peak EMF saturation on Earth. As more regions of the world become electrified, and as more technology evolves and spreads that produces EMF during its use, our exposure will only continue to grow.

INTRODUCTION OF X-RAYS FORETELLS EMF DANGERS

X-rays are among the best examples of society's blind trust in the ability of technology to improve lives, well before that technology's physical effects are understood or even examined. At the turn of the 20th century, Americans embraced X-rays just as their grandchildren would later welcome wireless technologies—with a near-total lack of health concerns.

X-rays were first discovered in 1895 by Wilhelm Conrad Röntgen, a physics professor at the University of Würzburg in Germany. Röntgen was experimenting with a cathode ray tube when he noticed that a wooden board covered in phosphorous resting on a nearby table glowed whenever the cathode ray tube was in operation.

Legend has it that he then covered the cathode ray tube in thick black paper, yet still the phosphorous-covered board emitted a subtle luminescence. Röntgen knew then that he had discovered some type of invisible ray that followed an unexpected path.

Because he didn't quite understand where the ray came from, or how it worked, Röntgen named this unknown ray an "X-ray," with the *X* representing its unknown origin.

X-rays quickly caught the attention and imagination of medical and scientific experts at the time. Thomas Edison was one of the early and enthusiastic experimenters with X-ray technology. In 1896, he even invited reporters to his lab to witness a series of experiments with X-rays.

Quickly believed to cure acne and heal other skin conditions, shrink tumors, and cure cancer, X-rays offered the promise of medical miracles without surgery. The media furthered this promise by running articles heralding X-rays' healing abilities, such as the 1896 *Chicago Daily Tribune* article that ran with the headline, "Is the X Ray a Curative Agent?"[25]

There was widespread fascination with the "magical" ability of X-rays to reveal the vast unknown that catalyzed and encouraged their widespread use. Salons used them for their ability to remove hair, photographers used them to craft a far more intimate portrait, and hobbyists made or purchased their own X-ray machines for personal experimentation.

By 1920, these magic rays were being used at airports (to inspect luggage), the art world (to authenticate paintings), and the military (to evaluate the structural integrity of ships, planes, and cannons). X-ray machines even pervaded rural areas well before the electric grid had spread to more remote regions. Generators, sometimes gasoline-powered, added to the sheer sensory spectacle that the early X-ray machines provided.

A well-known radiation martyr was Pierre Curie, who, along with his wife, Marie, discovered the radioactive element radium and coined the term *radioactivity*.

Although Pierre didn't die as a direct result of his radiation-triggered ailments, which included pervasive dermatitis and radiation sickness, he surely would have had he not been trampled by a horse in 1906 first. His wife, Marie, as well as their daughter,

Irène, and her husband, Frédéric Joliot-Curie, all died of radiation-induced illnesses.

Yet, the fact that people were dying because of exposure to X-rays did little to stifle their use. A 1926 *New York Times* article described the fate of Frederick Baetjer of Johns Hopkins University, who lost eight fingers and an eye, and endured 72 surgeries as a result of his work with X-rays.[26] Despite these obvious examples of X-rays' potential for danger, they soon expanded into use in, of all places, shoe stores.

ANOTHER EXAMPLE OF FAILED DANGEROUS TECHNOLOGY: THE SHOE-FITTING FLUOROSCOPE

One particular use of X-rays implemented shortly after their discovery was to provide an image of what the bones and soft tissues of feet looked like while wearing shoes.

This device was a wooden cabinet with a space at the bottom for customers to insert their foot inside the shoe they were considering buying. When peering into the viewer, one could see the shape of the bones and soft tissues of the foot while wearing the shoe and determine if the shoe fit properly.

The X-ray was located at the bottom of the cabinet, separated from the compartment for the customer's foot by a thin aluminum or lead lining. It pointed straight up, which meant that not only did the feet get irradiated, but so did the legs, pelvises, and abdomens of the people crowded around the contraption.

In fact, the entire body of the child being measured—along with the parent and the salesman—was bathed in radiation; others in the shop were also being irradiated through the walls of the machine.

The machine also irradiated the hands of the shoe salesman, who would often reach in to the compartment to squeeze the customer's foot during the X-ray procedure. There were many reported cases of shoe salesmen contracting dermatitis of the hands, and at least one shoe model had to have her leg amputated due to a severe radiation burn.[27]

Shoe stores rapidly adopted foot fluoroscopes from the 1920s to the late 1940s. By the early 1950s, it is estimated that there were 10,000 of these machines in use throughout the United States, with an additional 3,000 machines in the United Kingdom, and approximately 1,000 in Canada.[28]

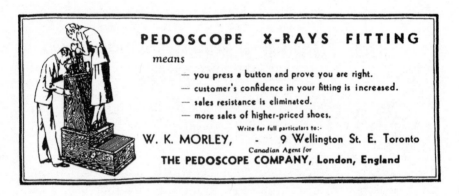

Fig. 1.3. Pedoscope Company Advertisement, *The Shoe & Leather Journal*, 12 June 1938, page 73.

The manufacturers of shoe-fitting fluoroscopes also deluded parents into believing that the machines could guarantee a better fit and, therefore, a lower chance of impaired foot development caused by shoes that were too restrictive. The whiffs of scientific truth gave confidence to moms who were largely responsible for making the purchasing decisions.

In this way, the shoe-fitting fluoroscope was a perfect example of science providing cover for naked capitalistic ambitions. Americans were lured into sacrificing their health by a concealed effort to increase sales for shoe retailers.

Similarly, today we're told we need ever-increasing exposure to wireless radiation in the name of faster download speeds and better connectivity, when what's primarily driving the industry's growth is a hunger to sell more products and services, no matter what the health costs may be.

What is important to note here is that the foot fluoroscopy craze happened well after American doctors and scientists knew that exposure to X-rays was dangerous. There had already been many well-publicized incidences of agonizing deaths from radiation exposure by so-called martyrs to science. There were some calls to abandon the foot X-ray machines, but it took decades for the message to be fully heard, and the machines to fall out of use.

It wasn't until after World War II and the dropping of the first atomic bomb that concerns over radiation exposure grew to such a point that governments and the public began in earnest to pursue a path toward banning foot fluoroscopy use. In March 1948, New York City became one of the first places to regulate the machines.[29]

A 1950 *New York Times* article noted that shoe store personnel and customers (both adults and children) who were repeatedly exposed to the fluoroscope throughout the year had an increased risk of suffering from stunted growth, dermatitis, cataracts, malignancy, and sterility.[30]

In 1953, the esteemed journal *Pediatrics* published an editorial that called for ending the practice of using shoe-fitting fluoroscopes on children.[31,32] By this time, the ball really started rolling. In 1954 the International Commission on Radiological Protection called for the curtailment of X-ray use for anything other than "medical procedures."[33]

It still took a few more years for legislative action to protect consumers. In 1957, Pennsylvania became the first state to outright ban the use of shoe-fitting fluoroscopes.[34] In 1958, New York City withdrew all the fluoroscope permits it had issued. By 1960, 34 states had passed some form of regulatory legislation.[35] By 1970, there were as few as two machines still in operation in the world.[36]

In the end, these radiation-spewing machines were unleashed on the public for more than three decades, despite the dangers being well known from the very beginning of their proliferation.

Overall, the 30-year use of deadly fluoroscopes to sell shoes is an undeniable example of how profit so often trumps common sense. We are living through another decades-long lag between the introduction of an exciting new technology and the regulation of said technology by the government.

I hope that my sharing the story of foot fluoroscopes with you here (and the eerily similar story of the rise and fall of the tobacco industry that you'll read in Chapter 3) will help convince you that we can't trust technology companies to protect their customers' health, we can't trust the government to protect consumer health, nor can we trust ourselves to consider the potential for harm when introduced to exciting new technologies.

We have to take measures into our own hands to protect ourselves from exposure, to educate ourselves as consumers, and to advocate for our health and the health of our planet to our lawmakers.

MICROWAVE OVENS USHER A MASSIVE UPTICK IN EMFS INTO HOMES

Another innovation that extended the influence of EMFs in daily life was the development of microwave technology. Microwaves were first predicted by mathematical physicist James Clerk Maxwell in 1864. The first practical application of microwaves was radar, which was first produced in 1935 by the British physicist Sir Robert Watson-Watt and came into more widespread use by the military during World War II.

The term *radar* is an acronym for radio detecting and ranging. The radar frequencies are in the microwave range of the electromagnetic spectrum: Some radar equipment operates in the same frequency range as does the cellular telephone, 800–900 MHz. Other radar systems operate at higher frequencies, around 2,000 MHz (or 2 GHz).

In 1945, radar began to be used in an entirely new way when an engineer named Percy Spencer discovered that a peanut-cluster candy bar that was in his pocket while he stood near a radar device known as a magnetron had melted. Quite by accident, he had discovered that microwaves were capable of heating food. The microwave oven has since evolved into one of the most popular household appliances in the world.

After Spencer demonstrated that higher frequency radar, around 2.45 GHz (the same frequencies now used by many cordless phones, cell phones, and Wi-Fi), could cook popcorn and eggs, his employer, Raytheon, agreed that they had a new mode of cooking on their hands. Raytheon and Spencer went on to patent the Radarange oven and brought it to market in 1947.

The first Radarange was as big as a refrigerator. It weighed 750 pounds and cost $5,000 (the equivalent of more than $57,000 in today's economy). Due to a combination of its steep cost, large size, and unfamiliar technology, the Radarange was a commercial flop. But the concept stuck around long enough to see the microwave oven enjoy a meteoric rise in popularity.

By 2015, the U.S. Census Bureau[37] estimated that 96.8 percent of American households owned a microwave oven. While microwaves undoubtedly shorten cooking times and can get dinner on the table much more quickly, this convenience comes at a high price in terms of EMF exposure and secondary health consequences, as your microwave, when it is on, is likely the biggest source of radiation exposure in your home. (Cumulatively, however, your Wi-Fi router creates a larger EMF risk.)

CORDLESS TELEPHONES AND CELL PHONES

Another novel use of microwave radiation was discovered in the 1950s, when researchers first developed the cordless phone. Although not widely available to consumers until the 1980s, cordless phones were quickly embraced. According to a 1983 *New*

York Times article,[38] 50,000 cordless phones were sold in 1980. By 1982, that number had jumped to just over a million.

Cordless phones worked by using radio waves to communicate between the base of the phone and the handset. They started out using lower frequencies, such as 27 MHz, and quickly grew to 900 MHz, then 2.4 GHz, and even as high as 5.8 GHz.

The rush to switch from traditional, corded household telephones to cordless versions meant the biggest introduction of EMFs to homes since the widespread adoption of the microwave. But there was more to come.

As cordless phones were swelling in popularity, cell phones were just getting started. On April 3, 1973, Martin Cooper, the Motorola engineer who developed the world's first working cell phone, placed the first wireless phone call. While Cooper was undoubtedly aware that his invention would change the way people communicated with each other, it's doubtful he could have ever imagined just how much the cell phone would change life as we know it.

It took another 10 years for Motorola to develop a cell phone that was available to the public. In 1983, the company debuted the DynaTAC—a model that weighed 1.75 pounds and cost $3,995,[39] or the equivalent of nearly $10,000 in 2019. It took several more years for the price and the size of cell phones to come down enough to become widely accepted.

Throughout the 1980s and early 1990s, mobile phones slowly gained acceptance—they were quite the status symbol in the early days. It wasn't until the late 1990s and 2000s that cell phones truly gained mass appeal. In 1998, 36 percent of American households owned a cell phone. By 2001, that figure was 71 percent.[40]

MOBILE PHONE USE EXPLODES WORLDWIDE

By 2005, 33.9 percent of the global population had a mobile subscription, according to a 2015 Information and Communications Technology (ICT) report.[41] Ten years later, that number was up to 96.8 percent.

By the second decade of the new millennium, cell phone use around the world had proliferated to the extent that mobile devices were more available than the Internet, landlines, and even running water.

According to the 2016 Household Survey on India's Citizen Environment & Consumer Economy, 77 percent of the poorest Indians had cell phones, while only 18 percent had access to tap water.

And their usage rates are still going up: according to a report from the research firm IHS Markit,[42] the number of global smartphones is expected to reach six billion by 2020, up from four billion in 2016.

Cell phone usage is dependent on towers that receive and transmit radio waves—your voice is converted into a digital stream of information that is sent to the nearest cell tower where it is received and then sent back out to the person on the other end of your call.

The incredible popularity of cell phones and constant desire for cell phone coverage means that more and more cell phone towers are needed to broadcast and receive radio waves (which are EMFs) over greater and greater areas.

According to the World Bank, 99.9 percent of Americans have mobile network coverage.[43] This is important because if you have a cell phone signal—even if you aren't using your phone at that moment, or don't even have a cell phone—you are being exposed to radiation. When you begin using the phone and hold it close to your body, you are being exposed to even more.

As demands for more functionality—such as watching videos—from mobile devices rises, the more these cell towers need to be expanded and strengthened, with new frequencies added in order to handle demand.

In addition to receiving and transmitting radio waves, cell phone towers are also sources of dirty electricity, as they must convert AC current from the grid into DC, which the transmitters use for power and which charges the backup batteries.

Of course, cell phones emit even more EMFs when you are using them to make a call or access the Internet (whether by Wi-Fi or the cellular network), and this exposure increases the closer you hold it to your body.

Even cell phone manufacturers admit this, because they state in their user manuals that cell phone users should always keep their phone at least 5 to 15 millimeters away from their body. Sadly, this information typically appears only deep inside the manual, which very few people ever read.

See How Many Cell Towers Are Near You

Cell phone antennas are pointed in all directions. This is why getting measurements from a qualified expert, especially those that measure the body for radio frequency (RF) as an antenna, is important. Directional meters measure only the frequencies that the RF meter is pointed at.

Your body is exposed from all angles, so it collects the micro-voltage from multiple frequencies as an antenna from all directions. Some antennas could potentially be aimed right at your home, while others could be aimed away or have obstructions that reflect the energy away.

To see how much cell phone radiation you are exposed to at your home, office, or school, I encourage you to visit AntennaSearch.com. This site is a useful tool to see the various types of frequencies and saturation that you are exposed to in your living situation.

The best way to search is to process and view the "antenna results" instead of focusing on the "tower results." The antenna results provide you with the frequencies that you are exposed to in addition to the location relative to your home. Once the antenna results are loaded, a list of companies appears under "multiple" and "single." The "multiple" are multiple antennas, or frequencies, that are installed on each tower.

There can be as few as two transmitters or as many as several hundred installed on one tower! Some people get a false sense of security using this site when they see only a few antennas yet fail to see how many transmitters are on each antenna. There could potentially be only five antennas near your home but several hundred transmitters when you add them all together.

In order to view the frequency and the number of transmitters you have to click on each company's name. When you do that the website will open up a new window with the information about the frequency, the power output, and the power radiated.

You must do this for each company that comes up in the search results in order to add up all the various frequencies and understand the true saturation of your home's location. The addresses of the towers are also listed, so you can drive by and see the antennas for yourself and try to determine if they are pointed toward your home or not.

It surprised me to find out that my daily beach walks were taking me past a grove of cell phone towers. When I investigated further, I discovered the EMF readings (which I will teach you how to take in Chapter 7) were 1,000 times higher on the beach than inside my house! Now I take a different route and head south on the beach instead of north because there are fewer cell towers there and the radiation levels test lower.

WIRELESS INTERNET

The seeds of Wi-Fi were sown in 1985, when the FCC opened up several bands of the EMF spectrum for communication purposes without requiring a government license.[44] The sections of the spectrum in question were 900 Hz, 2.4 GHz, and 5.8 GHz—what were referred to as "garbage bands"—that were already being used by devices such as microwave ovens.

It took the next 14 years for engineers and corporations to develop a regulated system that would enable devices made by different vendors to access a wireless broadband signal. To minimize interference between Wi-Fi signals and household appliances,

Wi-Fi was developed to transmit by bouncing between multiple frequencies.

Wi-Fi burst onto the market and into the public consciousness in July 1999, when Apple released its first laptops with Wi-Fi capability via an adapter made by Lucent Technologies called an AirPort.

These early adapters freed laptop users from needing to be plugged into an Internet connection while working at home, and the technology spread quickly. We have now come to rely on and expect wireless access to the Internet in our offices, homes, hotels, and coffee shops. Entire cities have established virtually ubiquitous and continuous wireless access to the Internet.

New classes of devices, such as tablets like the iPad, were developed primarily for their ability to connect wirelessly to the Internet and allow users to read books, play games, watch videos, and check e-mail without needing access to a full computer.

Unlike computers, these devices are often held just inches from a user's face, where the radiation exposure is exponentially higher than when it is an arm's length away (as with a desktop).

According to a report by the PEW Charitable Trusts, in 2010 only 3 percent of Americans owned a tablet; by 2016 that number was up to 51 percent.[45] And it's expected to rise to 62 percent, or 185 million people, in the U.S. by 2020.[46] What all this connectivity also delivers is constant exposure to radiation.

It's not just that more people have wireless access to the Internet; we're spending ever more amounts of time using this wireless connection—nearly three times as much as at the start of the 21st century.

The 2017 Digital Future Report by USC Annenberg's Center for the Digital Future found that Americans spend 23.6 hours per week online—up from 9.4 hours in 2000.[47] That's more than just a lot of screen time—it's a lot of time being bombarded by unhealthy EMFs.

5G AND THE INTERNET OF THINGS

Riding on the popularity of Wi-Fi is the development of appliances that use a wireless Internet connection to provide access to information, monitoring, and reporting.

These include thermostats that you can adjust by using an app on your smartphone; baby monitors, refrigerators, and "smart" utility meters that report your consumption to the utility company without needing to send a representative to read it; and virtual home assistants such as Google Home and Amazon's Alexa.

Collectively known as the Internet of Things, these so-called smart devices raise concerns about privacy and security as they are vulnerable to hacking.

But the other risk they pose is that they become yet another source of EMF radiation and dirty electricity in your home. There were 15.4 billion connected devices worldwide in 2015, a number that is predicted to go up to 75.4 billion by 2025.[48]

And to top it all off, in order to make the Internet of Things possible we will be forced to adopt 5G, which poses a huge risk to public health that I'll cover in Chapter 2.

WHAT ALL THIS CONNECTIVITY ADDS UP TO

Every scientific and technical development I've shared in this chapter brings with it a mixed blessing. On the plus side, the gadgets and technology offer greater convenience, enhanced capabilities, and a leap forward in our ability to expand our learning. On the negative side, they provide ever-larger exposures to EMFs in amounts that humans have never before experienced. It is only natural to think that there would be some health consequences of this.

One of the guiding principles I've used throughout my four decades of practicing natural medicine is to compare new research to our ancestral heritage to see how it reconciles.

Let's apply this thinking to EMFs and compare the type and amount of EMF fields your ancient ancestors were exposed to and the types and levels you are subjected to today.

Your ancestors did encounter electromagnetic radiation, from their own cells, the Earth's magnetic field, the atmosphere's electric field, lightning, and, of course, the sun.

To compare that to today, when, in addition to this natural radiation, we are continually exposed to more and more man-made electromagnetic radiation, really isn't a fair comparison since, as you just learned, man-made EMFs didn't exist until about 170 years ago. So let's compare the EMF exposure in the early 1900s to today.

To make an accurate comparison, we need to restrict our answer to a specific wavelength. So let's choose a pervasive one that nearly all of us are exposed to, 2.4 GHz, which is very close to the frequency your Wi-Fi and cell phones use.

So, how much of an increase in your exposure to EMF have you had in the last 100 years?

I have posed this question to thousands of individuals in many of the lectures I have given and no one has ever answered it correctly. In fact no one has ever come close—because the answer is truly mind-boggling. Typical answers are somewhere between 10 to 1,000 times more exposure now compared to 100 years ago. The rare, courageous soul will guess a million times more. But even this seemingly outrageous guess is off by many orders of magnitude.

The answer is well beyond a billion. It is larger even than one trillion. The truth is, we are exposed to *one billion billion more EMFs* now than we were just 100 years ago. (In case you were wondering, a billion billion is 10 with 18 zeros.)[49]

(For my scientifically minded reader: Even if small amounts of wideband frequencies existed as background radiation from the big bang that many theorize created the universe, the man-made frequencies we encounter today have a different shape and polarity—they are square and pulsed—than any naturally occurring frequency. As such, you could argue that we are exposed to infinitely more EMFs.)

Your body was never designed to be exposed to these levels of EMFs. It takes thousands and thousands of years for evolution to do its work and for humans to adapt to changing environments. One hundred years in evolutionary terms is not even a tiny fraction of the time required to adapt to this type of exponential change. Thus, it is perfectly reasonable to suspect that there will be some health consequences from persistent exposure to this level of radiation.

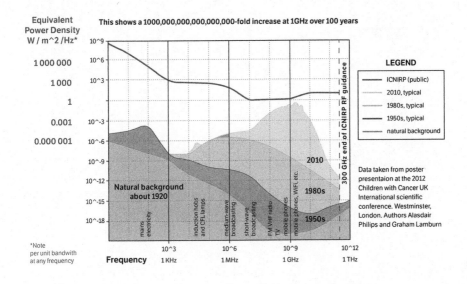

Figure 1.4: Typical daily human exposures over time of natural and manmade radio-frequency electromagnetic power densities, plus ICNIRP safety guidelines.

Essentially, our hunger for electronic devices and connectivity turns us into research subjects in a global health study; one that we never consented to be part of, and one that is getting increasingly more difficult, if not impossible, to opt out of. And one of the biggest reasons we won't be able to opt out is the widespread adoption of 5G—a topic we'll unpack in the next chapter.

CHAPTER 2

5G: THE SINGLE BIGGEST HEALTH EXPERIMENT EVER

Wireless devices, including cell phones and Wi-Fi routers, have been around for nearly two decades. You've had many years to integrate these useful technologies into your daily life. Yet suddenly it's very urgent that you change these behaviors. Why?

The answer is simple: 5G. This latest wireless technology is on the verge of completely changing your electromagnetic reality.

The term *5G* is an abbreviation for *fifth generation*, which makes it sound like it is a simple improvement on 3G or 4G technology. But this is a misperception, because true 5G is an entirely new creature that will use a different part of the electromagnetic spectrum than what is already in use.

The difference between 4G and 5G is the equivalent of the difference between a mountain stream of EMF exposure and a vast ocean of it.

This is because 5G will not replace existing wireless technology, but rather add to it. That means every single person, not to mention every microbe, insect, animal, and plant, will experience an exponential increase in EMF exposure, at a frequency that has not been tested for its long-term health ramifications.

ANOTHER CREATURE ALTOGETHER: MILLIMETER WAVES

There are some phones and devices that claim to be 5G now, but most of them are still using LTE (long-term evolution) technology, which uses the same underpinnings as 3G and 4G. Whereas LTE cellular service (and most current iterations of 5G) use radio waves that are 6 GHz or less, eventually 5G will add a bandwidth between 24 and 28 GHz, and later it is expected that a bandwidth above 30 GHz will be added as well.

These frequencies are structurally very different from the ones that power 3G and 4G networks.

Part of the frequencies that 5G will ultimately use will be *millimeter waves* (MMWs), so called because the length of one wave is less than 10 millimeters. This is opposed to the lower frequencies that are currently used (and will continue to be used), which have lengths that are measured in the tens of centimeters.

The main reason that telecommunications companies are turning to MMWs is that their bandwidth is significantly larger than the radio waves that current cell phone and Wi-Fi technologies use. That means a lot more information can be carried on them, enabling data to be transmitted in larger amounts, at a much faster speed, and with significantly shorter wait times.

With 5G, a large number of users in small geographic areas will be able to use MMWs at the same time much more efficiently than 3G or 4G technology is capable of. That means people in a packed stadium for an event will be able to make and receive calls and download data without lag time. It also means that hundreds of thousands of smartphones and appliances will be able to transmit and receive information within one small geographic area.

MMWs present some challenges, however. Primarily they are easily obstructed by physical structures such as buildings, trees, and the walls in your office or home. They can also be easily absorbed by rain and humidity.

This means that significantly more antennas will be required to provide consistent and reliable coverage—not just a few more, but literally *billions* of additional antennas compared to the 300,000 cellular towers that exist today.

THE SMALL CELLS ARE COMING

In order to ensure connectivity, the 5G network will require the installation of "small cell" stations every 300 feet or so, or every 3 to 10 houses in cities. They are called small cells because unlike the 90-foot cell towers that 3G and 4G technology use, which are usually spaced one to two miles apart, these antennas are small enough to be mounted on top of utility poles, lampposts, buildings, and bus stops.

Whereas existing cell phone towers each have a dozen antennas—eight for transmitting data and four for receiving—each small cell has enough room for about 100 antenna ports.[1]

Many of these small cell stations will have 4G transmitters that allow them to geolocate mobile devices with much more precision than what cell companies currently get from existing cell towers. Once located, the 5G antenna will then beam signals and information to that mobile device with very high speed; 4G and 5G technology work together, and many 4G transmitters will be updated to 5G over the years.

Ultimately many, if not most, homeowners can expect to end up with a 5G cell base mounted right outside or very near their home. Workplaces and educational institutions will also be saturated with small cells. Urban areas will be hit especially hard.

Because MMWs have a smaller wavelength than the frequencies used in 3G and 4G technologies, the antennas needed to broadcast them are also small. Each small cell antenna uses *multiple-input multiple-output* (MIMO) technology, which allows several users to send and receive information from each antenna simultaneously.

Because each antenna uses MIMO and each base has a hundred antennas, this is known as *massive MIMO*, which helps exponentially expand the number of users and bits of information the network can serve.

It also means that there is a high probability of interference with all those signals bouncing around in close proximity to each other. That's where a solution called *beamforming* comes in. Beamforming takes one signal and concentrates it into a beam that takes the most direct route to a user—kind of like GPS for cellular signals.

In fact, MMW signals cannot easily penetrate typical building materials like wood, brick, stucco, and even regular glass without being beamformed.

What is important to keep in mind is that these new signals from all these extra antennas and base stations will be *in addition* to the EMF swamp that we are all already swimming in. This is because 5G will not replace existing wireless technology, but will merely add to it.

Specifically, small cell stations will have never-ending 4G LTE antennas constantly spraying homes with RF signals used to geolocate mobile devices, although, granted, the power of the signal will be somewhat lower than that emitted by standard 4G cell towers.

But these small cell antennas will be so much closer to people's homes, especially second-story bedrooms, that RF from continuous 4G transmitters will be flooding bedrooms with strong RF signals, much stronger than the 4G signals from nearby existing macro cell towers.

Small cells will also send beamformed 5G signals into homes, but primarily when a device inside the home initiates a wireless connection (for example, when someone places a call). So the 5G data signals won't be constant like the 4G signals will be. When 5G data signals do come into your home, they will be strong, focused, and harmful.

Both the 4G and 5G signals emitted by small cells are highly problematic. As resistance to the widespread adoption of 5G and the infrastructure it requires grows (and it is already growing strong—see the list of groups opposed to 5G in the Resources section), 5G activists are focusing their efforts as much on preventing 4G transmitters on small cell stations as they are on preventing 5G transmitters on those same and additional standalone small cells from going up in residential neighborhoods.

THE PROMISE OF 5G

If 5G is so problematic, why are we racing to adopt it?

If you don't consider the health ramifications, 5G seems like a pretty appealing development. It promises to reduce many of the frustrations of current connectivity challenges, such as dropped calls and slow download times, and replace them with a long list of tempting benefits, including the following:

- **Faster connections.** The claim is that 5G will offer download speeds of 20 gigabytes (GB) per second as opposed to a limit of 1 GB per second with LTE. That means you can download a high-definition movie in about a second, compared to 10 minutes with LTE.

- **Greater bandwidth.** As I've mentioned, MMWs have larger bandwidth, which means more users will be able to use the network at the same time.

- **Low latency.** Latency is the time it takes a sent message to be received. Telecom companies claim that the optimal latency for 5G will be less than a millisecond, which can be up to 100 times faster than 4G. That means there will be virtually no delay in transmission and reception, which then enables all manner of technology that requires near-instantaneous communication, such as driverless cars communicating with each other in real time while driving so as to avoid accidents.

- **A massive Internet of Things.** The greater bandwidth will enable the Internet of Things—or the everyday devices and appliances that become Internet-enabled—to become truly massive. In fact, 20.4 billion devices are projected to be connected by 2020.[2]

   Thanks to 5G, we'll have washing machines that order their own detergent, refrigerators that monitor their supply levels, dialysis pumps that pump themselves, and robots that enable doctors to perform surgery remotely, among other technological developments that haven't even been imagined yet.

- **Smart cities.** The Internet of Things will extend beyond the walls of your home, into your city and onto your roads. Smart utility meters are already sending usage information from individual homes back to utility companies.

   In a 5G-enabled future, street lights, water mains, sewer systems, and runoff pipes will all be sending continuous information to utility companies so that the city's energy grid and infrastructure can be monitored on a minute-by-minute basis, as can traffic, parking spaces, and public surveillance.

   All this efficiency will require continuous transmitting and receiving of signals. The rollout of smart cities has been in the works since 2017, when Verizon announced its plans to roll out 5G in 11 cities, including Atlanta, Miami, Seattle, and Washington, D.C.,[3] while AT&T declared in 2018 it would pilot the technology in 12 cities, including Charlotte and Raleigh, North Carolina, as well as Oklahoma City and another 9 cities by mid-2019.[4,5]

- **A connected rural population.** As I'll discuss in greater detail later in the chapter, the FCC is talking a big game about how 5G will increase broadband access in rural areas of the country.

At its root, 5G is about ushering in a new era of computer-assisted living, as well as what's already being touted as a "fourth industrial revolution" as every part of manufacturing will also be impacted by the adoption of smart technologies.[6]

THE REAL REASON 5G IS BEING DEPLOYED— IT'S NOT FOR YOUR BENEFIT

The telecom industry is touting 5G as a necessity for modern life—something that will take us out of the "stone ages" of technology into a new frontier of appliances that do much of our everyday labor for us. But all this posturing about the public good is really just a ruse for creating ever-higher demand for connectivity and the products that are equipped to capitalize on that connectivity.

It's also about creating a captive audience. Not having to install cable saves money for the telecom companies. As the website TelecomPowerGrab.org put it:

> 5G will not necessarily bring broadband to underserved or rural communities. . . . It will not solve the digital divide. . . . And 5G will not immediately improve cell phone service, or assist first-responders in an emergency.
>
> Then what's the real purpose of 5G? This massive build-out of "small cell" wireless infrastructure is to enable telecom companies to beam their signals into homes and apartments without having to install a cable. It's that simple.

And that's all after 5G is a reality. Now, as it is being built out, there are vast amounts of money being spent and earned. The investment required to upgrade the infrastructure necessary to fulfill the promise of 5G connectivity is estimated at $200 billion a year according to a study by IHS Markit and commissioned by Qualcomm Technologies.[7]

Small cells, antennas, chips, satellites, and all-new hardware (phones, appliances, utility meters, and cars) will be required to communicate with the signals transmitted by the new hardware. For that investment, the same report estimates that 5G will produce $12.4 trillion in global economic output by 2035 and produce as many as 22 million jobs. Once 5G is up and running, it is predicted to produce $250 billion annually by 2025 just for providing the service.[8]

Make no mistake, 5G is absolutely big business. It isn't about human good; it's about the wireless industry's bottom line. Here's how former FCC Chairman Tom Wheeler described it in a speech at the National Press Club in 2016:[9]

> If something can be connected, it will be connected in the 5G world; but with the hundreds of billions of microchips connected in products from pill bottles to plant waterers, you can be sure . . . the biggest Internet of Things application has yet to be imagined. . . .
>
> To make this work, the 5G build-out is going to be very infrastructure intensive, requiring massive deployment of small cells. . . . The United States will be the first country in the world to open up high-band spectrum for 5G networks and applications, and that's damn important.

Chillingly, he added, "We won't wait for the standards."

YOU WON'T BE ABLE TO OPT OUT OF 5G COVERAGE— OR THE RADIATION THAT COMES WITH IT

A big piece of that "massive deployment" Wheeler referred to is low-orbit satellites. Because MMWs can't travel very far as they are absorbed by humidity and rain and can't penetrate buildings, satellites will be required to transmit and receive signals to and from users on the Earth in order to offer blanket coverage of urban and rural areas.

And not just a couple of satellites, either, but as many as 50,000, launched by companies including SpaceX, OneWeb, and Boeing.[10] Although it sounds futuristic, these satellites have already begun to be launched into space: The first operational satellites were launched by OneWeb in February 2019 and SpaceX in May 2019.[11]

These satellites will ultimately blanket the entire Earth in a field of MMW radiation that will be impossible to escape from.

In an open letter to medical organizations by the Global Union Against Radiation Deployment from Space (GUARDS), an international coalition against global Wi-Fi from space, scientists describe these satellites "flooding the planet with microwave radiation" as a violation of human rights:[12]

> Space-based microwave radiation deployments threaten to inundate the planet with RF radiation without informed individual consent or a meaningful option for individual avoidance.

5G ANTENNAS WILL EVEN INFILTRATE YOUR HOUSE

You may be thinking that since MMWs have difficulty penetrating through walls that you might be protected inside your home. Sadly, this is not the case. So-called smart appliances that use 5G technology will essentially turn your kitchen, laundry room, and outer walls into small cells.

Even the light bulbs in your home may become 5G transmitters. Starting in 2017, researchers at Brunel University London began developing light bulbs that use both *visible light communication* (VLC), also known as *Li-Fi*, which uses the rapid flickering of LED light to transmit digital communication, and MMW 5G technology to create high-speed home wireless networks.[13,14]

Even if you use non-LED light bulbs and don't purchase smart appliances, MMWs may be able to find their way into your house. As reported by Alasdair Philips, technical director of EMFields Solutions:

> Whether mm-waves will penetrate homes depends on many factors. Above 30 GHz the waves can slip through long slots such as those around PVC window frames as the metal cores are surrounded just by PVC extrusions. This makes it difficult to shield at the scale of housing.[15]

There truly may be no escape.

> Quiz: A primary physical effect of 5G, which relies primarily on the bandwidth of the millimeter wave, that many may be able to sense is:
>
> ☐ Coldness
> ☐ Paralysis
> ☐ Hallucinations
> ☐ Pain
> ☑ All of the above

THE HEALTH DANGERS OF MMW EXPOSURE

As of this writing, I am unaware of any studies that look at the effects of prolonged exposure to MMWs, much less at the effects of MMW exposure that happens at the same time as exposure to other common EMF frequencies (such as those emitted by 4G phones).

However, there are some things we already know about the health effects of MMWs. Ironically, MMWs have been used in Eastern Europe for years as a complementary therapy for ulcers, cardiovascular disorders, and cancer, and there are journals devoted to this subject in that part of the world.

Researchers have examined the health effects of this treatment. Their studies found that up to 80 percent of people can sense the presence of MMWs on their skin,[16,17] as well as increased electro-hypersensitivity,[18] particularly in postmenopausal women.[19]

Russian scientists also conducted research as early as the 1970s on the health effects of exposure to millimeter radiation. This research wasn't available for decades because the U.S. Central Intelligence Agency collected and translated the published research but did not declassify it until the 2010s.

A 1977 paper by the Russian researcher N. P. Zalyubovskaya, which was declassified in 2012, compared the effects of radiation in the range of 5–8 millimeters and density of 1 milliwatt/cm^2 on rats and mice that were exposed for 15 minutes a day for 60 days and people who worked with millimeter generators.[20] The study reported:

> Morphological, functional, and biochemical studies conducted in humans and animals revealed that millimeter waves caused changes in the body manifested in structural alterations in the skin and internal organs, qualitative and quantitative changes of the blood and bone marrow composition, and changes of the conditioned reflex activity, tissue respiration, activity of enzymes participating in the processes of tissue respiration and nucleic metabolism. The degree of unfavorable effects of millimeter waves depended on the duration of the radiation and individual characteristics of the organism.

In the minimal additional research recently conducted on the subject, MMW technology was linked to a number of potential health problems, including:[21-25]

- Eye problems such as lens opacity in rats, which is linked to the production of cataracts[26] and eye damage in rabbits[27,28]

- Impacted heart rate variability, an indicator of stress, in rats[29–31] and heart rate changes (arrhythmias) in frogs[32,33]

- Modified structure and function of cellular membranes[34]

- Suppressed immune function[35]

- Effects on bacteria, including depressed growth and increased antibiotic resistance[36]

No studies have been done to assess what might be a safe threshold for MMW exposure, a fact that led Washington State University biochemistry professor Dr. Martin Pall, one of the leading voices on the dangers of EMFs, to declare:

> Putting in tens of millions of 5G antennae without a single biological test of safety has to be about the stupidest idea anyone has had in the history of the world.[37]

Research compiled by the founder of ElectricSense.com and author of *EMF Practical Guide* Lloyd Burrell[38] and others[39,40] suggests the proliferation of 5G could turn into nothing short of a public health disaster.

MMW EXPOSURE CAN CAUSE PAIN

MMWs are known to penetrate human skin tissue at a depth of 1 to 2 millimeters,[41,42,] and to cause pain in the skin.[43] This is likely because MMWs trigger the nerve cells in the skin known as *nociceptors* that alert the brain of potentially damaging stimuli by eliciting a pain response.

Another suggested reason for the pain response is that sweat ducts in human skin act as antennae when they come in contact with MMWs.[44] In a 2016 letter to the FCC, Dr. Yael Stein of the Hadassah Medical Center in Jerusalem, Israel, who has studied 5G MMW technology and its interaction with the human body, wrote:[45]

> Computer simulations have demonstrated that sweat glands concentrate sub-terahertz waves in human skin. Humans could sense these waves as heat. The use of sub-terahertz (millimeter wave) communications technology (cell phones, Wi-Fi, antennas) could cause humans to percept physical pain via nociceptors. Potentially, if 5G Wi-Fi is spread in the public domain we may expect . . . more cases of hypersensitivity (EHS), as well as many new complaints of physical pain.

The U.S. Department of Defense knows very well that MMWs cause pain, because it uses these extremely high frequencies in crowd control weapons known as the Active Denial System (ADS).[46] The ADS has the ability to cause a severe burning sensation that feels almost as if the skin might catch on fire.[47] As a result, people exposed to the ADS will instinctively retreat.

5G COULD ALTER ALL BIOLOGICAL LIFE AND CHANGE THE ENVIRONMENT IN UNFORESEEN WAYS

As you'll learn more about in Chapter 4, it's not just human health that's at stake, but also insects, plants, animals, and microbes, especially since MMWs are absorbed by both plants and rain. Widespread MMW exposure could even pose a danger to the food supply via its potential absorption by plants. Studies have already shown that MMWs may invoke stress protein changes in plants such as wheat sprouts.[48]

Insects, being millimeter-size creatures, serve as mini-antennas for MMWs. A recent review of the world literature on plummeting insect populations predicts the extinction of 40 percent of the world's insect species over the next few decades, even without the implementation of 5G.[49]

Because humans and animals rely on plants for food, the use of 5G could well result in foods' nutritional value being degraded further than it already is, due to our industrial agriculture practices depleting soil nutrients and coating our environment with harmful pesticides. Or worse, it could result in a radical reduction of our ability to produce enough food.

And, as I will cover in Chapter 4, low levels of nonionizing radiation have already been linked to disturbances and health problems in birds and bees, with bees in particular being problematic for human health because of the crucial role they play in pollinating so many of the plants needed to provide our food.

In Addition to Being Potentially Deadly, 5G Infrastructure Is Unsightly

Although they have the name "small cell," the equipment that houses the transmitters and receivers of the 5G signal are not that small. While the antennas can reside at the top of a utility pole, other equipment must be housed in a box that is the size of a small refrigerator.

These boxes must either go on the ground near the pole (in concept designs they are often depicted as being disguised as a mailbox), or attached to the pole itself. With small cells needing to be placed within 500 feet of each other, that's a lot of visual and spatial real estate eaten up by 5G.

This has raised legitimate concerns about aesthetics and property values. A 2005 study published in The Appraisal Journal found that 38 percent of survey respondents felt that a cell phone tower being built in close proximity to their house would reduce their property value by 20 percent or more.[50]

Additionally, a 2014 survey of homebuyers and renters by the National Institute for Science, Law, and Public Policy (NISLAPP) found that 94 percent are less interested in and would pay less for a property located close to a cell tower or antenna. And 79 percent said they absolutely would not rent or buy property within a few blocks of a cell tower.[51]

With 5G, nearly everyone in urban and semi-urban areas is ultimately likely to have a small cell close to their house. This could precede a major correction in the housing market, one of the biggest drivers of economic stability.

THE FCC GIVETH, AND THE FCC TAKETH AWAY

In reality, the urgency the FCC claims to have about bringing broadband to underserved populations appears to be a cover for rushing through legislation that gives more power and money to the wireless industry and takes away autonomy and revenue from the states, cities, and towns that own the property that will house 5G infrastructure.

As FCC Chairman Ajit Pai said in a September 2018 press conference to announce the FCC's 5G Fast Plan, "We cannot let today's red tape strangle the 5G future."

In 2018, the FCC passed rules that cap the fees local jurisdictions can charge telecom companies for housing small cells to $270 per year—when municipalities had routinely been getting a few thousand dollars for each site. This new policy also set a constrictive timeline for cities and counties to approve the addition of small cells to existing structures (60 days) as well as newly constructed sites (90 days).

Worse yet, it virtually eliminated the rights of cities to say where 5G antennas are allowed and where they aren't. As a result, citizens will not be able to prevent installation of 5G cell bases outside their homes.

Multiple cities, including Los Angeles, sued to overturn these new rules. But in January 2019, the U.S. Court of Appeals for the 10th Circuit sided with the FCC and the wireless industry, essentially abandoning the public's health.[52]

EVEN TELECOMMUNICATIONS EXECS ADMIT THEY'VE DONE NO SAFETY STUDIES

Speaking at a press conference in December 2018 regarding 5G technology and its impact on the American people and economy, U.S. Senator Richard Blumenthal of Connecticut said:[53]

The stark simple fact is, the health hazards are unknown and unstudied, and that is a sign of neglect and disregard on the part of the Federal Communications Commission that seems unacceptable. . . . There have been no answers so far, the FCC has basically said everything's fine, but in order to reach a conclusion about the health and safety of this new technology, we need fact.

Two months later, during a February 7, 2019, hearing of the Senate Commerce, Science, and Transportation Committee, Blumenthal questioned telecommunications industry representatives about whether they'd invested any money into studying the health effects of their much-touted 5G rollout.

How much money has the industry committed to supporting additional independent research, and I stress independent research? And is that research ongoing? Has it been completed? And where can consumers look for it?

To which one of the lobbyists replied:

Safety is paramount. . . . We rely on the findings of the FDA and others . . . to keep all of us safe. There are no industry-backed studies to my knowledge right now. . . . We're always for more science. We also rely on what the scientists tell us.

So here we have the truth of the vicious cycle that the wireless industry has created. They have captured the Federal Communications Commission (FCC), as we'll discuss more in Chapter 3, and they use the FCC's claim of proof of safety as justification for the 5G deployment.

This is an absolutely brilliant business strategy but beyond devastating from a health perspective. (You'll learn more about the many tactics the telecom industry uses to present a narrative that its technologies are safe in Chapter 3.)

Blumenthal pressed: "So, essentially, the answer to my question—How much money?—zero."

And again, the concession: "To my knowledge there's no active studies being backed by industry today."

Ultimately, Blumenthal summed up our 5G travails quite succinctly: "We're kind of flying blind here, as far as health and safety is concerned."

THE SCIENTIFIC COMMUNITY IS SPEAKING OUT—BUT IS ANYONE LISTENING?

The scientific community is also concerned about the 5G roll-out. In fact, in 2017 more than 180 doctors and scientists from 35 countries signed a petition[54] that calls upon the European Union to enact a moratorium on the rollout of 5G due to the potential risks to wildlife and human health. In it, they wrote:

> We the undersigned, more than 180 scientists and doctors from 35 countries, recommend a moratorium on the roll-out of the fifth generation, 5G, for telecommunication until potential hazards for human health and the environment have been fully investigated by scientists independent from industry.

And as of October 29, 2019, 171,798 scientists, doctors, environmental organizations, and citizens from 201 nations and territories have signed an International Appeal to Stop 5G on Earth and in Space.[55]

SMALL REASONS FOR HOPE: A BRIEF HISTORY OF RESISTANCE TO 5G

Although 5G appears to be as unstoppable as a runaway freight train, there are some city and national governments around the world and in the U.S. who have at least constructed some speed barriers.

Around the World

Florence, Italy[56] April 2019	The mayor of Florence refused to grant permission for individual 5G towers until the city developed an overarching plan that considers the public health ramifications of such a plan, citing the precautionary principle and the "uncertainty of supranational and private organizations" (such as ICNIRP) that "have very different positions from each other, despite the huge evidence of published studies." The Italian government has been forced by its supreme court to inform its citizens about the health effects of EMFs and talk about precautionary measures, partially based on the actions of the Phonegate Alert association.[57]
Netherlands[58] April 2019	Members of the House of Representatives called for studies of the health effects of 5G before any rollouts begin.
Germany[59] April 2019	Nearly 55,000 Germans signed a petition asking Parliament (the Bundestag) to stop the rollout of 5G frequencies, due to "scientifically justified doubts about the safety of this technology."
Canton of Vaud, Switzerland[60] April 2019	The Grand Council of Vaud, in Switzerland's third-largest region, approved a moratorium on permits for 5G antennas until the Swiss Federal Office for the Environment conducts and delivers a final report on the health and environmental ramifications. One Swiss newspaper declared, in part, "[Telecom] operators are furious."
Geneva, Switzerland[61] April 2019	Following in Vaud's footsteps, the Grand Council of Geneva also voted to institute a moratorium on 5G rollout. They went one step further than their counterparts, however, by calling on the World Health Organization (headquartered in Geneva) to investigate and report on the health effects of such a rollout.
Rome, Italy[62] March 2019	In the face of the first 5G networks opening in Rome, a resolution of the XII municipality of the city, which passed with 11 votes in favor and 3 abstentions, asks "the mayor to stop the 5G trial and not to raise the limit values in the threshold of electromagnetic radiation avoiding the positioning of groups of mini-millimeter antennas on homes, schools, day centers, recreation centers, street lamps and more."

Russia[63] March 2019	The Russian Ministry of Defense refused to transfer frequencies for 5G to telecommunications companies, saying it was "too early" to do so.
Belgium[64] March 2019	The Environment Minister of Brussels called off the implementation of a 5G pilot program due to concerns about radiation exposure, saying "the people of Brussels are not guinea pigs whose health I can sell at a profit. We cannot leave anything to doubt." Many governing bodies of the European Union (EU) are headquartered in Brussels, including the European Commission, Council of the EU, and the European Council. Could it be that they don't want to participate in the 5G public health experiment?

American Cities and States Fighting Back

San Francisco, California[65] April 2019	In a unanimous decision, the California Supreme Court upheld a city ordinance from 2011 that requires a permitting process for antennas to be placed on utility poles and other city infrastructure.
Hallandale Beach, Florida[66] April 2019	A unanimous city resolution called on the Florida legislature and federal government to study the health effects of small cells and develop guidelines for the installation of 5G infrastructure that protects public health.
Montana[67] March 2019	The Montana House passed a resolution calling on Congress to amend the Telecommunications Act of 1996 to allow health considerations to be taken into account when determining the location of small cells in residential areas. As of this writing, a Senate version of the resolution was still in committee.
Portland, Oregon[68] March 2019	The city filed a lawsuit against the FCC over the commission's rules that limit how much cities can charge telecommunications companies to use city property as transmitter sites, saying that the low, FCC-approved fees (capped at $270 per site) would cost Portland up to $10 million in lost revenue, as other cities charge up to $3,000 per site. The city also voted on a resolution to require the FCC to investigate the health effects of 5G and to make that information available to the public.

Palos Verdes, California[69] January 2019	An update to the municipal code created stringent restrictions on where telecommunications towers and antennas can be located, unless an exception is granted.
New Hampshire[70] January 2019	A bill was introduced in the New Hampshire House of Representatives to study the environmental and health effects of 5G. It passed the House and, as of this writing, was being reviewed by a Senate committee. Language in the bill asked, "Why have 1,000s of peer-reviewed studies, including the recently published U.S. Toxicology Program 16-year $30 million study, that are showing a wide range of statistically significant DNA damage, brain and heart tumors, infertility, and so many other ailments, being ignored by the Federal Communications Commission (FCC)?"
Fairfax, California[71] January 2019	With an eye toward protecting public health, Fairfax passed an urgency ordinance to its municipal code that prohibits small cells in residential zones, requires a 1,500-foot separation between small cells, and requires the city to study the viability of a fiber-optic cable network as an alternative to small cell technology.
San Rafael, California[72] December 2018	This Bay Area city passed an ordinance to protect residential neighborhoods from small cells. This one requires a 500-foot setback from residential districts and 500 feet of separation between small cells.
Sonoma, California[73] November 2018	The Sonoma City Council passed an ordinance requiring a test by a licensed radio-frequency engineer to measure the frequency and power levels emitted by each small cell facility, and giving notice to all property owners within 500 feet of a proposed telecommunications infrastructure site. The ordinance also requires that pole-mounted antennas be no less than 1,500 feet apart.
San Anselmo and Fairfax, California[74,75] October 2018	Inspired by Mill Valley's ordinances, the Fairfax Town Council passed an ordinance requiring 1,500 feet between small cells and appointed a committee to explore alternatives to small cells. The San Anselmo Town Council passed an ordinance requiring notification to residents within 300 feet of a proposed small cell antenna.

Burlington, Massachusetts[76] October 2018	The city's small cell equipment committee created a policy that requires an application fee of $500 for each proposed small cell site and an annual recertification fee of $270. The policy caused Verizon to withdraw its applications, citing concerns about the precedent the policy set and questions regarding its legality.[77]
Booneville, Arkansas[78] September 2018	The city proposed an ordinance that would, among other things, restrict new cell towers to industrial areas.
Mill Valley, California[79] September 2018	The city council of this Bay Area enclave voted unanimously to prohibit new or updated towers in residential zones and to require a minimum distance of 1,500 feet between small cells.
Petaluma, California[80] July 2018	Petaluma updated its municipal code to protect residents against adverse health effects of 5G by station, including the provision that "no small cell shall be within 500 feet of any residence."
Monterey, California[81] March 2018	City planning commissioners voted 7 to 0 to deny Verizon's application for a small cell tower to be placed in a residential neighborhood.
Walnut, California[82] October 2017	One of the first cities in California to push back against the 5G rollout, Walnut updated its municipal code to say that "Telecommunication towers and antennas shall not be located within 1,500 feet of any school (nursery, elementary, junior high, and high school), trail, park or outdoor recreation area, sporting venues, and residential zones."
Pennsylvania[83] June 2017	The Pennsylvania Public Utilities Commission stripped antenna-distributing companies of their utility status, requiring them to go through a standard permitting process to install new poles and taking away their ability to use "certificates of public convenience" to put poles wherever they choose.

Palm Beach, Florida[84] May 2017	Palm Beach and a few other coastal communities lobbied to get a law passed that exempts them from another state law that places strong restrictions on local governments' influence over where 5G small cells are installed. Palm Beach Town Manager Tom Bradford was quoted as saying, "We have been carved out . . . That law does not apply to us." Palm Beach is home to Donald J. Trump's Mar-a-Lago resort. Could the fact that the president's home is exempted from requisite 5G coverage be mere coincidence?
Mason, Ohio[85] May 2017	It's not just cities on the coasts that are concerned about 5G; the town of Mason, Ohio, passed an ordinance that prohibits small cells in residential areas or within 100 feet of property that is used for residential purposes. It also established that small cells must be 2,000 feet apart unless collocated.
Warren, Connecticut[86] December 2012	The city adopted a special permit for telecommunications facilities and towers that urges the Connecticut Siting Council—which, according to state law, has jurisdiction over the placement of towers and antennas—"to locate towers and/or antennas in a manner which protects property values, as well as the general safety, health, welfare and quality of life of the citizens of Warren and all those who visit this community."

THE BEST ALTERNATIVE TO 5G—FIBER-OPTIC NETWORKS

To be clear, I'm not suggesting that we go back to our pre-Wi-Fi ways. Rather, I believe the best way for us to improve connectivity with safer, more reliable, and faster service for all Americans is to use fiber-optic cables instead of small cells broadcasting 4G and MMWs.

This isn't just a theory. Two American cities have introduced municipal fiber-optic broadband systems to great success: Chattanooga, Tennessee, and Longmont, Colorado. Chattanooga's municipal electric company, the Electric Power Board, built the system with assistance from federal grant money.

In the first three years of the broadband network's existence (2009–2012), home values in Chattanooga increased 14 percent and median household income rose 13.5 percent, even as the state government cut nearly 3,000 jobs.[87] In 2014, Longmont Power & Communications rolled out NextLight, its municipal broadband system that allows residents to download data at a rate of one gigabit per second for about $50 a month.[88]

A 2018 156-page report by the National Institute for Science, Law, and Public Policy provides an excellent, in-depth look at the benefits of a wired Internet system over the wireless one we seem hell bent on making the status quo for decades to come. In this report, the author, Timothy Schoechle, Ph.D., writes:

> Wired infrastructure is *inherently more* future-proof, more reliable, more sustainable, more energy-efficient, and more essential to many other services. Wireless networks and services are inherently more complex, more costly, more unstable, and more constrained. . . .
>
> Millimeter wave (e.g., 5G wireless) backhaul is at best an on-the-cheap solution favored by corporations looking for short-term profits. It is wholly inadequate for a number reasons, among which is that it depends on an invasive and unstable complex millimeter wave hardware/software prone to (sometimes-planned) obsolescence.
>
> This complex approach contrasts sharply with the simplicity of basic future-proof fiber/hardwired facilities. At the same time, the wireless approach provides fewer jobs (most of its jobs are in the area of technical/software) and is subject to line-of-sight limitations, interference, asymmetric service, slow data rates, congestion problems, and potential public health risks.

You may fear that wired connections are bound to be slower than the 5G speeds we've been promised by the FCC, Cellular Telecommunications Industry Association (CTIA), and telecommunications companies, but even ancient phone lines have been shown to be able to deliver gigabit data rates, and fiber-optic cables have a proven ability to deliver 1.4 terabits of data per second,[89] orders of magnitude higher than 5G.

Any reductions in speed and wait times that wired systems may have over 5G are well worth the trade-off in public and environmental health. If government—whether it be municipal, state, or national—invested in a wired infrastructure, we'd ensure that the Internet remains accessible to all, instead of at the mercy of a handful of companies determined to push their moneymaking agenda over concerns of the public good.

We simply need more resources directed to improve fiber-optic technology. Recent simple innovations of using a vibrating plow that requires only one person and equipment rental to hook up your home to the central neighborhood fiber-optic line will serve to minimize the cost of connecting fiber-optic cables in your home.[90]

The ray of hope here is that there *are* ways to have the connectivity you've come to love and rely on that don't inflict massive amounts of harm on living creatures on this planet.

Know that as you continue to read this book, you'll learn ways to protect your body from the threat of wireless technologies—including 5G—from the inside out, as well as ways to reduce your exposure, and the damage it can cause.

But first, I want to dive a little deeper into how we ended up living in such an EMF-saturated swamp in the first place. It will be even more of a wake-up call that we shouldn't allow the wireless industry to prioritize its profits over our health.

CHAPTER 3

CELL PHONES ARE THE CIGARETTES OF THE 21ST CENTURY

Perhaps right about now you are thinking to yourself, *If EMFs are so bad, why isn't anybody doing something about it?* Moreover, *Why are we only continuing to adopt more and more devices that have the potential to harm our health?*

I am so glad you asked because I find the truth to be quite a sickening tale. You might too when you learn how these companies have valued their profit over your health, and your family's health.

The story of how EMFs became such an integral part of our environment—despite mounting evidence that they harm human and environmental health—shares many parallels with the history of tobacco use.

Many tend to forget that the tobacco industry, like the wireless industry today, adopted a policy of denial and silence to the over-whelming science documenting the biologic damage and health hazards caused by cigarettes. It effectively stuck to this tactic for decades.

I believe that when you see the parallels between the tobacco and the wireless industries, you'll be motivated to reconsider how much you use cell phones and other wireless devices.

If you want to review all the sordid strategies the tobacco industry successfully and brilliantly deployed that prematurely killed millions of people, I encourage you to read Harvard University professor Allan M. Brandt's comprehensive review, *Inventing Conflicts of Interest: A History of Tobacco Industry Tactics*[1] and former assistant secretary of labor for occupational safety and health David Michaels' book *Doubt Is Their Product: How Industry's Assault on Science Threatens Your Health*.

THE TOBACCO INDUSTRY PURPOSEFULLY LIED TO THE PUBLIC FOR DECADES

As early as the 1950s, there was a powerful consolidation of scientific evidence showing smoking led to serious respiratory and cardiac diseases. Yet it took 50 years before health concerns about smoking became pervasive enough for smoking rates to drop significantly.

How did we stay in the dark for so long?

The tobacco companies' guiding light through it all was the public relations firm they hired in the 1950s, Hill+Knowlton Strategies. Rather than play the losing game of simply denying facts, Hill+Knowlton proposed brilliant strategies the wireless industry would later co-opt.

It is revealing to review the bullet points below from a leaked document outlining the objectives of tobacco company Brown & Williamson at the time:

- Objective No. 1: To set aside in the minds of millions the false conviction that cigarette smoking causes lung cancer and other diseases; a conviction based on fanatical assumptions, fallacious rumors, unsupported claims, and the unscientific statements and conjectures of publicity-seeking opportunists.

- Objective No. 2: To lift the cigarette from the cancer identification as quickly as possible and restore it to its proper place of dignity and acceptance in the minds of men and women in the marketplace of American free enterprise.

- Objective No. 3: To expose the incredible, unprecedented, and nefarious attack against the cigarette, constituting the greatest libel and slander ever perpetrated against any product in the history of free enterprise. . . .

- Objective No. 4: To unveil the insidious and developing pattern of attack against the American free enterprise system, a sinister formula that is slowly eroding American business with the cigarette obviously selected as one of the trial targets.[2]

Martin Blank, Ph.D., a leading expert on the health dangers of EMFs, suggests in his book *Overpowered* rereading these objectives while replacing *cigarette* with *cell phone* and *smoking* with *using cell phones*. The result is quite clarifying, and quite chilling.

FUNDING BIASED RESEARCH

By paying scientists directly to perform studies, the industry could hand-select researchers who were already biased toward believing that cigarettes were safe. By doing so, tobacco companies also created conflicts of interest, as even impartial researchers can be influenced by a desire to keep their funders happy.

As an example, a 1997 review by researchers at Washington College in Maryland looked at 91 studies that investigated a possible link between tobacco and cognitive performance. They analyzed the results of each study as well as the source of funding, and they saw a clear difference in findings of studies that received funds from the tobacco industry versus those that did not.

The study authors wrote, "Our analysis shows that researchers acknowledging tobacco industry support were considerably more likely to arrive at a conclusion favorable to the tobacco industry, versus those researchers not acknowledging industry support."[3]

By pumping out more studies, the tobacco companies could claim that the science regarding the health effects of tobacco use was inconclusive, all the while pretending to be committed to public well-being.[4]

Even a 1964 report by the U.S. Surgeon General that reviewed 7,000 articles relating to smoking and disease and concluded that cigarette smoking was a cause of lung cancer and laryngeal cancer in men and a probable cause of lung cancer in women didn't result in new government regulations or a decrease in public demand. That report cued the tobacco industry to fund even more studies.

A wide-ranging and long-lasting secondary effect of this approach was to introduce a culture of skepticism of science itself. Ultimately, by making science fair game in the battle of public relations, the tobacco industry set a destructive precedent that would affect future debates on subjects such as food, global warming, pharmaceuticals,[5] and, yes, EMFs.

SPENDING MILLIONS TO SWAY LEGISLATORS

Hill+Knowlton guided its tobacco clients to form a separate entity to lobby for legislation and regulatory rules that were friendly to their industry. The Tobacco Institute was formed in 1958 and quickly became one of the most powerful and well-funded lobbying organizations in Washington, D.C.

It empowered tobacco companies to buy favorable treatment by the government while evading the perception that they were doing so. After all, it was a separate entity. The Tobacco Institute went on to operate for more than 40 years.

Although the tobacco industry managed to escape liability and major regulation for more than four decades, eventually its stranglehold on the American public came to an end. In March 1997, nearly 30 years after smoking was strongly linked to the dramatic rise of lung cancer, Liggett Group, the smallest of the country's five leading cigarette makers, finally admitted that smoking causes cancer.[6,7] The other tobacco companies soon followed suit.

The admissions of harm were instrumental in swaying public opinion. For example, the first government-mandated warnings on cigarette packages appeared in 1965 when approximately 45 percent of Americans smoked, and that percentage did not decline significantly until 1977, when it reached 36 percent. It wasn't until 1989 that the number dropped below 30 percent. In 2018, the number fell to its lowest ever—16 percent.[8]

What makes all this history acutely tragic is all the lives that were lost. Even the conservative Centers for Disease Control and Prevention (CDC) estimated in November 2018 that nearly half a million people in the U.S. continue to die every year from cigarette smoking, despite the fact that the percentage of smokers had decreased by more than 50 percent from previous years.[9]

Therefore, the 50 years of tobacco industry denial easily resulted in tens of millions of needless deaths and suffering in the U.S. and many hundreds of millions worldwide.

This deeply saddens me, as my own mother was one of its victims. She smoked from a young age, and although she quit in her late 70s, the damage was done. She developed chronic obstructive pulmonary disease (COPD), required regular oxygen therapy with daily breathing treatments, and eventually died prematurely from complications.

CREATING CONFLICTS OF INTEREST

It seems that the wireless industry has carefully studied the strategies the tobacco companies used to deny the health risks associated with their products for more than 50 years. In fact, in the past two decades, many big players in the wireless industry have hired Hill+Knowlton, including Motorola and Virgin Mobile as well as a wide variety of other tech companies engaged in the wireless industry.

In that time, telecommunications companies have regularly funded studies to assess the health risks of their mobile devices, just as the tobacco companies did before them. Ostensibly, this appears to be an approach designed to help protect consumers. Yet we know that when a company funds research into its own products, it creates a powerful conflict of interest that distorts findings in favor of whomever financed the study.[10–12]

A major push to produce supportive research began in 1994 by the wireless industry trade group CTIA, which, at that time, was headed by Tom Wheeler (remember his name, as he went on to become chairman of the FCC in 2013).

This effort came about after David Reynard, a widower, filed a lawsuit against wireless phone manufacturer NEC Corporation of America. In late 1993, Reynard appeared on *Larry King Live*, where he shared how his wife regularly used an NEC wireless phone before developing the brain tumor that killed her.

In Reynard's mind, the connection between his wife's cell phone use and her cancer was clear, and he called for greater safety measures. His story went viral, and shares of telecom stocks plunged in the aftermath.

In order to produce a counter-narrative, the CTIA handpicked Dr. George Carlo, a scientist who was known for his industry-friendly scientific findings, to be the founding director of the Wireless Technology Research project (WTR), an industry-funded research group.

Before heading the WTR, Carlo had conducted research into the safety of breast implants as well as low levels of dioxin exposure. In both instances, Carlo's research was funded by the industries involved. And in both cases, Carlo found only minimal or no health risks.

He likely seemed to the CTIA to be the perfect person to further the wireless industry's efforts to at least muddy the scientific waters, if not refute any evidence of harm altogether—though that's not what came to pass, as Carlo would eventually warn wireless industry executives of the health risks of their products.

Throughout the late 1990s and early 2000s, the industry gave Carlo $27 million in funds to pay for research evaluating the health risks of EMFs, and hundreds of conflicted studies were produced during that time.

Ironically, over the course of this initiative, Carlo became disillusioned. In 2007, he admitted in a paper that "the industry strategy has been to fund low-risk studies that assure a positive result—then use them to convince the media and public that cell phones have been proven to be safe, even though the actual science proved nothing of the sort."[13]

Other researchers were coming to similar conclusions around the same time, including Henry Lai, a professor of bioengineering at the University of Washington who had conducted research of his own that found that exposure to radiation similar to that emitted by cell phones could cause DNA damage.

In 2006, Lai examined 326 studies on the safety of cell phone radiation conducted between 1990 and 2006 and discovered that 44 percent of them did not find harmful effects, while 56 percent did.

Here is where it gets interesting. When he categorized the studies by funding, the numbers told an entirely different story: 67 percent of the independently funded studies found a harmful effect, while only 28 percent of the industry-funded studies did.[14] This groundbreaking insight led others to investigate the link between funding and results.

In 2008, a team of Swiss researchers led by Dr. Anke Huss conducted a review of 59 studies evaluating the biological effects of exposure to wireless radiation. They found that 82 percent of the studies funded by governments and other independent agencies showed harmful effects, compared to only 33 percent of studies funded by industry.[15]

A 2009 review of 55 studies that compared human brain activity in the presence and absence of wireless radiation fields found that 37 of those studies concluded that there was an EMF-related effect on brain function, while 18 observed no effect.

What was conclusive was that industry funded a full 87 percent of the studies included, suggesting that the industry was seeking to increase the number of studies so it could claim there was no consensus in the scientific community.[16]

FUNDING STUDIES OF QUESTIONABLE DESIGN

It is not just the conflicting findings that can be problematic in industry-funded studies; it is also often the very design of the studies themselves. There are many variables in any scientific study—it is imperative that researchers construct their experiments in a way that doesn't inadvertently skew their results, which is not ordinarily the case in industry-funded research.

In a 2010 review of 23 studies designed to determine a connection between the use of cell phones and the risk of developing tumors, researchers at the University of California, Berkeley, analyzed not only the results of the studies, but also the initial design of the studies, and then compared that to the source of funding.

Their conclusion was that "among the 10 higher quality studies, we found a harmful association between phone use and tumor risk. The lower quality studies, which failed to meet scientific best practices, were primarily industry funded."[17]

One way industry-funded studies of EMFs are problematic from the outset is that they use simulated EMF exposures instead of real cell phones. They do this under the justification of seeking to control variables, but the reality is that a simulated cell phone is far safer than a real cell phone.

Real EMF signals vary unpredictably from moment to moment, especially in their intensity. Simulated EMF signals have fixed parameters, and thus are invariable and completely predictable.[18]

There is a dramatic difference between the results of studies using real exposures from commercially available devices and studies employing simulated exposures from test phones. While about half of the studies using simulated exposures with test phones do not find any effects, nearly all studies using real-life exposures from commercially available devices demonstrate adverse effects.[19-37]

BROADCASTING THE MESSAGE THAT THE SCIENCE IS INCONCLUSIVE

Once the wireless industry funds these studies it "counts up the studies and presents the issue to the public as a simple scoreboard," as Martin Blank, Ph.D., wrote in his book *Overpowered.*

If there are 100 studies done on the safety of cell phones and 50 of them (in most cases, those funded by the industry) find no harmful effects and 50 of them do, then the wireless companies can claim that "the science is mixed," when in reality the science that is not funded by the industry is actually quite clear.

The main vehicle for spreading these safety claims is the CTIA, which creates websites such as wirelesshealthfacts.com that contain statements such as "The scientific consensus, based on peer-reviewed evidence in the U.S. and a number of other countries, indicates that wireless devices do not pose a public health risk for adults or children."[38]

CTIA then feeds its position to the media. Here is a quote from a 2018 article in *Consumer Reports,* a periodical purported to protect the public. It is a classic illustration of how mainstream media often addresses the question of whether or not cell phone radiation is harmful:

When it comes to cell phones, scientists have looked at findings from animal research and cells in test tubes exposed to RF radiation in a lab, as well as observational studies in humans. These human studies have tried to see whether heavy users of cell phones have higher rates of brain cancers and other health problems compared with people who use cell phones less often.

All that research . . . has been mixed, with no definitive proof that cell-phone radiation harms human health, but also unable to completely clear it of any potential risk."[39]

Clear bias also shows up in coverage of major studies that find links between cell phone radiation and health. Let's look at an example: The National Toxicology Program's $30 million, multi-year study that evaluated the effect of exposure to radio frequencies, similar to those used in 2G and 3G cell phones, on rats.

In the study, researchers exposed rats to varying levels of wireless radiation for nine hours a day, seven days a week, for their entire life span. A control group of rats received no exposure to wireless radiation throughout their life span.

Final results, which were released in 2018, found "clear evidence" of malignant tumors, known as schwannomas, in the hearts of male rats and "some evidence" of malignant tumors, known as gliomas, in the brains of male rats. Interestingly, the cancer rates in the female rats were far lower.[40]

According to the National Institute of Environmental Health Sciences, approximately 150 reporters attended a press conference held via telephone to announce the study's preliminary findings in May 2016 and, as a result, the media wrote more than 1,000 news stories about the findings.[41]

Of these stories, there was a wide variance in how the media reported the findings of the study, as evidenced by coverage in *The New York Times* versus *The Wall Street Journal*.

The *Times* piece ran with the headline "Study of Cellphone Risks Finds 'Some Evidence' of Link to Cancer, at Least in Male

Rats," with the subhead, "Many caveats apply, and the results involve radio frequencies long out of routine use."[42]

The Journal ran a story with the headline "Cellphone-Cancer Link Found in Government Study," with the subhead, "Multiyear, peer-reviewed study found 'low incidences' of two types of tumors in male rats exposed to type of radio frequencies commonly emitted by cellphones."[43]

With such disparity in reporting on the same study, it's easy to see how the public remains largely unconvinced of the dangers of wireless radiation.

A LANDMARK LEGAL VICTORY FOR THE WIRELESS INDUSTRY: THE TELECOMMUNICATIONS ACT OF 1996

Just as the tobacco industry had the Tobacco Institute, the entity that lobbied lawmakers on behalf of cigarette manufacturers, the telecommunications industry has the CTIA and National Cable & Telecommunications Association (now called NCTA: The Internet & Television Association) to do its bidding.

Temptation is everywhere in Washington, where moneyed lobbyists and industry representatives throw the best parties and dinners. The industry's deep pockets enables it to exert its influence over lawmakers already in office, candidates running for office, and government employees and appointees who work at and run the agencies overseeing telecommunications.

It was lobbying that played a major role in the passage of the Telecommunications Act of 1996, which included a huge concession to the wireless industry that effectively silenced the public's say in where and how wireless infrastructure is built out. Section 322(c) (7) (B) (iv) reads, in part:

> No State or local government or instrumentality thereof may regulate the placement, construction, and modification of personal wireless service facilities on the basis of the

environmental effects of radio frequency emissions to the extent that such facilities comply with the Commission's regulations concerning such emissions.[44]

As a result, the industry was essentially given the blessing of the government to install cell towers basically wherever they like: school roofs and playgrounds, church spires, water towers, and trees all became fair game for hosting cell towers.

More than 300,000 such sites have been built since the act passed.[45] The public was left with little to no recourse to influence these decisions because of health concerns.

It was a huge victory for the telecom industry that came as a direct result of a massive lobbying push, reportedly with a price tag of approximately $50 million.[46] Larry Pressler, then a Republican senator from South Dakota, described it as the most lobbied bill in history.

Lobbyists lavishly rewarded congressional staffers who helped them write this new law, as 13 of 15 staffers later became lobbyists themselves.[47]

Since their founding, the NCTA and CTIA have been among Washington's top lobbying spenders annually. Take 2018, for example, when AT&T spent $18.5 million, Verizon spent $12 million, NCTA spent $13.2 million, and CTIA spent $9.5 million.[48] Consider this is in *only one year*. Overall, the communications/electronics sector is one of Washington's super heavyweight lobbyists.

While these numbers are large indeed, they are still getting bigger. In a 2019 interview, researcher Joel Moskowitz, Ph.D., who is on the faculty of the School of Public Health at the University of California, Berkeley, stated that the wireless industry is now investing $100 million dollars a year in its lobbying efforts.[49]

SMEARING SCIENTISTS WHO FIND PROBLEMS WITH CELL PHONES

Another tactic the wireless industry has used to sow seeds of doubt with the public is to handpick scientists it believes will be a source of supportive studies, and then discredit those same scientists if their findings suggest that the cell phones you rely on for so many things are found to be contributing factors to illness.

Let us start by looking at what happened to Dr. Henry Lai, whose research into the number of studies on the effects of wireless radiation I discussed earlier in this chapter.

In the early 1990s, Lai and fellow University of Washington researcher Narendra "N.P." Singh submitted a request for funding from the Wireless Technology Research project (WTR) to conduct research on the effects of exposure to low-intensity microwave radiation on the brain cells of rats.

As Lai and Singh recounted in a letter published in *Microwave News*, "WTR made two site visits to our laboratory, in June and July of 1994. During one visit, [George] Carlo said that he was interested in our data and would send a check to us the following week so that we could continue our research. The check never came." They secured funding from the National Institutes of Health instead. What they found was damning indeed.

Their results, published in the journal *Bioelectromagnetics,* found single-strand DNA damage in the brains of rats who were exposed to a mere two hours of both pulsed and continuous low-intensity microwave radiation of 2.5 GHz, a similar frequency to the one that is emitted by your 4G cell phone.[50]

Motorola, when it learned of Lai and Singh's findings, went into defensive mode. An internal company memo, dated December 13, 1994, discussed the best strategy to cast doubt on the study's conclusions. In it, executives suggested the following language:

While this work raises some interesting questions about possible biological effects, it is our understanding that there are too many uncertainties—related to the methodology employed, the findings that have been reported and the science that underlies them—to draw any conclusions about its significance at this time.

Without additional work in this field, there is absolutely no basis to determine whether [what] the researchers found . . . [had] anything at all to do with DNA damage or health risks, especially at the frequencies and power levels or wireless communication devices.[51]

It's not only industry that has sought to stifle research into the biological effects of EMFs—the military has done it too. One of the premier researchers in this area, Dr. Allan Frey, began researching how microwave frequencies affect the body in 1960. At the time, Frey was 25, a young neuroscientist working at General Electric's Advanced Electronics Center at Cornell University.

From these early days, Frey was interested in how electrical fields affect brain function. So when he received a call from a radar technician who made the incredible claim that he could "hear" radar, Frey eagerly went to the site to evaluate why this radar might be audible. Sure enough, he could hear it too—a low-level, persistent humming. "I could hear the radar going 'zip, zip, zip,'" he later reported.

Intrigued, Frey began an investigation that ultimately led him to realize that the ear did not record the radar sounds, the brain did. This is now called the "Frey effect" and caused quite a stir in the scientific community.

On the heels of this discovery, Frey began receiving funding from the Office of Naval Research and the U.S. Army, who were seeking to increase their use of radar in populated areas and wanted to evaluate its effects on public health.

For 15 years, Frey enjoyed the support he received from the military to test the potential effects of EMFs on the body. What he found was remarkable. He showed that rats became docile when exposed to radiation levels of 50 microwatts per square centimeter. Then he showed that he could change rat behavior at exposures to 6 microwatts per square centimeter.

Next, he stopped a frog heart—stopped it dead—at 0.6 microwatts per square centimeter. This is particularly remarkable when you consider that 0.6 microwatts per square centimeter is 10,000 times less than your cell phone emits when you have it pressed to your ear on a call.

Frey ran into trouble with his source of funding in 1975, when he published a landmark paper in the *Annals of the New York Academy of Sciences* that revealed how EMF exposure caused "leakage" of the blood-brain barrier.[52] During this particular study, Frey injected a fluorescent dye into the circulatory system of rats, then ran microwave frequencies over their bodies. After that exposure, the dye showed up in the rats' brains.

The blood-brain barrier is an extremely important means of protection for your brain; it prevents viruses, toxins, and microbes that may be in your bloodstream from penetrating the sanctity of your brain.

Frey later reported that the military instructed him to stop talking about his research or risk losing his funding.[53] Pentagon-funded scientists also claimed to have tried to replicate his results without success. This essentially shut down further research on the effects of EMFs on the blood-brain barrier for decades, at least in the U.S.

Frey certainly was not the first researcher to conflict with the military.

In the late 1950s, ophthalmologist Milton Zaret became one of the first scientists to warn of the potential for harm from exposure to nonionizing radiation. Zaret found a link between microwave radiation and the development of cataracts.

At the time, the primary exposure to microwave frequencies came through the military's use of radar. Microwave ovens were still in their infancy. Cell phones were decades off. As a result, most of Zaret's funding came from the military, including the Air Force, Army, and Navy.

Throughout the 1960s, Zaret published findings that established harmful effects at levels of exposure to EMFs well below current safety standards. In 1973, Zaret was the first medical doctor to testify in Congress about the dangers of microwave radiation. During his testimony, Zaret sounded the alarm.

> There is a clear, present, and ever-increasing danger to the entire population of our country from exposure to the entire non-ionizing portion of the electromagnetic spectrum. The dangers cannot be overstated because more nonionizing radiation injuries occur covertly, usually do not become manifest until after latent periods of years, and when they do become manifest, the effects are seldom recognized.[54]

Gradually, Zaret lost every one of his military contracts because of his findings. He was also the brunt of a campaign to discredit him.

There were some who gave Zaret the credit and credence he deserved. Paul Brodeur, an investigative science journalist who covered the health hazards of EMFs for *The New Yorker* and wrote the 1977 book *The Zapping of America: Microwaves, Their Deadly Risk, and the Coverup*, rightfully refers to Zaret as an "early prophet."

"CAPTURING" THE FEDERAL COMMUNICATIONS COMMISSION

There is one way that the wireless industry has surpassed Big Tobacco—and that is by using its money and influence to get insiders appointed to government agencies charged with regulating its products, namely the Federal Communications Commission (FCC).

Most people believe that our federal regulatory agencies, such as the Food and Drug Administration, the Environmental Protection Agency (EPA), and the FCC, are staffed with impartial experts who take a leading role in performing research and establishing safety standards with an eye toward protecting public health.

This is very often not the case. Typically, government agencies rely on the research community to produce findings that they then merely evaluate to determine regulatory action. And guess who is funding much of the research that determines product safety regulations? That's right, the industries who manufacture the products.

The FCC in particular is frequently referred to as a "captured agency" thanks to Norm Alster of the Edmond J. Safra Center for Ethics at Harvard University, who in 2015 wrote a short book titled *Captured Agency: How the Federal Communications Commission Is Dominated by the Industries It Presumably Regulates.*[55]

As a captured agency, the FCC is a prime example of institutional corruption. Corruption not in the sense that the higher-ups receive envelopes bulging with cash, but the regulatory system favors powerful private influences so much that even the most well-intentioned efforts to protect the public and the environment are often overwhelmed, typically at the expense of public interest.

A detailed look at FCC actions (and nonactions) shows that over the years the agency has granted the wireless industry virtually everything it has ever requested.

The wireless industry controls the FCC through a soup-to-nuts stranglehold on Congress that includes well-placed campaign donations to members of Congress; power over the House Energy and Commerce Subcommittee on Communications and Technology, which oversees the FCC; and persistent lobbying.

According to a 2019 article that appeared in *The Guardian,* the 51 U.S. Senators and their spouses are often heavily invested in public companies they are charged with regulating. And the Wireless Telecomm Group is the company with the single highest amount of stock owned by Republican U.S. Senators, to the tune of $3 million. Apple is the second highest, with Republicans owning stock worth nearly $1.5 million and Democratic Senators just shy of $1 million worth. As the article says:

It's not illegal for members of Congress to have personal financial stakes in the industries on which they legislate. But such investments raise questions about lawmakers' motivations. If a representative on the House financial services committee owns hundreds of thousands of dollars worth of stock in Bank of America, how might this investment affect their questioning of Bank of America's CEO in a hearing? Could it influence how they legislate and vote on banking issues?[56]

The wireless industry has spun a web that embraces Congress, congressional oversight committees, and Washington social life. The network ties the public sector to the private through a frictionless revolving door, really no door at all.

Recent FCC chairmen, including Tom Wheeler (who held the office from 2013 to 2017) and Ajit Pai (who assumed the role in 2017), have worked directly for the industry they were then tasked with overseeing. Pai was once a general counsel for Verizon; Wheeler was the CEO of the CTIA and president of the NCTA.

HOW THE WIRELESS INDUSTRY INFLUENCES GOVERNMENT POLICY

A natural consequence of all the efforts to sow confusion about the true risks of wireless radiation and to infiltrate regulatory agencies is that the government as well as nongovernment organizations charged with safekeeping public health falter.

They seesaw on whether or not there are health hazards in the first place, and then on how serious those hazards are. A perfect example of this has been the long and winding road for EMFs to be classified as a potential, possible, or probable carcinogen.

In 1989, the EPA assigned a team in its Office of Health and Environmental Assessment (OHEA) the task of carefully examining the known biological effects of exposure to microwave radiation.

While the team's work continued for several years, in March 1990 the OHEA issued a draft of its initial findings suggesting that the EPA designate all EMFs "probable human carcinogens." *The*

New York Times reported on the draft and drew a fair amount of public attention.[57] It seemed like the tide of both public opinion and governmental oversight might turn toward caution.

Alas, the moment did not last long. The OHEA draft inspired the White House to order its Committee on Interagency Radiation Research and Policy Coordination (CIRRPC) to create its own report. The CIRRPC report stated that there was "no convincing evidence in the published literature" to link extremely low frequency EMFs to any "demonstrable health hazards."[58]

Following the lead of the executive branch of the government, the OHEA team issued another draft of its report later in 1990 in which it walked back its earlier recommendation, stating that it would be "inappropriate" to compare EMFs with chemical carcinogens.

Even though the OHEA draft report did not result in an official EPA designation of EMFs as any kind of carcinogen, it did contribute to other branches of government taking action to investigate the health risks. In 1992, Congress passed the Energy Policy Act, part of which funded a five-year research initiative to investigate the potential health risks of EMFs.

A working group of nearly 30 scientists appointed by the National Institute of Environmental Health Sciences (NIEHS) carried out this research. In 1998, NIEHS produced a 532-page report in which the experts voted 19 to 9 in favor of designating EMFs a "possible carcinogen."[59]

Again, there was backlash to the report, and it triggered another important investment into further research. In 2000, the International Agency for Research on Cancer (IARC), a division of the World Health Organization (WHO), began a 10-year, $30 million, 13-country Interphone Study that looked specifically at the effects of the radiation emitted by cell phones and its potential role in the development of brain cancer.

When the Interphone Study results were finally released (years behind schedule), they appeared inconclusive. They found no overall increased risk of brain tumors for cell phone users—something that most of the mainstream press latched on to when reporting the findings.

However, the study group did acknowledge that "heavy users" of cell phones had an approximately *80 percent increased* risk of glioma, a life-threatening and often-fatal brain tumor, after 10 years of cell phone use.

What was the definition of a heavy user?

About two hours—per month!

When this study was conducted (1999–2004), cell phone use had not yet exploded to the extent it has today. Now, after two decades have passed since the study began, the average American uses their cell phone more than three and a half hours *per day.*[60]

This significant finding did not garner much attention, except by the IARC, which went on to host a working group of 31 scientists from 14 different countries in May 2011.

This committee reviewed all available scientific literature, looking specifically for studies that examined the effects of consumer exposure to wireless telephones, occupational exposure to radar and microwaves, and environmental exposure to radio, TV, and wireless signals.

This review included the Interphone Study, as well as another study published by Lennart Hardell, a leading brain tumor researcher and professor of oncology and cancer epidemiology at Örebro University Hospital in Sweden. Dr. Hardell found that the risks of brain tumors doubled or even tripled, depending on the type of tumor, in cell phone users after 10 years of cellular phone use.[61]

Largely because of its review, the IARC finally concluded that exposure to cell phone radiation is "possibly carcinogenic to humans" and gave it a Group 2B classification. This is the same category as the pesticide DDT, lead, gasoline engine exhaust, burning coal, and dry-cleaning chemicals, to name just a few.

While this was an important piece of progress in establishing the potential for harm, it stopped short of designating microwave radiation and EMFs as category 2A—"probably carcinogenic to humans"—which is the next step up from "possibly."

Since then, the U.S. government has dithered on warning the public about the hazards of cell phone use: In 2014, the CDC updated its website to state: "We recommend caution in cell phone use."

That's pretty strong language from an agency that had previously said any risks "likely are comparable to other lifestyle choices we make every day." It only lasted a few weeks, however, before the language was removed, along with text that specifically warned against the heightened health risks for children.[62]

The most consistent voice of reason has come from the scientific community. In 2015, 190 EMF scientists from 39 countries issued the International EMF Scientist Appeal to the United Nations calling for the WHO to adopt "more protective exposure guidelines for non-ionizing electromagnetic fields (EMF) in the face of increasing exposures from many sources."[63]

The late spokesperson Martin Blank, Ph.D., announced the appeal.

> We are scientists engaged in the study of biological and health effects of non-ionizing electromagnetic fields (EMF). Based upon peer-reviewed, published research, we have serious concerns regarding the ubiquitous and increasing exposure to EMF generated by electric and wireless devices.

Thankfully, some people *are* listening to the science. In 2016, in the wake of the release of the first round of findings of the National Toxicology Program, Dr. Otis Brawley, chief medical officer of the American Cancer Society, released an official statement.

For years, the understanding of the potential risk of radiation from cell phones has been hampered by a lack of good science. This report from the National Toxicology Program (NTP) is good science. The NTP report linking radiofrequency radiation (RFR) to two types of cancer marks a paradigm shift in our understanding of radiation and cancer risk.[64]

This was an about-face for the American Cancer Society, which has long been a denier of risk. Of course, we need more than just talk. We need action.

HISTORY IS REPEATING ITSELF

History has shown that an admission of the potential health hazards of EMFs will not happen without considerable legal pressure, and that it can take many decades for widespread changes in behavior to occur.

In many of the iconic movies and television programs of the late 20th century, the main characters smoked incessantly—Marlon Brando in *A Streetcar Named Desire*, James Dean in *Rebel without a Cause*, and the TV series *The Twilight Zone*, in which Rod Serling was the smoking moderator who ultimately died from lung cancer.

Watching these programs now, the smoking looks odd—a time stamp of a different era, when ignorance about the health effects of smoking was pervasive.

Perhaps at some point two or three decades down the road, the memory of everyone staring at their cell phones all day will seem outdated too. Perhaps this book will help that future come true on a faster timeline than the five decades it took for cigarettes to lose their widespread allure.

Once you review the mechanisms by which EMFs cause damage (which I cover in Chapter 4) and the science that links them to several diseases (which I will walk you through in Chapter 5),

I believe you will realize that EMFs deserve the designation of a Group 1 carcinogen, the same as cigarettes.

However, there are strong arguments that EMFs are even more pernicious than cigarettes, because you can substantially control your exposure to cigarette smoke; the same cannot be said about your EMF exposure since EMFs are emitted by infrastructure such as ubiquitous cell phones, power lines, electrical wiring, Wi-Fi routers, and cell towers.

If the 50-year timeline of cigarettes' rise and fall pertains here, that would put us at 2045–2050 before the overwhelming evidence comes crashing down on the wireless industry as it did to tobacco in 1998.

By the time those decades have passed, how many people will have become ill, or even died, due to their EMF exposure? Especially considering that, just as with cigarettes, it can take decades for damage to manifest. As Robert N. Proctor, a professor at Columbia University, explained in his submitted written expert testimony in the 2002 federal court case *United States v. Philip Morris USA*:

> It might take 20, 30, or even 40+ years for a tobacco cancer to develop after onset of exposure (this is the so-called "time lag" or "latency").[65]

Exposure to EMFs also has a long time lag. Brain cancer, in particular, can take 40 years to develop. Survivors of the atomic bombs dropped on the Japanese cities of Hiroshima and Nagasaki, for example, are still developing malignant tumors more than 65 years after their radiation exposure.[66] One can only imagine how high the prevalence of cell phone and Wi-Fi related diseases will be in another 20 or 30 years.

A 1969 memo written by an executive at Brown & Williamson, a large tobacco company at the time, concisely sums up this strategy by the phrase "Doubt is our product."[67] Doubt is the wireless industry's product as well.

It has learned, from Big Tobacco's example, that it needs not disprove the idea that its products carry health risks; it only has to provide enough evidence to the contrary that consumers are lulled into a false sense of security. This tactic not only ensures sales, it also wards off regulatory measures and deflects blame for any illnesses or deaths from its products.

While the world waits for the evidence to be deemed conclusive, you, your family, and our entire society are all guinea pigs in an experiment that has the potential to handicap future generations with potentially insurmountable health consequences.

The wireless industry, just like the tobacco industry before it, will continue its strategies and claim that the science is not yet settled and we need more research. It will continue to deny any link between its products and cancer while the evidence to the contrary slowly and steadily piles up, just as it did for cigarette smoking. If you value your health, you simply must act now to protect yourself and your loved ones.

CHAPTER 4

HOW EMFS DAMAGE YOUR BODY

As I wrote about in the introduction, I first became aware of the dangers of EMFs about 20 years ago. I realized that there was likely some biological merit to the arguments but, perhaps like you, I didn't fully believe them. I have always embraced technology and didn't want to limit my access to the wonderful conveniences it provides.

That is why I have written this chapter, to help you understand the biology of precisely how these "safe" wavelengths are damaging your body. I'm hopeful that this information will accelerate your understanding of the very real threat that electromagnetic frequencies expose you to.

I admit that it is fairly complex. I have attempted to make the science as digestible as possible so that you too will be motivated to change the way you interact with these alluring technologies that are deeply embedded in our daily lives.

STUDIES SUPPORTING THE DANGERS OF EMFS

The wireless industry has long held that radiation from its devices produces no thermal damage in humans. This assumption is precisely what the existing safety standards are based on.

Yet this assumption is incorrect and myopically focused, because cell phones *do* have heating effects. Literal hot spots in the brain have been shown to occur as a result of exposure to the radiation emitted by cell phone antennas, largely as a result of the structure of your skull.[1]

You have probably experienced a sensation of heat from holding your phone to your head. That's because your skin is actually being heated, as well as your brain beneath.

It appears that even the FCC knows this, because its exposure limits were formulated to prevent a rise in brain temperature of more than one degree Celsius. The guidelines should have been designed to maintain baseline brain temperature instead; after all, a one-degree rise in temperature is usually called a fever.

It's just that the increase in temperature is not the primary source of the damage they cause—that honor goes to the oxidative damage that cell phone radiation triggers, which is similar to the harm caused by ionizing radiation such as X-rays.

The U.S. government first published documents acknowledging the existence of the harmful effects of EMFs nearly 50 years ago. This included the 1971 U.S. Naval Medical Research Institute report[2] and a follow-up report from the National Aeronautics and Space Administration (NASA) in 1981.[3]

The science documenting the health effects of EMFs that have emerged since these early papers were written has been cataloged in the *BioInitiative Report*, published in 2012 by the BioInitiative Working Group, a collective of 29 authors from 10 countries, including 10 M.D.s, 21 Ph.D.s, and an M.Sc., M.A., and M.P.H.

The group released an update in 2017, a massive 650-page report that contains 1,800 new studies. If you are interested, I suggest downloading it at https://bioinitiative.org.

An even more comprehensive collection of studies on EMFs is compiled at the EMF-Portal (emf-portal.org/en). It lists nearly 30,000 studies with more than 6,300 summaries and you can view a list of the publications for the last 30 days.

If you don't want to pore through hundreds and hundreds of pages of research, Dr. Martin Pall prepared a summary of some of the best literature in this area,[4] and I have included a list of the studies Pall summarizes in Appendix B of this book. Perhaps these are two better places to start a serious review of the science.

As important as these tens of thousands of studies are because they show that cell phone exposure is connected to many different diseases in your body,[5] they were largely observational and none of them illuminated a solid mechanism of how EMFs actually affect your biology.

Thankfully, recent research has elucidated some of the mechanisms of how exposure to nonionizing EMFs may impact your biology other than thermal damage. A lot of this work dovetails with the past 15 years of cancer research, which has focused on intermediary cellular metabolism, expanding our understanding of how basic cell function is a central driver of an ever-growing number of human diseases.[6]

Since understanding the mechanism was so profoundly foundational to my taking action on EMF remediation, I will walk you through it in this chapter. Let's get started.

A NEW UNDERSTANDING OF EMFS AND YOUR BIOLOGY: IT ALL STARTS WITH CALCIUM

One of the prevailing theories on how EMFs impact human health was proposed by Martin Pall. It rests on a mineral you are likely very familiar with: calcium. Calcium is the most abundant mineral in your body, making up approximately 2 percent of your body weight.

Your body uses about 98 percent of its calcium to keep your bones and teeth strong,[7] thereby supporting your skeletal structure and function. You likely believe this is calcium's sole function in your body.

But calcium has many other roles that are each absolutely essential to your health, including:

- Cell signaling

- Regulating enzyme and protein functions

- Muscle contraction

- Blood clotting

- Nerve function

- Cell growth

- Learning and memory

It is calcium's role as a biological signaling molecule that is affected by EMF exposure. To understand how this occurs, we need to dive a bit deeper into the details of how calcium actually works as a chemical messenger.

The first important fact to understand is that calcium is far more concentrated outside of your cells than inside. In fact, the amount of calcium outside your cells is 20,000 to 100,000 times higher than the level inside your cells.[8]

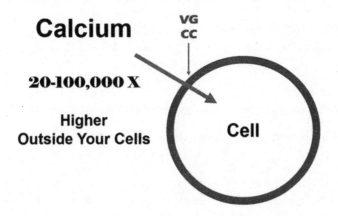

Figure 4.1: Relative calcium levels inside the cell versus outside the cell.

It's also important to note that calcium doesn't flow freely from outside to inside your cells. Rather, your cells have evolved a very elegant way to tightly regulate and control their level of calcium. This fine tuning of calcium levels is necessary to allow the mineral to maintain precise control over the many areas of your body that it is responsible for.

If this highly regulated system is distorted, it can wreak metabolic havoc in your body. And this is precisely what happens when you are exposed to excessive EMFs.

This finely tuned control of calcium from outside your cells to the inside occurs through tiny ion channels embedded in your cell membranes.

Scientists have given these ion channels a more technical term that we will use throughout the rest of this book: *voltage-gated calcium channels* (VGCCs). There's a popular class of drugs that works on the VGCCs known as calcium channel blockers. They are used primarily to relax blood vessels for individuals with high blood pressure, and to help normalize certain types of abnormally rapid heart rhythms.

THE CONNECTION BETWEEN EMF EXPOSURE AND CALCIUM

It seems quite clear that the way EMFs damage your cells is by increasing oxidative stress in your cells, and that this damaging process involves intercellular calcium.

The discovery that exposure to EMFs increases calcium levels inside the cells dates back to the early 1990s.[9]

More recent studies have also confirmed the role of increased calcium inside your cells following EMF exposure.

In 2013 Martin Pall published a study (updated in 2018)[10] in which he described his theory of the mechanism of how EMF exposure increased calcium inside the cell. Pall came to his conclusions by reviewing 26 studies where investigators used calcium channel-blocker drugs, the same drugs that are prescribed to patients with high blood pressure, to examine their effects on VGCCs when EMFs were present.

These studies were not done in humans but in in vitro cells and in animals at a low-frequency EMF of 50 or 60 Hz, which is the typical electrical field exposure.[11]

Amazingly, research confirmed that when calcium channels were blocked, the damage that the EMFs caused was radically reduced, providing very compelling evidence that the calcium channels were responsible for facilitating the damage from the EMF.

The researchers found that when EMFs activated the VGCCs, after about five seconds the channels opened up and flooded the inside of the cell with an unhealthy amount of calcium ions at the rate of about one million per second.

EMFs also disrupt the flow of calcium once inside your cells, allowing too much of it to pass into your mitochondria.

You might remember from high school biology—or from one of my previous books, *Fat for Fuel* or *KetoFast*—that your mitochondria are tiny organelles inside most of your cells, and each cell normally has several hundred mitochondria inside.

Your mitochondria are generally referred to as the energy producers of your cells as they have the enzymes and machinery to create *adenosine triphosphate* (ATP), which is the primary energy currency of your cells.

When calcium inside your mitochondria increases, it leads to a series of damaging states, including a lowered ability to generate ATP and increased oxidative stress that eventually contributes to premature cell death.[12] There are many, many reasons to avoid unnecessary EMF exposures, but keeping your mitochondria healthy is one of the most important ones.

Humans are not the only species who have channels allowing calcium to flow in and out of cells.[13] They are in all plants and animals. The VGCCs in plants are constructed differently, but they function very similarly to the ones we have, essentially serving as ways to regulate the flow of calcium into and out of cells.

As I'll discuss more later in this chapter, the fact that VGCCs exist in both plants and animals is a powerful illustration of how EMFs impact virtually all forms of living things exposed to them, and therefore have enormous environmental consequences.[14]

Despite the number of studies showing a direct relationship between EMF exposure and VGCC activation, it is still a theory, and not one that everyone agrees with.

Dr. Henry Lai, a prominent EMF researcher whose work has shown evidence of EMFs' ability to cause DNA damage, agrees that VGCCs are an important area to investigate, but he maintains that there are many unanswered questions about the theory, which I won't delve into here as they are highly technical. You can read about them on Dariusz Leszczynksi's blog, *Between a Rock and a Hard Place*.[15]

THE PROBLEM WITH EXCESS CALCIUM IN YOUR CELLS

Remember that in addition to providing support for your physical structure, calcium is a very important biological signaling molecule with vital biological roles. When too much calcium is released into your cells it can trigger a chain of events that can increase your risk of diseases, especially cancer, and premature aging.

So what happens when excess calcium floods into your cells?

The answer has to do with free radicals, which are any molecules that have been damaged and, as a result, have an unpaired electron. Unpaired electrons are what make free radicals highly reactive and potentially very damaging.[16]

The broad strokes of how EMFs do damage is that they release excess calcium into your cells, which then initiates a cascade of molecular events that ultimately result in an increase in free radicals. These highly reactive molecules then proceed to travel and damage your cell membranes, proteins, mitochondria, and stem cells, and not only your mitochondrial but also your nuclear DNA.[17]

Interestingly, this is the precise end result that sources of ionizing radiation, like X-rays and gamma rays, produce, as I reviewed in Chapter 1.

Although it means we will wade fairly deep into the waters of science, I would like to uncover the details of these molecular events.

Why? Do we really need to break it down at a molecular level?

We do, because the media and the wireless industry will try to tell you that the information in this book is simply not true. This is why I want to provide you with the detailed biological impacts so you can confront these sources with the science that will refute their assertions of wireless safety.

So strap on your life vest, here we go.

When extra calcium ions rush into your cells, they cause an increase in both *nitric oxide* and *superoxide*. At first glance this may not seem like a bad thing, because although these two molecules are free radicals, they are relatively benign and each plays many important roles in your body (I will explain more about those functions in just a moment).

But once you unleash loads of them all at once and they come very close to each other, they will spontaneously combine and can instantly form one of the most damaging molecules in your body, *peroxynitrite*.

Therefore, it's not nitric oxide and superoxide themselves that are the issue, it's the fact that when they occur in large amounts in close proximity to one another they produce the dangerous molecule peroxynitrite, which is harmful.

And they don't produce just a little of it. Even a modest increase in nitric oxide and superoxide results in an exponential rise in peroxynitrite. A tenfold increase in nitric oxide and superoxide will increase peroxynitrite formation a hundredfold.

Once it is formed, peroxynitrite starts attacking important biological molecules that damage your cells, cause disease, and lead to premature death. Peroxynitrite can damage nearly every significant tissue in your body, such as your precious cell membranes,[18] proteins,[19] mitochondria,[20] stem cells,[21] and DNA.[22]

Peroxynitrite-induced damage cues an inflammatory response from your immune system. Once your body is inflamed, even higher concentrations are possible, increasing nitric oxide and superoxide a thousandfold, which means a potential millionfold rise in the formation of peroxynitrite![23]

Because it inflicts damage on so many of your vital tissues, you can begin to understand how peroxynitrite is one of the most pernicious toxins you can be exposed to. Keeping your levels of this toxin low will radically decrease your risk of chronic degenerative diseases and will slow down the aging process in your body.

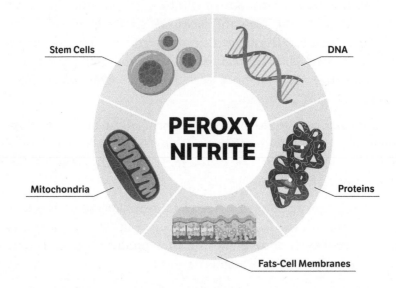

Figure 4.2: The reactive nitrogen species (RNS) damages vital parts of your cells.

SUPEROXIDE: A BENEFICIAL FREE RADICAL WITH A DARK SIDE

Let's back up a moment and learn a little more about the two molecules that combine to form peroxynitrite: nitric oxide and superoxide. We'll start with the latter.

Superoxide is an important biological signaling molecule.[24] It is also a free radical. From its name, it sounds like it would be a super-oxidizing molecule. But the truth is that superoxide is actually relatively weak because it is more likely to surrender its electron than to accept an additional electron from another molecule.

Under good health conditions, superoxide is not particularly toxic because your body has efficient means to minimize its accumulation—namely, scavenging enzymes such as *superoxide dismutase* (SOD), which quickly remove superoxide from circulation—and you don't produce all that much of it during the regular course of metabolizing food into energy.

The problems arise when your health is less than optimal because you are burning carbohydrates as your primary fuel instead of fat. In other words, if you're eating too many carb-rich foods and rarely go longer than a couple hours without eating.

If you read my book *Fat for Fuel*, you probably recall that your body can burn either carbs or fat in order to make energy, and that burning carbs produces far more free radicals than burning fat. So when you eat—and therefore burn—primarily carbs, you expose your mitochondria and your cells to significantly more free radicals, including superoxide.

While I go into great detail about how to tell if you are burning fat or carbs in *Fat for Fuel*, I'll give you the brief version here. For a general idea of whether you are burning fat or carbs, answer the following questions:

1. Are you overweight? (Is your body mass index higher than 25?)

2. Do you have diabetes?

3. Do you have, or have you had, heart disease?

4. Do you have high blood pressure (130/80 or higher)?

5. Is your waist-to-hip ratio greater than 1 (men) or 0.8 (women)?

To find your waist-to-hip ratio, measure the smallest part of your waist with a tape measure. Don't hold in your belly while you measure! Now measure the biggest part of your hips—the part where your buttocks stick out the most. Divide your waist measurement by your hip measurement. The answer is your waist-to-hip ratio.

If you have answered yes to any of these conditions, odds are good that you are burning carbs. If you don't have these diseases and are healthy, then it is likely that you have the capacity to burn fat as your primary fuel—although, consider that this is probably only about 15 percent of the total population. But if you are a member of this small group, the amount of superoxide that your mitochondria produce is probably in a healthy range.[25]

THE RELATIONSHIP BETWEEN THE FOOD YOU EAT AND DAMAGE CAUSED BY EMFS

The process of converting the food you eat into energy, in the form of adenosine triphosphate (ATP), is not 100 percent efficient. Even if you are healthy, it is still only somewhere between 95 and 97 percent efficient.

Meaning, some electrons will leak out of the energy-generation mechanism known as the electron transport chain in your mitochondria and form what are called *reactive oxygen species* (ROS). ROS are unstable oxygen atoms that have gained one or more unpaired electrons and can damage your tissues. Superoxide is an ROS.

When you rely on burning carbs for fuel you will generate 30 to 40 percent more ROS, including superoxide, as the process of burning carbs leaks far more electrons into your mitochondria than burning fat does. The more superoxide you make through poor dietary choices and timing of your meals, the more damaging peroxynitrite your body will create.[26–28]

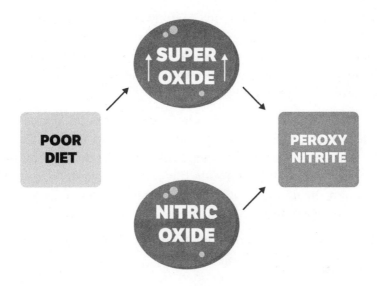

Figure 4.3. How a poor diet increases oxidative stress.

HYDROXYL FREE RADICALS

Now that you understand how your food is broken down to supply your body with energy, let's examine the ROS that are produced during this process in more detail as they impact what happens to your body when you are exposed to EMFs.

Because superoxide has a limited reactivity, there was considerable controversy among researchers in the 20th century about what role it plays in cell toxicity.[29] They were perplexed as to what could cause most of the oxidative damage inside the cells if it wasn't superoxide. They eventually learned that the true villain was actually a cousin, the *hydroxyl free radical.*

Hydroxyl radicals are hyperreactive and will combine with virtually any biological molecule within a very short distance. Because they were known to be so biologically damaging researchers believed that the hydroxyl radical was the major toxin produced in cells. It rapidly became widely accepted that hydroxyl radicals were the primary mechanism of free radical damage.

Similar to superoxide, hydroxyl radicals are normally made in your mitochondria in the process of burning food for fuel. There is a slight difference between the mechanisms that create these two different molecules though, as iron is required as a catalyst to form hydroxyl radicals.

Like most things in life, the hydroxyl radical theory only lasted so long. While hydroxyl radicals do play a role in oxidative stress, they are very short lived, lasting only about a billionth of a second. This radically limits the distance they travel, usually less than the diameter of the typical protein, before they perish and cease their destructive damage.

Since the vast majority of hydroxyl radicals are created in your mitochondria and they can only travel very short distances, they simply do not have enough time to pass out of the mitochondria and into the nucleus, where they could damage your nuclear DNA. Therefore, most of the damage they cause is limited to your mitochondria.

We now realize that the biological relevance of hydroxyl radicals is seriously limited because of its incredibly short life span. Yet the hydroxyl free radical theory is still widely described in many pathology textbooks.

A far better explanation of superoxide toxicity became apparent with the discovery of nitric oxide. It is now widely appreciated that when both superoxide and nitric oxide are produced within a few cell diameters of each other, they will combine spontaneously to form the highly pernicious peroxynitrite.[30] And peroxynitrite seems to be a champ at causing cellular destruction in your body, as we will cover in the following section.

MEET NITRIC OXIDE, ANOTHER BENEFICIAL FREE RADICAL WITH A DARK SIDE

Very few molecules can compete with the magnitude of impact that nitric oxide has had on biology since its discovery in

1980.[31] When scientists finally started to understand the biology of nitric oxide it challenged some of the foundations of biological thinking.

In 1992, *Science,* one of the most prestigious scientific journals in the world, named nitric oxide "Molecule of the Year." Six years later, in 1998, three researchers responsible for the major discoveries surrounding nitric oxide won the Nobel Prize. Since then the field of study of nitric oxide has grown immensely with 160,000 publications that touch on all aspects of health and disease.

So, what is it?

Nitric oxide is a small molecule comprised of oxygen and nitrogen atoms that readily crosses your cell membranes as a colorless gas. (It is not to be confused with *nitrous oxide,* the so-called laughing gas used in your dentist's office.)

Even though nitric oxide is a free radical, it has many beneficial effects in your body:

- It regulates the tone of your blood vessels through its ability to relax them and help normalize blood pressure.[32]

- It plays a crucial role in controlling infections.[33]

- It decreases platelet aggregation or the tendency of blood to clot, thus decreasing the risk of blood clots leading to stroke or heart attack.[34]

- It promotes new blood vessel formation, a process called angiogenesis.[35]

- It helps prevent erectile dysfunction.[36]

Many people are actually deficient in nitric oxide and therefore benefit from strategies to increase their levels. Rather than taking potentially dangerous drugs such as Viagra, which increase nitric oxide, you can increase your intake of plant-based dietary nitrates from foods such as arugula, or take nitric oxide precursors, like arginine or citrulline malate, as supplements in order to achieve healthy levels of this beneficial molecule.

Nitric oxide is mostly made in the inner layer of your blood vessels; since your blood vessels are the primary users of nitric oxide, this is where the bulk of it is produced and stored until it is needed. The important point to recognize here is that nitric oxide is not ordinarily stored inside your cells, nor does it float around just waiting to be used. It is far too reactive to do that.

Rather, it is bound to molecules like glutathione, heme, and other proteins. This is where EMF exposure is such a major concern, because one of the results of all the extra calcium that rushes into your cells when exposed to EMFs is that it causes this stored nitric oxide to be released, increasing the levels of nitric oxide inside your cells.

This EMF-induced nitric oxide increase might seem beneficial, but nitric oxide's positive effects occur only when it is produced naturally *outside* your cells. The problem with elevated levels *inside* your cells is that nitric oxide is highly reactive, meaning it quickly combines with superoxide, the other free radical that increases when there is excess calcium in your cells.

This combination then forms peroxynitrite, and this process is radically accelerated when you are eating an unhealthy diet as described earlier, because you have more superoxide for the nitric oxide to react with and form peroxynitrite.

PEROXYNITRITE MAY BE ONE OF THE MOST DAMAGING MOLECULES IN YOUR BODY

The primary reason peroxynitrite is more biologically pernicious than hydroxyl free radical is because it lives about 10 billion times longer, meaning it has loads more time to damage your tissues.

Peroxynitrite is not technically a free radical. Rather, it is a strong oxidant that reacts relatively slowly with most biological molecules. It also is not classified as a reactive oxygen species (ROS) because unlike ROS it has nitrogen in its structure. So, it is called a *reactive nitrogen species* (RNS).

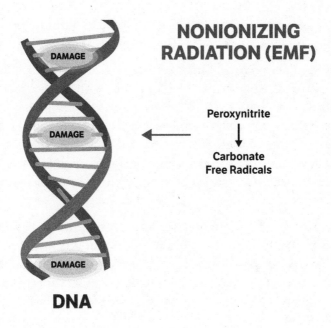

Figure 4.4: How your cell phone and Wi-Fi router damage your DNA.

The damage peroxynitrite induces is the result of its primary breakdown product, *carbonate free radicals*, which likely causes far more serious damage to DNA than hydroxyl free radical.

The carbonate free radical lives much longer than the hydroxyl free radical, albeit only thousands of times longer, not billions like peroxynitrite. When you combine the half-lives of these free radicals, you can begin to appreciate why the cascading domino of free radicals resulting from EMF exposure is so damaging.

In fact, peroxynitrite is the only known molecule that has both a long enough half-life to travel within and between cells and the ability to break DNA bonds.[37] It lives more than long enough to travel relatively great distances and can easily cross cell membranes and penetrate the nucleus where it creates carbonate free radicals to trigger breaks in the strands of your DNA.

As if that weren't reason enough for concern, peroxynitrite accelerates the damage to your body by inhibiting superoxide dismutase (SOD). This is the scavenging antioxidant enzyme that neutralizes superoxide and converts it to another free radical, hydrogen peroxide, which is then typically converted to water.

When peroxynitrite inhibits SOD it has the effect of increasing available superoxide to combine with nitric oxide and creating a vicious cycle of even more peroxynitrite, because peroxynitrite is formed nearly every time superoxide and nitric oxide get close to each other. Nitric oxide and superoxide do not even have to be produced within the same cell to form peroxynitrite, because nitric oxide can readily move through membranes and between cells.

No enzyme is required to form peroxynitrite; in fact, no enzyme can possibly catalyze a reaction that quickly. Nitric oxide is the only known biological molecule that reacts with superoxide quickly enough and is produced in high enough concentrations to outcompete SOD, which would otherwise normally break superoxide down.[38]

Even the generation of a moderate amount of peroxynitrite over long periods of time will result in substantial oxidative damage. This leads to the impairment of critical cellular processes. It disrupts important cell signaling pathways and damages your mitochondria, which then decreases your ability to create energy in the form of ATP.

Long term, peroxynitrite causes inflammation and ultimately damages your tissues, contributing to cardiovascular disease, neurodegenerative disease, diabetes, and many other conditions, most of which have been scientifically linked to EMF exposure, as I'll explain in the next chapter.

WHY YOU LIKELY HAVE NEVER HEARD OF PEROXYNITRITE

If this molecule is so dangerous, why haven't you heard about it before? Peroxynitrite was only discovered shortly before the turn of this century. It was first described in 1990.[39]

This is why nearly every doctor who went to medical school in the 20th century, and most thereafter, were not taught about peroxynitrite. Pretty much the only people who are aware of this pernicious molecule are either biochemists or molecular biology science geeks.

Thankfully there is a great resource for those with science training who want to learn more about peroxynitrite, and best of all it's free. It is an epic paper called "Nitric Oxide and Peroxynitrite in Health and Disease"[40] that has nearly 1,500 references and can be reviewed at no charge by typing the title into your favorite search engine.

This paper was written by three leading scientists funded by the National Institutes of Health (NIH). It is a 140-page, landmark comprehensive review documenting how elevated levels of peroxynitrite cause extensive cellular damage that disrupts at least 97 critical biological processes and, as a result, are associated with more than 60 chronic diseases. The beginning of this article is a must read for any serious student of EMFs.

NONIONIZING RADIATION ALSO DAMAGES YOUR DNA

As I explained in Chapter 1, it is widely accepted that ionizing radiation—like X-rays and gamma rays—damages your body and greatly increases your risk of cancer. This is because ionizing radiation has short wavelengths and high frequencies that carry enough energy to directly break the covalent bonds holding your DNA together.

Contrary to popular belief, most of the damage that ionizing radiation causes is not by breaking your DNA's covalent bonds directly, it is actually a result of interacting with the water in your cells, and more specifically your nucleus.

When ionizing radiation hits the water in your nucleus it creates dangerous hydroxyl free radicals. As you learned in the section above, hydroxyl radicals are unable to travel very far, but since the ionizing radiation can create these radicals in the nucleus right next to your nuclear DNA, they are able to inflict damage on your DNA and cause single- and double-stranded breaks.

This is called *indirect ionization* and likely results in the vast majority of the damage that ionizing radiation causes to DNA. This is illustrated in the graphic below.

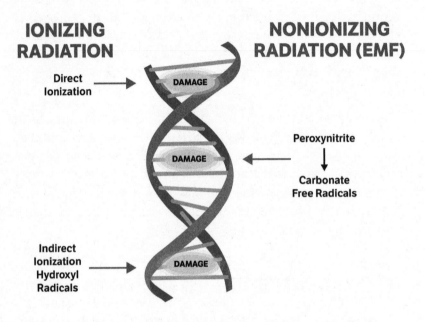

IONIZING RADIATION

Direct Ionization → DAMAGE

Indirect Ionization Hydroxyl Radicals → DAMAGE

NONIONIZING RADIATION (EMF)

Peroxynitrite ↓ Carbonate Free Radicals → DAMAGE

Figure 4.5: Similarities of how X-rays and your cell phone cause DNA damage.

It is true that nonionizing radiation, like that emitted by your cell phone and Wi-Fi, has lower frequencies than ionizing radiation and simply doesn't have enough energy to create hydroxyl radicals or cause significant thermal damage.

But it is not true that nonionizing radiation is incapable of damaging DNA. It can, and it does, through the production of peroxynitrite and its secondary creation of carbonate free radicals. It has become clear that peroxynitrite production is the missing link that connects the dots as to why nonionizing radiation can be every bit as damaging as ionizing X-rays.

The German EMF researcher Franz Adlkofer used a comet assay, which is a very sensitive test for DNA damage, in a 2008 study.[41] He found that very low intensity EMF exposure at 1.8 GHz produced large numbers of DNA breaks. It actually produced more DNA damage than 1,600 chest X-rays.[42]

Adlkofer did another comparison study[43] and from this comparison, it seems clear that nonionizing radiation similar to 3G radiation can be much more dangerous to the DNA of your cells than a similar energy of ionizing radiation.

Now we know that the reason EMF exposure can result in extraordinarily high levels of peroxynitrite is that there are three steps in the process, each of which has high levels of amplification. When you have three amplification steps in sequence (see below), you can get a very large response from a very small initial signal:

- When the VGCC channels are open, they allow the influx of about a million calcium ions per second into the cell.

- That elevated calcium inside your cells then activates the synthesis of both nitric oxide and superoxide.

- Peroxynitrite is formed in proportion to the product of nitric oxide concentration times the superoxide concentration.

These three steps occur more frequently in some cells than in others. That is because all your cells have VGCCs, but certain tissues have far higher concentrations of them, as they rely more on calcium to regulate their function. These tissues include your brain, your heart, and your reproductive organs—the very tissues that are impacted most when you are exposed to EMFs.

This is likely why neuropsychiatric diseases like anxiety, depression, attention deficit/hyperactivity disorder (ADHD), and autism; neurodegenerative diseases like Alzheimer's; and declining fertility rates have exploded in the past two decades. And, as I'll discuss later in this chapter, the risks of EMF exposure to children are even greater than they are for adults. But first, you need to understand that humans aren't the only beings who are negatively impacted by EMF exposure.

ALL LIVING THINGS ARE VULNERABLE TO EMFS

Humans exist within a broader ecosystem of other living things. Just as EMFs affect our biology, they do the same to all life forms. EMFs affect the function of cell membranes and can lead to DNA dysfunction: they have an impact on anything with DNA. And that includes plants, animals, insects, and even microbes.

There have been at least two major reviews of studies that have evaluated the biological and ecological effects of EMFs on all life forms. One, published in 2012 in *Biology and Medicine*, examined nearly 1,000 research papers on birds, bees, plants, animals, and humans. Negative impacts were discovered in 593 studies, while only 180 showed no effect and 196 were inconclusive.[44]

A 2013 review of 113 studies found that 65 percent of those studies reported significant negative effects from EMFs, whether at high or low dosages. Half of the studies demonstrated harmful effects on animals, and 75 percent showed negative influence on plants, with the most pronounced effect on the development and reproduction of birds and insects.[45,46]

Existing science confirms the negative health implications of EMFs. You must broaden your view and take in how they relate to the environment at large.

INSECT POPULATIONS ARE BEING DECIMATED

EMFs are believed to have a major role in colony collapse disorder (CCD), the widespread collapse of bee colonies around the world. Where there were 6 million honeybee colonies in the U.S. in 1947, by 2012 only 2.6 million remained,[47] a number that has held fairly steady since then.[48,49]

And it's not just the total number of bees, but the number of species. For example, in 2013, Oklahoma had only half the number of bumblebee species that it had in 1949.[50] The decline in bees coincided with the rise in man-made EMFs, as most of the decrease has happened in the 21st century.

In the winter of 2006–2007, bees began experiencing CCD. During this winter, beekeepers reported losing anywhere between 50 and 90 percent of their hives. The following effects of EMFs on bees—whether individually or as hives—have been recorded:

- Exposure to mobile phones instigated worker bees to emit a piping signal, which is typically used only to cue a swarm or as a distress signal.[51]

- Bee colonies exposed to cell phone radiation experienced a significant decline in colony strength. The queen laid fewer eggs. And the colony did not have pollen or honey in it when the experiment concluded.[52]

- When an experiment was conducted on 16 different hives—8 exposed to a nearby cordless phone, and 8 not—only 7.3 percent of bees came back to the irradiated hive, compared to 39.7 percent returning to the non-irradiated hive.[53]

- In another, similar experiment, the bees in irradiated hives built 21 percent fewer cells within the hive than in non-irradiated hives.[54]

Bees aren't the only insects to demonstrate such precipitous declines. In 2014, researchers conducted 280 different experiments where they exposed fruit flies to varying sources of nonthermal radiation, including Wi-Fi, baby monitors, Bluetooth, and both mobile and cordless phones. At every level, the exposure resulted in significant detrimental effects on reproduction and apoptosis (programmed cell death).[55]

It's gotten to the point that a 2019 review of scientific literature documenting insect populations around the globe found that if the current rate of insect population decrease continues, all insects could be radically decreased if not totally wiped off the face of the earth within 100 years.[56]

A co-author of the review, Francisco Sánchez-Bayo, an environmental biologist at the University of Sydney, told the *Guardian*:

> It is very rapid. In 10 years you will have a quarter less, in 50 years only half left and in 100 years you will have none. If insect species losses cannot be halted, this will have catastrophic consequences for both the planet's ecosystems and for the survival of mankind.[57]

PLANTS AREN'T EXEMPT EITHER

Just as EMFs wreak havoc in the human body by activating voltage-gated calcium channels, allowing excess calcium to flow into cells, they do the same to plants.[58] This is because plants have calcium channels that respond very similarly to our VGCCs.

As you likely recall from earlier in this chapter, activating VGCCs is the trigger for the oxidative stress caused by EMFs. That means plants experience oxidative stress and DNA damage similar to what humans and animals experience, as well as thinner cell walls, smaller mitochondria, and increased emissions of volatile compounds.[59]

Tomato plants have even been shown to react to EMFs at 900 MHz. In an elegant experiment, researchers showed that leaves exposed to these EMF frequencies reacted with stress signals; shielded leaves did not. When a calcium channel blocker was applied to the leaf surface, the leaf did not respond to the EMFs.[60]

This likely explains why trees and trembling aspen seedlings that are near cell towers are experiencing damage.[61,62] A 2017 study found that many important food plants seem more susceptible to EMF-induced damage than others, including maize, peas, tomatoes, and onions.[63]

DISEASE-CAUSING BACTERIA APPEAR TO BE EMBOLDENED BY EMF EXPOSURE

Since EMFs can effect changes even at the cellular level within the bodies of living things, it makes sense that they can also have an impact on bacteria. Especially when you learn that bacteria communicate with one another using electronic signals.

You have trillions of bacteria residing inside your body, some good and some bad. The friendly bacteria play a huge role in your health, contributing greatly to your ability to digest and extract nutrients from the food you eat, your immunity, and even your mental health, as they manufacture many of the neurotransmitters that relate to mood and emotions, such as serotonin.

The not-so-friendly bacteria are viruses and other pathogens that can make you sick and contribute to your overall toxic load with their waste products. The bad news about EMFs is that they impair function in the good guys, while actually increasing the ability to cause damage in the bad guys. For example:

- Exposure to household wiring has been shown to activate Epstein-Barr virus bacteria that had been dormant.[64]

- One of my early mentors, Dr. Dietrich Klinghardt, founder of the Sophia Health Institute in Woodinville, Washington, has research that demonstrates that bacteria such as candida (aka yeast) and mold produce exponentially more toxic byproducts when in the presence of non-thermal radiation—perhaps in an attempt to protect themselves from the invisible assault.[65]

- Research has also found that yeast strains seem to grow more quickly when exposed to EMFs.[66,67]

- And it appears that cell phone and Wi-Fi signals could play a role in certain types of bacteria—in the case of this study, *E. coli* and listeria became resistant to antibiotic treatment.[68]

The effects of EMFs on bacteria are an important secondary means by which human health is compromised through the ever-increasing soup of electromagnetic radiation that our society swims in every day.

THE ANIMAL KINGDOM IS ALSO AFFECTED

There are multiple mechanisms by which EMFs interfere with the animal world. Because many animals navigate by following the Earth's magnetic fields, the rise in EMFs can disrupt their innate navigating abilities. This is as problematic for bees seeking their way back to the hive after foraging for pollen (as I discussed earlier) as it is for migrating birds,[69] wood mice trying to remember where they made their nests,[70] and even lobsters traversing the ocean floor.[71]

EMFs have also been implicated in reducing the number of tadpoles that grow into frogs,[72] the amount of milk produced by dairy cows,[73] and the areas where bats willingly fly.[74]

So the good news is that when you make efforts to protect yourself from EMFs, you are also helping the environment. But to make an even more dramatic impact, you will need to play an activist role and participate in movements to limit the spread of EMFs. I hope that thinking of the current and future health of our children will help motivate you to get into action.

THE POPULATION MOST VULNERABLE TO EMF DAMAGE

As dangerous as EMFs are to adults, plants, bees, microbes, and animals, they pose a dramatically greater health risk for children, primarily because of the duration of exposure. The youth of today will be exposed to EMFs for a much longer time than adults. As a result, the opportunity for them to experience greater mitochondrial damage over time is exponentially higher.

Children under 12 years of age also have higher body water content than adults, which allows them to absorb considerably more radiation. Additionally, a child's bone marrow absorbs 10 times more wireless frequency radiation than an adult's.[75,76]

Perhaps their biggest vulnerability, however, is all in their head.

CHILDREN'S BRAINS ARE PARTICULARLY AT RISK OF DAMAGE

There are no two ways about it: EMF radiation from cell phones penetrates more deeply into kids' brains than it does into those of adults. There are several reasons for this:

- Children's skulls are thinner than adults' skulls, which means more radiation is able to penetrate this protective barrier.

- Children have smaller heads in general, meaning there is less distance for radiation to travel in order to penetrate more deeply into the brain.

- Children's brains are still developing; they aren't fully myelinated yet, which means they have more water and less fat than adults and are more susceptible to radiation absorption.

- Their ears are smaller, and since the ear acts as a buffer between a cell phone and the skull, this means when children use cell phones the devices are closer to their skulls than when adults use them.

Regarding the use of cell phones within the pediatric population, Ronald L. Melnick, scientific adviser for the Environmental Health Trust, said, "The penetration of the cell phone radiation into the brain of a child is deeper and greater. Also, the developing nervous system of a child is potentially more susceptible to a damaging agent."[77]

The California Department of Public Health's Environmental Health Investigations Branch concurred, finding: "EMFs can pass deeper into a child's brain than an adult's. The brain is still developing through the teen years, which may make children and teens more sensitive to EMF exposure."[78]

It's important to take precautions now to protect your children, especially because the damage done by EMF radiation can take years, and sometimes decades, to develop.

We have known about these heightened risks for children since 1996, when researcher Om P. Gandhi released his groundbreaking study that showed 5- and 10-year-old children had higher peak spatial specific absorption rates than adults.[79]

He confirmed his findings again in 2002,[80] and they were cited by the World Health Organization (WHO) in 2013, when it classified cell phone and wireless radiation as Class 2B Possible Human Carcinogens. In the monograph that lays out their reasoning, the WHO's International Agency for Research on Cancer stated:

> The average radio frequency radiation energy deposition for children exposed to mobile phone RF is two times higher in the brain and 10 times higher in the bone marrow of the skull, compared with mobile phone use by adults.[81]

Gandhi's research not only highlights the heightened risks to children, but also the negligence of America's safety guidelines for radiation exposure, which are based on the specific absorption rate (SAR) of a 220-pound, six-foot-two male.

EXPOSURE STARTS IN UTERO

Depending on the habits of their parents, especially their mothers, many children are affected by exposure to radiation from EMFs when they are still in the womb—from their mother's use of laptops, cell phones, tablets, or cordless phones, or simply as a result of their mother's daily lifestyle.

While there is no reliable way to predict the long-term effects on children who are exposed while still in utero, one study involving more than 13,000 mothers revealed some sobering potential effects. As compared to children born of mothers who did not use cell phones during pregnancy, children born of mothers who did experienced a

- 49 percent increase in behavioral problems;
- 35 percent increase in hyperactivity;
- 34 percent increase in peer-related problems; and
- 25 percent increase in emotional issues.[82]

Two Danish studies have documented an association between cell phone use in the mother and ADHD in children. In looking at two different groups—one made up of more than 13,000 children, the other of nearly 29,000 children—researchers found that if a mother talked on a cell phone while pregnant, her child would go on to have a 50 percent higher risk of ADHD. And if the mother kept the cell phone on continuously, that increased risk was 100 percent higher.[83,84]

Human studies also have found a link between the use of cell phones by pregnant mothers and higher rates of obesity,[85] asthma,[86] and yes, behavioral and attention challenges.[87]

It's not just cell phone radiation that poses a risk; it's all EMFs. Researchers at Kaiser Permanente in California have conducted multiple studies in which they have asked pregnant women to carry meters that measured their magnetic field exposure for 24 hours during their pregnancy, and then followed the birth outcomes as well as the babies for as long as 13 years.

They have found that women with higher exposures have 2.72 times the risk of miscarrying,[88] and their babies had a higher risk of having asthma, being obese, and suffering from thyroid problems.[89–91]

If you are pregnant or plan to become so in the future, please be certain to limit your exposure to EMFs, especially your cell phone, and magnetic fields—both for your own health and the health of your baby. Visit the website babysafeproject.org for specific guidelines on protecting your baby from EMFs.

A LINK BETWEEN EMF RADIATION AND ADHD?

Many studies, including those I mentioned above, suggest that perhaps the rising rates of ADD (attention deficit disorder) and ADHD in children are at least partly attributable to increased EMF exposure.

A 2010 German study followed children who wore a radiation meter for 24 hours; those who had the highest levels of exposure had an increased risk of displaying more boisterous and uncontrollable behavior, similar to that displayed by kids who have been diagnosed with ADHD.[92]

In fact, ADHD shares many symptoms with electrohypersensitivity, including:

- Memory loss
- Brain fog
- Difficulty focusing
- Blunted learning abilities

The Kaiser Permanente researchers I referenced in the previous section also found that babies born to mothers with higher magnetic field exposure during pregnancy also had 2.9 times the risk of developing a neurodevelopmental disorder such as ADHD.[93]

In 2018, researchers theorized that the common denominator between EMF-related ADHD and autism is damage to DNA and changes to gene expression (known as *epigenetics*).[94]

EMFS AND INCREASED AUTISM RISK

A number of researchers have found EMFs are quite capable of contributing to autism spectrum disorder (ASD) too. Martin Pall, whose work elucidated the molecular mechanism of how EMFs damage you, suggests that the dramatic rise in autism rates is "probably caused by EMF exposure."

Pall theorizes that EMFs contribute to autism through the opening of voltage-gated calcium channels (VGCCs), flooding cells with calcium, contributing to damaging oxidative stress (as I outlined earlier in this chapter), and disrupting the formation of healthy synapses in the brain, all of which contribute to the physiological environment that fosters the development of autism.[95]

Further support for this position comes from the observation that there are genetic mistakes (called SNPs or *single nucleotide polymorphisms*) that involve the VGCCs, such as *CANA1C*, that appear to increase the risk for a child to develop autism.[96] Other genetic variations that can impair the body's ability to deal with oxidative stress likely contribute as well.[97,98]

There are other well-documented effects of EMF exposure that align with established biological conditions found in children with ASD. EMFs also cause damage to stem cells,[99–108] which, in children, can impair brain development in a way that likely contributes to autism.[109,110]

Dr. Martha Herbert of Harvard Medical School wrote a 2013 review elaborating on the biologic factors that could contribute to this, including "oxidative stress and evidence of free radical damage, cellular stress proteins, and deficiencies of antioxidants such as glutathione."[111]

In addition, many other researchers have been studying a possible link between EMF exposure and autism.[112-121] It would certainly seem rational to conclude that this is one of the reasons why autism rates have spiked so precipitously in the past 20 years: skyrocketing from 1 in 150 children in 2000, to 1 in 59 in 2014 (according to the CDC)[122], to 1 in 40 in 2016 (according to a study appearing in the journal *Pediatrics*).[123]

As further clues point to a link between autism and EMFs, many health-care practitioners report placing their young patients with autism on a low-EMF-exposure program (turning Wi-Fi off at night, unplugging cordless phones and baby monitors, and even turning off the circuit breaker to the bedroom) resulted in dramatic improvements in behavior.[124]

Dr. Dietrich Klinghardt first linked autism in children to excessive EMF exposure in 2001 when he noticed that children of employees of the software giant Microsoft headquartered outside Seattle, in Bellevue, Washington, seemed to have significantly higher rates of autism.

Klinghardt conducted a pilot study in which he evaluated EMF exposure in mothers of children with autism and their autistic children, as well as mothers of healthy children and their healthy children. Specifically, he measured:

- Body voltage of mothers where they slept while pregnant

- Body voltage of children in their current sleeping location

- Microwave power density in sleeping locations of the mothers while pregnant

- Total microwave exposure of children's sleeping environment

It turned out the average exposure of an autistic child to high-frequency EMFs from household currents and microwaves from cell phones and other wireless technologies was 20 times that of the non-autistic children. Unfortunately, the study never made it into publication, but it convinced him that EMFs were an unacknowledged factor that contributes to autism.[125]

The real-world impact of EMFs is also evident in Klinghardt's clinical practice, as families with autistic children who take EMF remediation seriously report significant improvements in their children's behavior, while those who fail to take steps to reduce EMF exposure fail to notice improvements.

If you or your child display ADHD-like behaviors, or have autism, there is a protocol developed by California pediatrician Toril Jelter that guides you to turn off Wi-Fi and electricity to your child's room at night. Turn off all cordless phones and baby monitors, and keep mobile devices at least six feet away from your child for two weeks, and notice which of their behaviors and symptoms improve during that time. (I also offer a full breakdown of how to minimize your EMF exposures in your own home in Chapter 7.)

Of course, you'll have to also monitor their exposure to frequencies outside of the house—particularly in school, where Wi-Fi use is prevalent.

EMOTIONAL EFFECTS OF EMFS ON KIDS

Cell phones, wireless-enabled tablets, laptops, and Bluetooth devices affect kids emotionally, and it starts when they are very young. Many parents have done it; maybe you have too: Your toddler starts melting down and you hand him a phone to pacify him.

This shuts down eye contact and communication between parent and child. It can also teach the child to distract himself rather than endure unpleasant situations or emotions and develop necessary coping skills. Both these things can stunt development, according to sociologists and psychologists.

As reported in a 2018 *New York Times* article: The social scientist Sherry Turkle analyzed 30 years of family interactions in her book *Alone Together: Why We Expect More From Technology and Less From Each Other.* She found that children now compete with their parents' devices for attention, resulting in a generation afraid of the spontaneity of a phone call or face-to-face interaction. Eye contact now seems to be optional, Dr. Turkle suggests, and sensory overload can often mean our feelings are constantly anesthetized.[126]

Once children are old enough to have their own phones, it becomes a bone of contention between them and their parents. A Common Sense Media survey found that 25 percent of American parents say they fight with their child *every day* about phone usage.[127]

That same survey also reports that 29 percent of kids keep their phones in bed with them; worse yet, 36 percent of teens wake up to check their phones in the middle of the night.

This has a strong connection to mental health, as the blue light and radiofrequencies emitted from the phone as well as the mental stimulation of responding to notifications interrupts their sleep, reducing the length of time spent asleep as well as the quality of that sleep. Without sleep, the body can't restore itself properly, and this shows up in many factors of health, including mental health.

A 2018 Australian study of 1,101 high school students found that kids whose sleep was impaired by late-night phone use were significantly more likely to experience depressed moods, lowered self-esteem, and a lowered coping ability.[128]

No matter which hours of the day kids spend on their phones, the resulting reductions in their mental health from using the phone can lead to devastating results: In 2017, San Diego State University psychology professor Jean Twenge published a study in *Clinical Psychological Science* for which teens in 8th through 12th grades were surveyed and compared those results to national statistics on adolescent depressive symptoms and suicide rates.

She found that teens who spent more than three hours a day on screens were 35 percent more likely to have a risk factor for suicide than those who spent one hour or less. When teens spent five or more hours a day on their phones, that risk increased by 71 percent.[129]

And suicide among young people is rising precipitously. According to the CDC, the suicide rate among males 15–24 rose nearly 20 percent between 2000 and 2016. For females, it's worse: In that same time period, suicide among girls ages 10–14 skyrocketed 183 percent, and for 15- to 24-year-olds, the increase was 80 percent.[130]

APPLE CHANGED ITS SCREEN TIME GUIDELINES FOR CHILDREN

In 2018, Twenge's study prompted representatives of the hedge fund JANA Partners and the California State Teachers' Retirement System—major investors in Apple, to the tune of $2 billion at the time—to write an open letter to members of Apple's leadership team, begging them to consider the ill effects their products were having on the emotional health of kids and teens and develop better parental controls to limit kids' screen time.

The letter cited "a growing societal unease about whether at least some people are getting too much of a good thing when it comes to technology," and focused on the risks to children.[131]

The letter may have contributed to Apple including a feature in iOS 12 called Screen Time, released later in 2018, that allows users to see how much time they—or their children—are spending on all connected Apple devices and how much of that time is being spent on games, web browsing, e-mails, social media, and texts. Parents can then utilize a feature called Downtime to set time limits on their child's app use on those Apple devices."[132]

While all this is helpful, the best solution is to delay your child having a cell phone or tablet as long as you possibly can, then teaching them how to use the device responsibly. Perhaps most important, parents have to model appropriate use of their own devices.

At this point, responsibility for children's health and safety when it comes to EMF exposure must come from their parents, as the government is doing so little to regulate the industry. There are a few glimmers of hope, however.

SOME COUNTRIES RECOGNIZE THE RISK

Unlike the U.S., several countries have developed a deep concern regarding the risk that EMF exposure poses to children and have implemented laws to address it.

In late 2018, France imposed a cell phone ban in schools for students in first through ninth grades.[133] Those students are not permitted to use their phones even at breaks, during lunchtime, or between classes. Russia has also implemented laws to minimize Wi-Fi exposure in schools,[134] and Switzerland, Italy, Austria, Luxembourg, Bulgaria, Poland, Hungary, Israel, and China have set radio frequency exposure limits that are up to 10,000 times lower than in the U.S.[135]

The evidence makes it abundantly clear that EMF exposure is a significant health hazard for today's youth. Schools need to take a step back and begin to implement strategies to protect students while in the classroom, such as eliminating Wi-Fi and converting to wired connections. Parents also need to establish firm guidelines around children's use of technology. There's simply no reason to flood children with wireless signals from dusk till dawn.

Sadly, most children in the U.S. and in Europe have widely and wholeheartedly adopted a wireless lifestyle and are growing up completely enveloped in EMFs. They carry cell phones at younger and younger ages, have nearly continuous exposure to Wi-Fi at home and at school, and use wireless computers and tablets beginning in the early school years.

In late 2016, a Nielsen survey found that nearly half of American kids ages 10–12 have a cell phone with a subscription plan (and not just a wireless connection), and a 2017 census by Common Sense Media found that almost half of U.S. kids 8 and younger have their own tablet.[136]

Rates of cell phone use among children are similar in Europe, where 46 percent of kids ages 9–16 own a smartphone.[137] A British survey found that 25 percent of kids 6 and younger already have their own phones, and that 8 out of 10 parents don't restrict the amount of time kids can spend on their phones.[138]

In 2018, the Pew Research Center reported that 45 percent of teenagers are "almost constantly" online, up from 24 percent in 2015, and that 95 percent of teens have access to a cell phone.[139]

As noted by Devra Davis, Ph.D., an epidemiologist and author of the book, *Disconnect: The Truth about Cell Phone Radiation, What the Industry Is Doing to Hide It, and How to Protect Your Family*, children have never before been exposed to this level of pulsed radiation, and it's still too early to determine the exact extent of harm. Still, mounting evidence suggests damage is indeed occurring, so it would be foolish to wait to respond until we're in the midst of a global catastrophe.

If we hope to protect children, we must first understand the magnitude of these dangers so that we can teach them to protect themselves now and over the course of their lifetimes. Reviewing the evidence of the link between EMF exposure and disease, which we'll do in the next chapter, should help convince you to take steps to protect your children.

CHAPTER 5

EMFS AND DISEASE

In the previous chapter, you learned how EMF exposure damages your body. Now let's take a look at the results of those mechanisms and see how regular exposures have been linked to the development of specific diseases.

Of course, disease doesn't take root overnight. You don't install a smart meter on your home and wake up the next morning, or even the next week or month, with heart disease. It starts with subtle shifts in your body, things you're not likely to think about too much.

Perhaps you notice that you're not sleeping as well as you once did and you're a little tired. Or you catch a cold that you would have otherwise fought off. But those symptoms could be explained by any number of things, so you don't connect the dots back to EMFs.

Because the damage that EMFs wreak is happening far below the level of your awareness, you simply aren't cognizant of the need to lessen your exposure. After all, nobody else seems to be concerned, so why worry?

The problem is that the effects of EMFs—particularly when it comes to brain cancer, which has a minimum 10-year latency period—usually take quite a while to manifest as a disease that you recognize. This makes it easy to dismiss any concerns you might have about the health risks of EMF exposure.

Yet research has firmly established that EMFs contribute to many diseases. I will review the major ones in this chapter. Please understand that it would take hundreds, if not thousands, of pages to comprehensively document the evidence for the damage that EMFs can cause to your biology. But I hope this concise summary will help you understand how EMF exposure can create and contribute to disease.

RINGING IN YOUR EARS (TINNITUS)

Tinnitus is the perception of sound described as ringing in the ears, with the absence of any source. While this is certainly not a life-threatening problem, it is a common ailment, affecting an estimated 1 in 10 adults. Interestingly, humming or ringing in the ears is one of the most common symptoms of those who are impaired by or suffer with EMF hypersensitivity.[1]

Tinnitus may also be a sign of some other, more serious underlying condition such as ear injury or circulatory system disorder.[2] Worse still, it may be a sign of permanent nerve damage that could predict future hearing impairment.

Tinnitus occurs when cells inside your inner ear, or cochlea, are damaged. These malfunctioning cells end up sending signals to your brain even in the absence of audible sound. Your brain translates these signals into what has been described as ringing, buzzing, hissing, clicking, chirping, screeching, static, roaring, pulsing, whooshing, and/or whistling sounds.[3]

The pitch can be either high or low and may change intermittently. The volume may also be high or low, depending on surroundings and other factors. Oftentimes the sound is most noticeable at night, which is why tinnitus is frequently associated with sleep disturbances and depression. Many people with this problem report that it negatively impacts their quality of life.

Most of those who suffer from tinnitus have no idea that it may be related to EMF exposure. In early 2019, I had mold damage in my home. The lead remediator for the damage had long-term ringing in his ears. When he shared this with me, I recognized it as a common side effect of EMF exposure and took him to my completely RF-shielded bedroom. (More on shielding in Chapter 7.) When I shut off the electricity in the room, his ringing disappeared for the first time in more than 15 years.

Ears appear to be highly susceptible to the influence of EMFs, and thus they can be early indicators of EMF damage—sort of the canary in the coal mine. Perhaps this is because ears don't have the protection of the skull, as your brain has, and are therefore more on the front lines of exposure.

The link between EMF exposure and tinnitus is likely related to the way your body uses electrical signals to transmit information. In your brain, nerves communicate with each other via tiny electrical charges, and external EMFs can interfere with these signals. There is substantial evidence from electrophysiological studies showing EMFs, especially from cell phones, influence your brain function[4] and nerve processing in the auditory system of your brain.[5-7]

A 2010 study published in *Occupational and Environmental Medicine* compared 100 patients with tinnitus to 100 patients without it, in pairs matched by sex and age. While the researchers did not see a significant increase in tinnitus based on regularity of cell phone use or duration of calls, they did find an increase based on long-term cell phone use of four years or more.[8]

A pair of identical studies in Göteborg, Sweden, done nine years apart showed that tinnitus is increasing dramatically in young children. In 1997 just 12 percent of the seven-year-old schoolchildren studied had tinnitus.[9] In 2006, 42 percent of seven-year-old schoolchildren had tinnitus.[10]

There is also a link between tinnitus and electrohypersensitivity, which I cover later in this chapter.

CATARACTS

Cataracts aren't discussed much as side effects of EMF exposure because they are not life threatening and there are relatively easy and inexpensive surgical solutions available. Nevertheless, they are some of the most well-documented ailments linked to EMF exposure.

As you'll recall from Chapter 3, ophthalmologist Milton Zaret conducted research on military personnel who were exposed to radar and other similar radio frequencies as part of their work in the late 1950s. What he found was that exposure to low-grade microwave frequencies contributed to the formation of cataracts in a different location of the eye than cataracts typically form.

In 2008, Israeli researchers set out to assess the effects of 1.1 GHz radiation on the eye. They observed two types of damage in the lens: a reduction in optical quality of the lens, which was reversible, and structural and biochemical damage to the epithelial cell layer of the lens that was irreversible.[11]

A 2010 review of 45 studies on the nonthermal effects of nonionizing radiation on the lens of the eye found evidence that low-power microwave radiation alters cell proliferation and apoptosis (also known as programmed cell death, where impaired or damaged cells die off), impairs intercellular communication, and causes genetic instability and a stress response in the cells that make up the epithelial lining of the lens.[12]

The type of cataract that most of us are familiar with occurs with age, when proteins in the lens of the eye start to clump together and cloud the lens. Microwave-associated cataracts actually form in the capsule of the eye, which is the membrane that surrounds the lens.

DISRUPTION TO YOUR BLOOD-BRAIN BARRIER

One of the most concerning perils of cell phone radiation is the damage it can cause in your brain.

Your blood-brain barrier (BBB) forms a protective shield around your brain. This barrier is composed of cells that have such tight junctions between each other that there are no openings for items in the blood vessels to escape into the brain. The existence of the BBB was discovered in the late 19th century by the German bacteriologist Paul Ehrlich.

Your BBB exists to protect your brain from any toxins—alcohol, environmental pollutants, viruses, or bacteria—that might be circulating in your bloodstream. It also serves to selectively allow nutrients and neurotransmitters in so your brain has what it needs to function properly, as well as maintain constant pressure inside your head so you don't have a stroke.

The increased oxidative stress triggered by EMFs and peroxynitrite production can cause an increased permeability in your BBB. When your BBB is damaged in this way it can contribute to a wide variety of problems, including cancer and neurodegenerative processes like Alzheimer's disease.[13]

The first researcher to demonstrate a link between EMF exposure and permeability of the blood-brain barrier was Allan Frey, who conducted research for the military in the 1960s and '70s on the physiological effects of exposure to radar.

In the ensuing decades, Swiss neuroscientist Leif Salford conducted several studies into the effects of microwave radiation on the BBB of rats. In a study published in 1994, his team exposed rats to 915 MHz in continuous and pulsed signals for two hours. One hour later, the rats were sacrificed and their brains examined. In 56 out of 184 exposed rats, there were two proteins, which are normally filtered out by the blood-brain barrier, still present in their brains (as opposed to in only 5 out of 62 brains of rats who were not exposed).[14]

In 2009, Salford conducted a similar experiment, although this time the rats' brains were tested seven days after the two-hour exposure, and got similar results.[15] Other studies had failed to replicate these findings, but in 2015, Chinese researchers were able to do so. They exposed 108 rats to 900 MHz at an intensity of 1 milliwatt per square centimeter for three hours a day over the course of either 14 or 28 days, and compared their brains to rats who had not been exposed. The rats who had been exposed for 28 days showed significant leakage of the BBB.[16]

For more specific details of how our knowledge of the impact of EMFs on the blood-brain barrier has evolved, you can review the BBB section of the *BioInitiative Report*, which I referenced in Chapter 4 as a comprehensive review of the science on the physiological effects of EMFs, as it contains a very detailed analysis and explanation as to precisely how EMFs impact your blood-brain barrier.[17]

Suffice it to say here that EMF exposure figuratively pokes holes in a vital protective mechanism producing consequences we are only beginning to understand.

IMPAIRED SLEEP AND REDUCED MELATONIN

One of the most common symptoms reported by people who are experiencing a new EMF exposure is insomnia. Extremely low frequency EMFs (such as those emitted by power plants and electric wiring)[18] and radio-frequency EMFs such as those emitted by cell phones[19,20] have been shown to impair sleep.

One reason why this may be so is that EMFs excite the cortical region of the brain, which makes it harder to relax into sleep.[21] Another likely reason is that EMFs reduce melatonin levels.

Melatonin is a hormone primarily produced in your pineal gland, which is essential for establishing a healthy circadian rhythm.

When your melatonin levels are disrupted, you tend to experience a decrease in duration of deep sleep, which is essential for your body to function properly. Sadly, sleep is a seriously overlooked strategy to optimize your health. For a detailed discussion and increased appreciation of the importance of sleep to your health, I strongly recommend reviewing UC Berkeley professor Matthew Walker's book *Why We Sleep*.[22]

But melatonin is related to far more than just sleep. The sheer number of places in your body that have receptors for melatonin indicate just how important it is to whole-body function. It is used by nearly every organ, including your brain, liver, intestines, kidneys, cardiovascular system, and gallbladder as well as in immune cells, fat cells, and even in your skin.

In addition to optimizing your circadian rhythm, melatonin has powerful antioxidant properties, helping to suppress excessive harmful free radicals and reduce markers of brain aging and degeneration.

The negative impact EMFs have on melatonin has been known for decades.[23] A 2002 review found 17 existing studies proving nonionizing radiation lowers melatonin.[24] Because melatonin has a role as an antioxidant and has been shown to protect against the oxidative stress caused by EMF exposure,[25] lowered levels are doubly problematic.

EMFs ALSO DISRUPT YOUR INTESTINAL BARRIER

Similar to how EMFs degrade your BBB, they also weaken the integrity of another important barrier, your intestine. EMFs weaken the tight junctions between the cells that line your intestinal tract, creating a condition known as *leaky gut*.

While a leaky gut is primarily associated with inflammatory bowel diseases such as Crohn's and ulcerative colitis, healthy people can also have varying degrees of increased intestinal permeability, which can lead to a wide variety of symptoms.

Once the integrity of your intestinal lining is compromised, toxins and foreign proteins can enter your bloodstream. This results in many problems, including an increase in inflammation. Chronic inflammation can also contribute and/or lead to other health conditions such as arthritis and heart disease.

This compromise in your intestinal barrier may also cause your immune system to become confused and begin to attack your own body as if it were an enemy, which is a hallmark of autoimmune disorders.

Another way EMFs sabotage your gut health is by interfering with the function of the friendly microbes that live in your digestive tract and play an important role in many vital functions, including immunity.

As Dietrich Klinghardt puts it, the human microbiome is "hugely and directly damaged by the electromagnetic waves we're exposing them to."

INCREASED TOXIN ABSORPTION

When EMFs increase the permeability of your BBB, toxins are allowed easy access to your brain. This results in an increased toxic load in your brain.

Not only is your toxic load increased, your detoxification systems are impaired largely as a result of the increased oxidative stressors. And as I mentioned previously, EMF exposures can also reduce your deep sleep, which then disrupts the glymphatic drainage system in your brain that would normally help eliminate toxins while you sleep.

Another way EMFs can contribute to your overall toxic load is if you have any "silver" or mercury amalgam fillings. EMFs have been shown to significantly increase the amount of mercury leaching from any metal fillings you have in your teeth.[26] One theory as to why this is so is that there are tiny pockets of saliva trapped between the tooth and the amalgam.

Because the amount is so small, the radiation from a cell phone call can heat the saliva enough to create a "hot spot," which then causes the saliva to bubble, and these bubbles then cause the mercury in the amalgam to leak.[27] Regardless of the mechanism, this is yet another reason why I continue to advocate for stopping the use of mercury amalgams.

CANCER

While the wireless industry and its captured federal regulatory agencies would have you believe there is no relationship between cancer and EMFs, this is simply not true. There are a large number of peer-reviewed studies documenting an association.

One of the probable links between EMFs and cancer is the increase in oxidative stress; that contributes to mitochondrial dysfunction that is a major cause of DNA damage and cancer. There are a few types of cancer that currently have a stronger scientific connection to EMFs than others.

Brain Cancer

Perhaps the most conclusive association between EMFs and cancer belongs to brain cancer. There is now overwhelming evidence of the link between EMF exposure and brain cancer; here, I will highlight just a few of the many studies that show this connection.[28-33]

If you would like to examine the evidence more thoroughly, you can consult the *BioInitiative Report* I introduced in Chapter 4, which has compiled hundreds of studies in four PDFs on the use of wireless phones and the evidence for an increase in brain cancers.[34]

The type of malignant tumor most associated with EMF exposure is the glioma, which forms in the glue-like tissue of the brain that supports the neuron. It is a rare and highly aggressive form of brain cancer.

As with lung cancer caused by smoking, glioma has a long latency period in humans—more than 20 years[35]—so it is frequently not recognized as being associated with cell phone use, and epidemiological studies only recently have started showing a connection between the two.

Though glioma is a fairly rare disease that only accounts for a bit over one percent of all cancers,[36] there have been some high-profile cases of it in recent years; for example, U.S. Senators John McCain and Ted Kennedy both died of glioblastoma. These tumors are difficult to detect; by the time they are diagnosed, the typical survival time after discovery is only about a year.

Though few people connected these men's cancers to cell phone use, it is highly likely that their use of cell phones did contribute to their disease, as senators tend to do a good deal of business by phone, especially when they're in Washington, D.C., and away from their constituencies. (What's more, as *The Washington Post* reported, Verizon and AT&T installed portable cell towers on McCain's ranch near Sedona, Arizona, in 2007.[37])

Research finding a link between cell phone use and brain cancer has been around for decades. Several studies have also found an increased risk of developing brain tumors for cell phone users,[38] including many from the past few years that point to cell phone radiation exposure as a cause of brain cancer.

In 2016, for instance, a National Toxicology Program study (which I described in detail in Chapter 3) exposed male rats to radio-frequency radiation at frequencies and modulations used in the U.S. wireless industry. Rats exposed to cell phone radiation for about nine hours a day over a two-year period were at increased risk of developing malignant gliomas in the brain, as well as another type of tumor, schwannomas of the heart.[39]

Meanwhile, a 2017 systematic review looking at cell phone use and glioma risk, while noting that current evidence is of poor and limited quality, also found that long-term cell phone use (minimum of 10 years) may be associated with an increased risk of glioma.[40]

Another concerning study, published in 2015, looked at data from two previous case-controlled studies on Swedish patients diagnosed with malignant brain tumors during the periods of 1997 to 2003 and 2007 to 2009.[41] The patients were between the ages of 18 and 80 years old at the time of their diagnosis.

Regression analysis showed that the odds of developing glioma rose concurrently with increased cell phone use. The more hours the subjects spent with a cell phone pressed to their ears, and the more years they'd spent using cell phones, the higher the odds of developing brain cancer were.

The risk of brain cancer is even higher for children. In 2009, Swedish oncologist Lennart Hardell compared the cell phone and cordless phone usage of Swedish residents with malignant brain tumors, benign brain tumors, and healthy controls. He found that anyone who began using a cell phone at an age younger than 20 had the highest risk of developing glioma.[42]

Hardell also published subsequent studies strengthening the link between cell phone and cordless phone usage and brain tumors. They found that tumors were most likely to form in the area of the brain closest to where a cell phone rests while on a call, and that risks of developing malignant brain tumors spiked in association with three risk factors: number of years of use, total number of hours of use, and age at first use.[43,44]

There is also some very clear evidence of troubling *spikes* in brain cancer. In particular, a doubling in the incidence of glioblastoma tumors in England was documented in a 2018 paper published in the *Journal of Environmental and Public Health*.[45] The increase in malignant tumors was overwhelmingly found in the front and temporal regions of the brain, precisely where a cell phone is held during a call.

Breast Cancer

Breast cancer is one of the other common cancers associated with cell phone use. The *BioInitiative Report* has compiled nearly 50 studies providing evidence that EMFs can promote breast cancer.[46]

One of the plausible reasons why EMFs are connected to breast cancer is that some women carry their cell phones in their bras. In fact, in 2013 researchers at the University of California, Irvine, studied four young women who had no known risk factors for breast cancer—such as family history or genetic predisposition—who regularly carried their cell phones in their bras and developed tumors in the upper inner quadrant of the breast.

This spot, which was directly where the cell phones rested against their skin, is a very unusual location for breast tumors, which more often form in the upper outer quadrant of the breast.[47]

Conversely, a 2017 epidemiological study of women in Central Africa found that the habit of *not* keeping a cell phone in one's bra resulted in a significantly decreased risk of developing breast cancer.[48]

A 2015 study looked at how the distance from different EMFs emitted by cell phones affected human breast cancer cells in a test tube. It found that when the antenna was less than 10 centimeters away, there was excessive production of reactive oxygen species and increased apoptosis (natural cell death).[49]

A similar study exposed healthy human breast fibroblast cells to short exposures of a 2.1 GHz signal, which is emitted by some smartphones. The radiation led to a significant decrease in cell viability and induced higher levels of apoptosis.[50] And numerous other studies have found an increased risk of breast cancer in people who are subject to occupational exposure to EMFs.[51]

In addition, there is evidence linking breast cancer to exposure to extremely low frequency (ELF) EMFs, such as those emitted by power lines and electrical wiring. A 2016 meta-analysis of 42 studies that included more than 13,000 women with cases of breast cancer found that exposure to ELF EMFs is associated with breast cancer, especially in the United States.[52]

Childhood Leukemia

There are few things more heartbreaking than a child battling cancer. Sadly, there is a well-established link between ELF-EMF exposures and childhood leukemia, the most common cancer in children.

Evidence linking EMF radiation emitted by power lines and childhood leukemia has existed since 1979, when Dr. Nancy Wertheimer and physicist Ed Leeper published their findings that children in Colorado who lived close to power lines—p ELECTROMAGNETIC HYPERSENSITIVITY SYNDROME articularly those who resided at the same address close to power lines their whole lives—had a higher incidence of developing leukemia than those whose homes were farther away.[53]

At first, their findings were dismissed or met with confusion. Then, in 1988, a study sponsored by the New York State Department of Health supported their findings.[54] Now childhood leukemia has one of the strongest scientific records of being connected to EMF exposure. The *BioInitiative Report* has compiled nearly 100 studies providing evidence of the link between EMF exposure and childhood leukemia.[55]

The International Agency for Research on Cancer (IARC), an agency of the World Health Organization (WHO), classified EMFs as a possible carcinogen in 2002 in large part due to the strong evidence supporting the link between ELF magnetic fields from our use of electricity and childhood leukemia. In fact, the 2007 *Environmental Health Criteria*, a WHO publication, stated:

The IARC classification was heavily influenced by the associations observed in epidemiological studies on childhood leukemia.[56]

A 2008 Chinese study uncovered a plausible mechanism by which EMF exposure may contribute to childhood leukemia: A genetic variation is believed to be present in up to 6 percent of the population that prevents the repair of DNA strands that are damaged by EMF exposure.[57,58]

This finding could explain why Mexico City has one of the highest incidences of childhood leukemia in the world:[59] Not only are EMF exposures higher there than in other countries,[60] but also people of Hispanic descent appear to be much more likely to have the genetic variant that makes them more susceptible to this damage than people of European or African descent, according to statistics compiled by the Centers for Disease Control and Prevention (CDC).[61]

HEART DISEASE

Your heart has one of the highest densities of voltage-gated calcium channels (VGCCs) and as a result is highly sensitive to EMFs, especially the pacemaker cells of your heart. This may be why EMFs tend to trigger the following heart conditions.

- **Cardiac arrhythmias:** Arrhythmia is an irregular heartbeat; it may beat too fast, too slow, too early, or just irregularly. Most arrhythmias are not serious, but some can predispose you to a stroke or a heart attack and can even lead to sudden death. In fact, arrhythmia is responsible for about half of all deaths from heart disease each year. Arrhythmias can take the following forms:

  - Slow heartbeat: bradycardia

  - Fast heartbeat: tachycardia

  - Irregular heartbeat: atrial flutter or fibrillation

- Early heartbeat: premature contraction

Martin Pall believes that the rising rates of sudden cardiac death could very well be related to the increase of EMF exposure as a result of excessive (VGCC) activation.[62,63]

So if you, or anyone you know or love, has a cardiac arrhythmia, it is vital to put an aggressive EMF remediation program in place. Worst case is that it will only lead to better health; best case, it could save a life.

- **Blood pressure:** A study published in 1998 in *The Lancet* found that using a cell phone can lead to a 5–10 milligrams Hg (mercury) rise in blood pressure.[64] And in 2013, Italian researchers presented at the annual meeting of the American Society of Hypertension their findings that answering and talking on a cell phone raised blood pressure in patients with an average age of 53 by an average of 5–7 milligrams Hg.[65]

When you consider that medication to reduce high blood pressure has been linked to a significantly increased risk of developing skin cancer in a 2017 study published in *The Journal of the American Association of Dermatology*[66]—and this medication might be less needed if EMF exposure were reduced—you will hopefully be even more open to the idea of reducing blood pressure via EMF remediation.

If you have any of these conditions, it is important to understand that EMF exposure may be a major contributing factor. Therefore, it would be prudent to take immediate steps to remediate the harm you've sustained from your exposure (as I outline in Chapter 7).

NEUROPSYCHIATRIC ILLNESSES

Another vital part of your body that has a high density of VGCCs and thus a significant vulnerability to EMFs is your brain. I've already discussed the link between EMFs and a disruption of your BBB and brain cancer. But exposure to electromagnetic fields can affect your brain in other ways that are far more common—including mental health challenges, which have become pervasive and epidemic, such as anxiety, depression, hostility, and difficulty concentrating.

Anxiety disorders are the most common mental illness in the U.S., affecting more than 40 million adults ages 18 and older—nearly 20 percent of the population—annually.[67] Americans and residents of other higher-income countries are significantly more likely to experience and be impaired by anxiety, according to a 2017 study published in *JAMA Psychiatry* than people who live in less wealthy countries.[68]

In America, anxiety is clearly on the rise. In 2017 the American Psychiatric Association (APA) polled 1,000 U.S. residents, and a full two-thirds of respondents said they were "extremely or somewhat anxious about health and safety for themselves and their families."[69] On top of that, more than a third of them said that their anxiety had increased compared to the year before. In 2018 the APA ran the poll again, and this time self-reported anxiety had risen by another 5 percentage points.[70]

Americans are no strangers to depression, either: An estimated 17.3 million adults in the United States have had at least one major depressive episode, which is more than 7 percent of all adults in the U.S.[71]

And cell phones are notoriously linked to increased distraction, particularly among adolescents.[72] A 2014 study found that a full 94 percent of study participants who were told to walk down a Chicago sidewalk while interacting with their phones failed to notice the dollar bills that the study authors had conspicuously hung from a tree along the walking route.[73]

You don't even need to be interacting with your phone for it to negatively impact your ability to focus. A 2017 study published in the *Journal for the Association of Consumer Research* found that students performed worse on tests of memory and attention when their smartphones were near them—even though the phones were set to silent—than if the phones were outside the room.[74]

The researchers theorized that the more dependent you are on your smartphone, the more working memory it takes up, even when you're not directly interacting with it. It's likely that radiation emitted by your cell phone also plays a role. Radio-frequency radiation has long been known to impair memory.[75]

EMFS AND THE MECHANISMS OF MOOD

Once you know that EMFs may overactivate your VGCCs, it's no surprise that exposure can affect your cognition and mental health. After all, VGCCs play a major role in your thinking and your mood. As Martin Pall wrote in his review of studies that found a demonstrable link between EMFs and neuropsychiatric effects:

> VGCC activation has been shown to have a universal or near universal role in the **release of neurotransmitters** in the brain and also in the **release of hormones** by neuroendocrine cells . . . .[76,77]

Neurotransmitters, such as dopamine, serotonin, and norepinephrine, are the chemical messengers that keep your mind and mood running smoothly. If their delicate balance is upset—which is highly likely when your VGCCs are artificially activated by the presence of EMFs—it becomes more difficult to steady yourself when you have anxious thoughts, or to get a good night's sleep that helps to clear your head, or to focus on a task. Anxiety and depression can settle in as a "normal" way of feeling.

As I discussed earlier in this chapter, EMFs also suppress melatonin, and this important neurotransmitter and antioxidant plays a key role in mental health too, as low levels of melatonin have been shown to be related to a greater likelihood of depression.[78]

The studies linking anxiety and depression to EMF exposure are numerous. For example, a 1994 study found that workers exposed to broadcast radio frequencies experienced increased anxiety, social anxiety, sleeplessness, and hostility.[79] And a 2011 study found that high mobile phone use among adolescents led to increases in stress, sleep disturbances, and depression.[80]

Even U.S. government reports validate the link between EMF exposure and mental performance and health. Three government reports have listed multiple neuropsychiatric effects.

The earliest of these was a 1971 research report by the Naval Medical Research Institute that listed 40 neuropsychiatric changes produced by EMF exposure.[81] Ten years later researcher Jeremy K. Raines was contracted by NASA to document known biological effects of EMFs on humans. His report reviewed extensive literature based on occupational exposures to microwave EMFs and found 19 neuropsychiatric effects associated with microwave frequency EMFs.[82]

A third U.S. government report—written in 1994 by Scott M. Bolen and put out by the Rome Laboratory of the U.S. Air Force—also acknowledged the role of microwave EMFs on humans.[83]

In addition, there are at least 26 different epidemiological studies that show a wide range of neuropsychiatric effects aside from anxiety and depression that are produced by exposure to various nonthermal microwave frequency EMFs.[84] These other common neuropsychiatric illnesses are:

- Sleep disturbance/insomnia
- Headaches
- Fatigue/tiredness
- Dysesthesia (vision/hearing/olfactory dysfunction)

- Concentration/attention/cognitive dysfunction

- Dizziness/vertigo

- Memory changes

- Restlessness/tension/anxiety/stress/agitation/feeling of discomfort

- Irritability

NEURODEGENERATIVE DISEASES

Unfortunately, the cognitive effects of EMFs don't stop with neuropsychiatric illnesses.

As we just saw, when your brain VGCCs are overactivated, they produce excess free radicals that cause oxidative damage to the cells in your brain, spinal motor neurons, and elsewhere. Hence, consequences of excessive EMF exposure can lead to neurodegenerative diseases.

Indeed, studies dating back to the 1950s and '60s from the Soviet Union and the West (which were reviewed in a seminal 1973 paper[85]) show that the nervous system is the tissue that is most sensitive to EMFs. Some of these studies show massive changes in the structure of neurons, brain cell death, and synaptic dysfunction.[86]

Many studies have found that occupations with high EMF exposures—including seamstresses, hairdressers, utility workers, and welders—are associated with an increased likelihood of developing a neurodegenerative disease, such as Alzheimer's, Parkinson's, or amyotrophic lateral sclerosis (ALS), also known as Lou Gehrig's disease.[87]

But exposure doesn't have to come from work to have a negative effect. Research that analyzed mortality and census data on nearly 5 million residents of Switzerland found an association between living within 50 meters of power lines and an increased risk of developing Alzheimer's, and the risk rose significantly for every five years spent living in close proximity.[88]

In 2003, Leif Salford, the Swedish neurosurgeon who furthered Allan Frey's research into EMFs' effect on the blood-brain barrier, conducted a study to see if exposing rats to EMFs emitted by cell phones also affected the neurons in their brains. What Salford found was that the cell phone exposure for just two hours outright killed some brain cells and caused damage to their brain in a pattern consistent with Alzheimer's.[89]

Chinese researchers, in a study published in the *Archives of Medical Research* in 2013, looked at the effects on rats' brains when exposed to either 100, 1,000, or 10,000 electromagnetic pulses (at a strength of 50 kilovolts per meter with a repetition rate of 100 MHz). The exposed rats had a noticeable cognitive and memory impairment compared to rats who were not exposed. The test group also had increased levels over the control group of beta amyloid protein, a sticky substance in the brain that is a prime suspect in the development of Alzheimer's.[90]

ACCELERATES AGING

EMF exposure and the secondary cellular stress it creates can increase the number of senescent cells in your body.[91] Senescent cells are merely aged and senile cells that have stopped reproducing.

Senescence has its benefits: It plays a role in tumor suppression, wound healing, and tissue regeneration. As we age, however, senescent cells take on a less beneficial role as they accumulate in tissues and secrete numerous pro-inflammatory mediators.[92] Avoiding EMFs and avoiding excessive body fat are the two best ways you can limit the accumulation of senescent cells as you age.

ELECTROMAGNETIC HYPERSENSITIVITY SYNDROME

Electromagnetic hypersensitivity syndrome (EHS) is an umbrella term used to describe a variety of symptoms reported by patients that seem to have no other identifiable cause. These symptoms include:

- Disrupted sleep

- Confusion/poor concentration and/or memory loss

- Headaches

- Fatigue and muscle weakness

- Cardiac arrhythmia

- Skin itch/rash/flushing/burning and/or tingling

- Tinnitus

As you can see, these symptoms align closely with the conditions and diseases that I have already covered in this chapter and that have well-established research to support their connection to EMF exposures. Other reported symptoms include:

- Panic attacks

- Dizziness

- Ear pain

- Paralysis

- Seizures

- Irritability, even hostility

- Feeling a vibration in the body

As an illness, EHS is highly controversial; it is not recognized as a disease by the medical establishment. Yet studies from around the world have found that an average of 3 percent of the population experience its symptoms and have no other condition that would produce these symptoms.

Globally, in 2020 numbers, nearly 300 million people suffer from EHS.[93] This number is likely a gross underestimation, as far more people may experience EHS without connecting their symptoms to EMF exposure. And this tip-of-the-iceberg number will only increase as 5G is rolled out across the country and the globe, significantly adding to the number of EMFs you will encounter on a daily basis.

A recent study attempting to find objective methods for EHS evaluation discovered that about 80 percent of EHS self-reporting patients were found to present oxidative stress biomarkers in their peripheral blood, which is strongly related to DNA damage.[94]

EHS bears many resemblances to multiple chemical sensitivity syndrome (MCSS). This is likely because, as Annie Hopper reviews in her book *Wired for Healing: Remapping the Brain to Recover from Chronic and Mysterious Illnesses*, both conditions are presumably a result of injury to the limbic system, which is a complex network of nerves among the areas of your brain that are concerned with instinct and mood. The limbic controls basic emotions such as fear, pleasure, and anger, and basic drives such as hunger, sex, dominance, and care of offspring.

Often, those suffering from EHS will also be highly sensitive to chemicals or have MCSS.[95] This makes logical sense since your nervous system is a primary site impacted by both chemicals and electromagnetic fields, and if your nervous system has been damaged from toxic exposures, it may render you more susceptible to EHS as well.

People with specific genetic variants that decrease defenses to oxidative stress also appear to suffer from EHS at a much greater rate.[96]

Dr. Beatrice Golomb, a professor of medicine at the UC San Diego School of Medicine, has published research that indicates it is a web of cofactors, including low levels of certain antioxidants (including melatonin), genetic variations that result in impaired defense against oxidative stress, and oxidative stress-induced impairments to mitochondria, the blood-brain barrier, and VGCCs that contribute to EHS.[97]

The research of Dr. Yoshiaki Omura, a prolific medical researcher and educator and member of the Alumni Council of the College of Physicians and Surgeons of Columbia University, shows that the more your system is contaminated with heavy metals—due to things like having silver amalgam fillings, eating contaminated fish, living downstream from coal-burning power plants, and so forth—the more your body becomes a virtual antenna that concentrates radiation, making it far more destructive.[98]

Other groups at risk for developing EHS include those with:

- Spinal cord damage, whiplash, brain damage, or concussion

- Impaired immune function, lupus, or chronic fatigue syndrome (CFS)

- Bacterial and/or parasitic infections such as Lyme disease

- Electromagnetic, physical, chemical, and biological trauma as well as impaired immune system

- The very young and the very old. In children, EHS most typically presents as headaches, brain fog, and difficulty learning.

- Tinnitus. Evidence actually hints at a shared pathophysiology between EHS and tinnitus.[99] In one 2009 study, nearly 51 percent of EMF hypersensitive patients had tinnitus, compared to just 17.5 percent of participants in a control group.

Some countries are starting to recognize EHS as a legitimate disability. In 2013, Australia awarded workers' compensation benefits to a claimant who suffered from nausea, disorientation, and headaches due to exposure to EMFs during the course of his work as a scientist for the Commonwealth Scientific and

Industrial Research Organization, an agency of the Australian federal government.[100]

In 2015, a French court ruled that a woman was eligible for monthly disability benefits as a result of her EHS. This was significant because the court actually named EHS as the reason for its ruling.[101]

As of 2020, the United States has yet to give EHS any legal bearing. As an example, in 2018 a Massachusetts family sued their son's elementary school after he developed symptoms of EHS in the wake of the school's adopting a new Wi-Fi system. Rather than being given compensation for the damages, as happened in Australia and France, their case was dismissed from U.S. District Court.[102]

In one sense, people with EHS have an advantage, as the distinct discomfort that exposure to EMF causes strongly motivates them to take proactive steps to avoid exposures, as everyone else remains oblivious while still incurring biologic damage. Whether you feel it or not, damage is occurring.

INFERTILITY

There are estimated to be at least 48 million couples worldwide who are infertile,[103] which is approximately 7 percent of all men and women.[104] In couples who are having problems conceiving, approximately 40 percent of the issues are due to male impairments, while the remaining 60 percent is the result of fertility issues in the women.[105]

Men are facing a worsening trend of factors that contribute to infertility, particularly lower sperm counts, lower sperm motility, and sperm that have irregular shapes. This is likely because a man's genitals have a very high density of VGCCs, and men tend to keep their cell phones clipped to their waistband or in their pants pockets, very close to the genitals. It's a double whammy of exposure.

Since 1986, when the first study investigating the impact of electric blankets on fertility potential was conducted, there has been an increasing interest in studying the effects of exposure to nonionizing electromagnetic radiations on reproductive functions.[106] A significant decline in sperm quality from 1940 to date has been well documented.[107]

The beginning of the decline in male fertility precedes the rise of EMFs. A 1992 study published in *The British Medical Journal* found that there had been a significant decline that had started at least 50 years prior.[108] While there are undoubtedly many factors at play, including increasing toxic chemical exposures through pesticide use and air pollution, it is also clear that EMFs are playing a major role in the loss of male fertility.

Studies have established that exposure to wireless radiation reduces sperm motility,[109] total sperm count,[110] viability,[111] and quality[112] as well as increasing oxidative stress leading to infertility.[113] In fact, at least six meta-analyses that evaluated more than 200 separate studies have determined that cell phone radiation is indeed significantly harmful to sperm.[114]

Peter Sullivan, founder and CEO of Clear Light Ventures, a prominent funder of environmental health research, who also reviewed the science in this book, shared these insights on the importance of research examining the effects of EMF on sperm health:

> I think this is an area where the industry failed to fund any "fake science" until very recently. Also, unlike cancer, which has a long lead time and a range of complex mechanisms, sperm damage can be immediate and the research cycle can be very quick. So, it's harder for "merchant of doubt" tactics to blur these consequences.

A 2018 review showed that EMFs affect cell physiology by influencing reactive oxygen species (ROS) production, antioxidant response, and mitochondrial functionality, which plays an enormously important role in the acquisition and maintenance of the biological competence of the egg and sperm. It appears that EMFs impair mitochondrial function of the eggs and sperm thus impairing fertility.[115]

Interestingly, EMFs have been shown to decrease fertility in rats by lowering their testosterone levels. Merely exposing the rats to cell phone frequencies of either 900 MHz[116] or 2.45 GHz[117] for two hours a day for 45 days significantly reduced the rats' testosterone levels. This is far less than the five hours the typical American spends on a mobile device every day.[118]

Women's fertility is also susceptible to EMF exposure, in part because EMFs disrupt the delicate balance of a woman's repro-ductive hormones. This is supported by a 2008 study of women who were exposed to EMFs on the job—just as you likely are. Researchers found that the women experienced reduced pro-gesterone levels and significant disruptions in their menstrual cycles, including heavy bleeding.[119]

Oxidative stress is another mechanism by which EMFs are thought to impair female fertility. Free radicals can damage tissues, including oocytes (which are immature eggs) and embryos.[120] This may also explain why EMFs have been found to reduce the num-ber of follicles—the small fluid-filled sacs found on the outside layer of ovaries that contain one oocyte each—in rats.[121]

Two studies showed that the EMFs from living within 100 yards of a cell phone tower raise salivary levels of alpha-amylase, an enzyme that is released as part of the stress response.[122] Women with high levels of alpha-amylase have been found to have a nearly one-third lower chance of getting pregnant than women with the lowest levels.[123]

Not only is it harder to get pregnant when you are exposed to EMFs, but the risk of having a miscarriage also increases. A 2017 Kaiser Permanente study followed 913 pregnant women; those who were exposed to higher levels of EMFs had a nearly three times higher risk of miscarrying than those with lower exposures,[124] confirming the findings of previous similar studies.[125]

And it gets even worse. A 2017 study from China suggests that EMF exposure reduces fertilization and embryo implantation, a risk that increases as the length and intensity of the exposure increases.[126]

If the reduction in fertility rates as a result of EMF exposure continues to increase, as it very well could with the introduction of the 5G experiment, EMFs could serve as a potent existential threat to the very existence of our species.

Not only will we have an impaired ability to reproduce, but the children conceived at this time will face the very real, vastly unknown risk of the illnesses outlined in this chapter, as well as autism (as I discussed in Chapter 4), making it tremendously challenging to have a functioning society.

Although EMFs do appear to be playing a clear role in many diseases and conditions, it is possible to protect yourself. In the next chapter, you'll learn how to repair the cellular damage that EMFs can inflict so that you can prevent these diseases from occurring, or aid your body in mitigating these diseases if you already have one or more of them.

CHAPTER 6

HOW DO YOU REPAIR EMF-RELATED DAMAGE?

I know it may not feel like it at this point in the book, but there is good news here: Now that we have established how EMF exposure can damage your DNA through the peroxynitrite-induced creation of free radicals, we have a framework to remediate the damage.

And there is even better news: Although there is no way your ancestral biology could have predicted the enormous exposure you would have to MHz and GHz radiation from the wireless industry, you do indeed have a built-in repair system that can at least partially remediate the damage. It is called the *poly (ADP-ribose) polymerase* (PARP) family of enzymes. (I know that is a mouthful, but this is a really important group of enzymes.) PARP1 is the most common in the family of 17 PARP enzymes and is best known for its ability to repair DNA damage.[']

Note that in 2019 the PARP1 name was changed to ADP-ribosyltransferase diphtheria toxin-like 1 (ARTD1).[1] PARP enzymes function as DNA damage sensors and signaling molecules. These enzymes bind to both single- and double-stranded DNA breaks.[2]

Once these enzymes bind to damaged DNA, they form a matrix of long branches of ADP-ribose polymers.[3] This matrix of ribose polymers created by PARP then allows different specific DNA repair enzymes to come in and repair the DNA damage.

This process does come with a few downsides, however. The biggest one is that PARP requires fuel to work, and that fuel is one of the most important coenzymes in your body: *nicotinamide adenine dinucleotide*, or NAD+ for short.

You will get to know NAD+ better in a bit, but for now let's dive into how EMF exposure can lead to an inability to fuel PARP repair, and why this is one of the most important negative consequences of EMF exposure.

PARP enzymes are voracious consumers of NAD+. Every time you have a DNA break, PARP actually sucks ADP molecules from NAD+ to form long branches of polymers that create the matrix for the DNA repair enzymes to work.[4] PARP uses as much as 100 to 150 molecules of NAD+ for every DNA repair it facilitates.

Moderate levels of PARP formation facilitate efficient DNA repair and prevent the proliferation of abnormal cells that could lead to cancer.[5] A moderate degree of cell damage can be managed by PARP without overly depleting NAD+ and the energy molecule adenosine triphosphate (ATP). However, exposure to severe DNA stress eats up so much NAD+ that cell death can result.[6,7]

EMF exposure can cause your cells to become NAD+ depleted. PARP is ordinarily the largest consumer of NAD+ in your body, and if you have a large EMF exposure you can radically reduce your NAD+ levels. And when your cells become NAD+ depleted, it also impacts your mitochondria by lowering an NAD coenzyme called NADH, which is necessary for your mitochondria to produce ATP.

Another consequence of PARP sucking up most of your NAD+ is that it depletes the supply for other vital longevity proteins, called *sirtuins*, that require NAD+ to function.[8,9] If PARP is consuming most of your NAD+, your sirtuins will not have enough NAD+ to run and your aging will be accelerated dramatically.

There is also one other downside to PARP: When it is called to repair your damaged DNA it also activates proinflammatory pathways that will increase your risk for virtually every chronic disease.[10]

So while PARP is a powerful DNA repair mechanism, and thus an important line of defense against EMF exposure, you need to keep your NAD+ levels high in order to fuel it, and prime your body's ability to use antioxidants to fight inflammation. Let's look at how to do just that.

THE HISTORY OF NICOTINAMIDE ADENINE DINUCLEOTIDE

Nicotinamide adenine dinucleotide (NAD+) was first discovered in 1904 by British biochemist Arthur Harden as a cofactor for fermentation.[11] NAD+ has received abundant attention in research, including from four Nobel Prize laureates, one of whom was Otto Warburg, the German biochemist who discovered that cancer cells metabolize energy differently than healthy cells and whose work I discussed in my book *Fat for Fuel*.[12]

Since its discovery, NAD+ has been established as an important coenzyme involved in the energy-production process that occurs in your mitochondria known as *oxidative phosphorylation*.

Even though we've known about NAD+ for well over a century, we've only recently become aware of NAD+'s many important and diverse metabolic functions. This was largely a result of work at the Massachusetts Institute of Technology around 2000 demonstrating that the sirtuin proteins, which play a role in cellular health and longevity, required NAD+ to function;[13] this heralded a whole new era in NAD+ research.[14]

The more we learn about NAD+, the more it has come to be appreciated as an essential cofactor for a wide variety of vitally important cellular processes. As you will see, this makes it a key player in repairing EMF-induced damage. But before we get to that direct connection, it's important that you understand the many roles NAD+ plays in your body, and its many forms.

SOME OF THE MOST IMPORTANT MOLECULES IN YOUR BODY

NAD+ is a coenzyme, part of the NAD family of coenzymes, which also includes NADH, NADP+, and NADPH.

Coenzymes are small molecules that cannot by themselves catalyze a reaction. Rather, they bind with an enzyme and enable that enzyme to trigger a reaction. NAD coenzymes are central regulators of metabolism and thus probably some of the most important and necessary molecules in your body.

They are indispensable cofactors in more than 700 enzymatic redox reactions central to most metabolic processes in your body, including burning fuel in your mitochondria to generate ATP, making glucose, fats, DNA, RNA, and steroid hormones, and support detoxification of free radical species.[15–18]

What is common to all these molecules is that they all contain *adenosine monophosphate* (AMP), which is the precursor of ATP, the energy currency of your cells. For the sake of our focus on remediating the physiological damage caused by EMF exposure, we'll focus on NAD+ and NADPH.

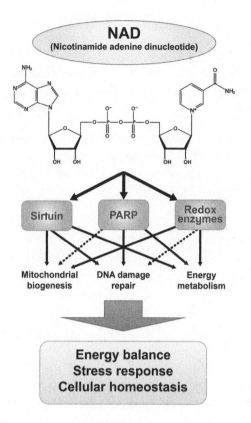

Figure 6.1: Biochemical structure of NAD+ and some of its important biological functions.

What has recently been appreciated is that the ratio of NAD+ to NADH inside your cells may be one of the key metrics to determine how healthy you are. High levels of NAD+ and NADPH are essential for maintaining cellular health. Decreased levels of these valuable molecules have been linked to a variety of conditions such as cardiovascular disease, cancer, aging,[19] traumatic brain injury-induced inflammation,[20] seizure disorders, and neurodegenerative diseases.[21]

OTHER NAD COENZYMES

In addition to helping your body produce energy, NAD coenzymes are necessary for your genes to be optimally expressed and for your immune and detoxification systems to function properly.

They help recharge your body's antioxidants, in a process I'll explain in just a bit, so you can lower free radical damage. And, perhaps most important, they are essential to slow down the aging process[22] and radically reduce your risk of chronic degenerative diseases and increased frailty.

Structurally, NADP is identical to NAD except for the phosphate (which is what the "P" stands for). NADK is the enzyme that attaches a phosphate group to NAD+ and NADH to form NADPH, which we'll discuss next.[23]

NADPH, THE BATTERY OF YOUR CELL

NADPH provides a reservoir of electrons and can thus be thought of as a stable form of storage of electronic-reducing potential. In simpler terms, NADPH is your cell's battery.[24] Yes folks, NADPH is the true battery of your cell—not your mitochondria, as some people believe. That is one of the reasons it is one of my favorite biological molecules.

NADPH is involved in keeping your antioxidants in tip-top shape by regularly supplying them with electrons so they can do their job and lower damage from oxidative stress.[25]

It does this by using its electrons (from hydrogen, the "H" in NADPH) to recharge your body's antioxidants like glutathione and vitamin C,[26] and convert them to their active functional forms.[27]

This is important because once glutathione performs its job by donating its electrons to help eliminate free radicals, it becomes oxidized and useless. It is only restored to its functional state through a series of enzyme-catalyzed reactions, in which

NADPH donates its electrons to make glutathione ready to go and tackle more free radicals.

ANTIOXIDANTS WITHOUT NADPH AREN'T AS HELPFUL AS YOU MIGHT THINK

After the free radical theory of aging was initially proposed by gerontologist Denham Harman[28] in the 1950s, supplementing with antioxidants became a popular strategy to slow down the aging process. There is an overwhelming amount of evidence showing that this is likely not a wise strategy.[29] In recent years it has been shown that taking antioxidant supplements, such as vitamins C30 or E,[31] does not extend life span.

This does not mean you should avoid taking vitamins or supplements, you just need to be careful about taking excess quantities of supplemental antioxidants as they may cause more harm than good by indiscriminately suppressing beneficial free radicals.

The main problem is that antioxidants like vitamins E and C and glutathione are charged molecules, and because of their charge they do not readily cross your cell membranes and enter your cells. This is why you want to leverage NADPH levels to recharge the antioxidants already in your cells.

Antioxidants work by donating an electron to neutralize free radicals. Once they donate that electron they become useless or, even worse, actually start to function as pro-oxidants. To work as antioxidants again they need to be recharged, very similar to the way an electric car needs to be recharged after being used.

NADPH is what recharges your antioxidants to their active forms. Without NADPH, antioxidants aren't all that helpful. In fact, research has shown that antioxidants provide little longevity benefit in elderly people whose NADPH levels have declined to such an extent to prevent their efficient recycling.[32]

For these reasons, it makes far more sense to increase your NADPH levels than to swallow antioxidants that will simply stop working after they donate their initial supply of electrons.

HOW TO INCREASE YOUR NADPH LEVELS

When it comes to boosting your available NADPH, you have several possibilities available to you.

Reduce Your EMF Exposure

One cause for the aging-related loss of NADPH and the increase in oxidative stress that comes with aging is the decrease in the levels of cellular NAD+.[33] This is because NAD+ is required for the synthesis of NADPH.

Minimizing your EMF exposure can radically increase your NAD+ levels, because when you are exposed to EMFs and your DNA strands break, PARP uses 150–200 molecules of NAD+ in an effort to repair that damage. Chapter 7 is going to show you a variety of ways you can reduce your EMF exposure.

Avoid Eating at Least 3–4 Hours Before You Go to Sleep

If you have read *Fat for Fuel* or *KetoFast*, or if you regularly read my website, you know the importance of not eating at least three to four hours before going to bed to optimize your health. I personally strive for a six-hour fasting window before going to sleep. While writing this book I learned that NADPH has a lot to do with why this is such a powerful health practice.

More generally, this is called "time restricted eating." Since 90 percent of people eat from the time they awaken to the time they go to sleep (more than 12 hours each day), there are quite dramatic and beneficial results when food consumption is restricted to a smaller window of 6 to 8 hours. This allows your body to activate the powerful process of autophagy that recycles your damaged cellular parts. On many days I only eat within a four-hour window.

The largest consumers of NADPH are the enzymes used for converting excess calories you eat to store them as fat.[34] If you eat a large meal close to your bedtime there is simply no way for your body to burn those calories as energy, so it must store the calories by creating fat.

This process consumes enormous amounts of NADPH. With your NADPH levels lowered this way, you will be unable to keep your antioxidants optimally recharged while you sleep. As a result, you will have far more oxidative damage from the free radicals that can't be neutralized (due to low NADPH levels) than if you had eaten those calories earlier in the day.

Inhibit NADPH Oxidase

The enzyme *NADPH oxidase* (NOX) is another major consumer of NADPH. It has many roles including supplying your white blood cells with the ability to destroy invading pathogens, cellular signaling, and the regulation of gene expression.[35] NOX in your blood vessels also generates reactive oxygen species (ROS), important for maintaining normal blood pressure.[36]

One of the other rarely discussed benefits of limiting EMF exposure is that it will also decrease NOX activation. The NOX enzymes don't work constantly, and they require a signal to cause them to turn on. Guess what that signal is? You are pretty sharp if you guessed it is increased calcium coming into the cell,[37] which is precisely what EMF exposure creates.

When you understand why calcium flooding into a cell activates NOX, you'll see how this process reinforces the EMF damage mechanism. Let me explain.

When NOX eliminates a viral or bacterial threat, it also increases superoxide in your white blood cells. This large localized production of superoxide will form a major way to trap nitric oxide produced by any cell in the region. The nitric oxide will then combine with superoxide to form peroxynitrite, which will form the highly reactive carbonate free radical to destroy the invading germs.[38]

Therefore, assuming you don't have a raging infection that needs to be battled with NOX by your white blood cells, you can increase NADPH by inhibiting excessive activation of NOX, and you can do that by limiting your EMF exposure.

You can also inhibit activation of NOX by using *molecular hydrogen*. Molecular hydrogen (H_2) is the lightest element and is the smallest molecule in the universe. It is extremely bioavailable, not only because of its size, but also because it does not carry a charge. It can easily penetrate your cell membranes and other subcellular structures.

H_2 can rapidly diffuse into your tissues and cells without affecting important signaling processes.[39] When H_2 enters into the subcellular compartments, it slows down the effects of excessive reactive oxygen species (ROS) and reactive nitrogen species (RNS) generated when you have a disease.

H_2 protects your DNA, RNA, proteins, cell membranes, and mitochondria from damage.[40] In addition to lowering oxidative stress and inhibiting excessive NOX activation, it is also a potent stimulus of the Nrf2 pathway, which I will discuss in just a few pages.[41]

H_2 has been shown to have therapeutic benefits in more than 170 different animal and human disease models. Several animal studies have shown that H_2 is effective at increasing resilience and mitigating the negative effects of acute and chronic stress such as inflammation and elevated ROS.[42]

One of the reasons why H_2 is so interesting is that it works to lower NOX levels when NOX is excessively activated.[43] This is ideal, as indiscriminate suppression of NOX may impair your immune function and the ability of your white blood cells to eliminate pathogens effectively.

H$_2$ functions this way because hydrogen does not directly scavenge ROS, rather, it decreases excessive levels of ROS. H$_2$ also reduces excessive ROS production and has mild pro-oxidant benefits similar to those produced by exercise.[44]

Interestingly, two human studies have shown that using hydrogen water helps mitigate side effects of radiation therapy in cancer patients.[45,46] Further studies on molecular hydrogen and its protection against radiation are in process, but more research is needed.

There are many ways to take molecular hydrogen therapeutically. Sadly, many methods deliver inadequate dosages. One of the most effective methods to take it is in the form of tablets that release the gas once dropped in water.

There are a wide variety of tablets out there, but you will want ones that have a concentration of 9 milligrams per liter, as they give you the most hydrogen. You can find these in our online store at mercola.com as well as through other outlets. If you take molecular hydrogen by dissolving it in water regularly throughout the day, many of its benefits diminish, as pulsing the hydrogen provides the best benefits. Once or twice daily dosing seems ideal.

Increase NAD+ Levels Directly

When you increase your NAD+ levels with NAD+ precursors you can help to restore your body's ability to repair the damage from EMF exposure by fueling the PARP enzymes.[47] Scientists have reported that NAD+ can also greatly reduce X-ray-induced radiation damage in tissues exposed to ionizing gamma radiation,[48] and that NAD+ deficiency is a key factor in ionizing radiation–induced tissue injury.[49]

This is a very important point because, as I reviewed in Chapter 1, we know that ionizing and nonionizing radiation cause virtually identical damage to your DNA. They just do it in different ways. If the damage is similar, it stands to reason that the precautions and post-damage remediation are similar as well.

After limiting your exposure as much as possible to EMF, which is clearly the most important step (discussed extensively in Chapter 7), the next best strategy will be to increase your NAD+ levels. This will not only help you fight EMF damage, but it's also likely one of the most powerful antiaging strategies we now know of.

Before we review the strategies to increase your NAD+ levels, it is important to understand that these strategies are not a magic bullet. They are in no way, shape, or form a replacement for sleep, exercise, minimizing processed food, and avoiding EMFs, as these, along with the time-restricted eating discussed above, are the foundations of health that will allow your body to take advantage of your increased NAD+ levels.

To determine how much NAD+ your body requires, you need to know how much you are currently using every day. If you weigh about 165 pounds, you will use about 9 grams (9,000 milligrams) every day. Although less than two teaspoons, that sure is a lot to replace with a supplement. The good news is that under normal conditions your body will recycle 99 percent of its NAD+, so you only need to replace roughly one percent, or about 90 milligrams.[50]

Please note that is under *normal* conditions. Remember, PARP is one of the primary consumers of your NAD+. If you are under constant EMF stress and damaging your DNA, you will deplete your NAD+ far more than one percent, meaning your replacement levels could easily exceed that one percent by many times.

No one knows for sure just how much EMF exposure reduces NAD+ levels, as virtually none of the researchers working on NAD+ recognize EMF as a cause of PARP activation and NAD+ depletion and they have not specifically studied the impact of EMF on NAD+ levels.

So, how do you go about replacing depleted NAD+?

There are two primary options.

The first is to make it from scratch, a process called *de novo synthesis*. This process typically uses the amino acid tryptophan. Unfortunately, it is very inefficient; it takes about 70 milligrams of tryptophan to make 1 milligram of NAD+.[51] This means you would need more than 6 grams of tryptophan to meet your daily needs, and the average intake is less than 1 gram per day.

What's more, if you are subject to excessive EMF exposure, you could easily deplete your body's tryptophan stores as it seeks to keep up with the increased NAD+ demand. This could contribute to neuropsychiatric and sleep disorders, as tryptophan is the precursor for both serotonin and melatonin. Supplementation with tryptophan might be appropriate to address the deficiency that NAD+ is creating.

The second way to produce more NAD+ is to make it from what is called a *salvage pathway*, in which you recycle its breakdown product, *niacinamide*, and convert it back to NAD+. This process takes niacinamide through a series of enzyme reactions to re-create NAD+.

This is the way the vast majority of your NAD+ is replaced. Unfortunately, with modern EMF exposures and nearly continuous PARP depletion, this pathway is not nearly enough to keep up with your daily demand. You can, however, enhance this pathway and keep your NAD+ depletion and replacement in balance, as I will now explain.

HOW TO KEEP YOUR NAD+ LEVELS HIGH

Another factor that can diminish your NAD+ levels is simply getting older—as they decline quite dramatically with age.

It remains unclear why the breakdown and synthesis of NAD+ do not stay in balance as we grow older, but it appears that synthesis becomes outpaced by consumption, which is likely related to increased inflammation and excess oxidative stress that has been especially accelerated in the 21st century by PARP activation through EMF exposures.[52]

Unfortunately, at this time NAD+ levels are not something that can be measured in a commercial lab. It requires a liquid chromatography and mass spectrogram to analyze. My guess is after awareness of the clinical importance of NAD+ becomes more widely known this will eventually be available in commercial labs.

One of my friends, James Clement, is an NAD researcher and has mass spectrometry equipment in his lab that can accurately measure NAD+ levels. He wrote a landmark paper with the leading NAD expert, Dr. Nady Braidy, in 2019 that was the most viewed article of the entire year in *Rejuvenation Research*.[53] It was an epic paper, as it was the first study to clearly document the radical and shocking decline in NAD+ levels that occur with aging.

Clement found that typical levels in healthy people under the age of 30 were around 40 nanograms per millileter ng/ml in the blood. Levels dropped progressively as individuals reached the age of 80, to less than 1 ng/ml.

There were some exceptions, though, as one 85-year-old who exercised aggressively had a level of 9 ng/ml. This is likely due to the fact that exercise is one way to activate the rate-limiting enzyme for NAD+ formation, NAMPT, from its degradation product nicotinamide. If you fail to exercise regularly as you age and grow old, not only will your NAD+ levels drop but your nicotinamide (NAD+ precursor) levels will rise; high levels of nicotinamide, in turn, will inhibit the sirtuin longevity proteins.

This information makes it very clear that there is not a generic one-size-fits-all approach to improve NAD+ levels. The older you are, the more aggressive the augmentation therapy needs to be.

If you are between 30 and 40 years old, or even younger, you need to do very little other than to make sure you are implementing the NAD+ basics that nearly everyone needs, such as:

- Getting enough niacin every day (around 25 milligrams—I explain more in the next section).

- Doing regular bouts of high-intensity exercise, as this will increase NAMPT and secondarily NAD+. Aerobic and resistance exercise training reverses the age-dependent decline in NAD+, as both forms of exercise increase NAMPT.

  The most exciting exercise development is the use of Blood Flow Restriction Training that allows the use of low weights and high repetitions to produce incredible metabolic benefits, including NAMPT activation.

  It is my absolute favorite way to increase NAD+. Not only will it increase NAD+ but it will also prevent and treat sarcopenia, or age related muscle loss, and osteoporosis. It will also help prevent heart attacks and strokes. It requires a full chapter to explain. As such, it is beyond the scope of this book, which is why I have placed the material that you can access for free at BFR.mercola.com.

- Implementing time-restricted eating also increases NAD+.

- Having your last food at least three to four hours before you go to sleep. If you eat closer to the time you sleep, you will likely store most of the energy from that food as fat, a conversion process that requires NADPH.[54]

NIACIN THERAPY

One of the most straightforward strategies for increasing your NAD+ balance is supplementing with its precursors. Oral NAD precursors have been shown to restore NAD levels in aged tissues and show beneficial effects against aging and aging-related diseases.[55–58]

Niacin is one of those precursors. I believe that low-dose niacin therapy, around 25 milligrams, is a therapy that most people would benefit from, as it is very low cost and has no serious side effects.

Niacin has been shown to efficiently increase intracellular NAD+ levels, especially in your brain where it counts.[59] And a deficiency in niacin can cause very serious health problems in addition to contributing to NAD+ depletion.

Prior to food supplementation with niacin, people died from pellagra, a disease caused by a niacin deficiency whose hallmark symptoms are skin rashes, diarrhea, mouth sores, and dementia, which at that time was endemic in the United States.[60,61] Niacin deficiency also has been shown to cause DNA damage and unstable chromosomes.[62–65]

Since timed-release niacin eliminates the flushing reaction, many believe it is a better choice. Unfortunately, a high-quality study tested this strategy and the results appear far inferior,[66] so inexpensive non-timed release niacin seems to be the preferred choice. You can purchase it in pills, capsules, or powder.

Niacinamide

Another vitamin B_3 precursor that can be used is *niacinamide* (also called *nicotinamide*). This is actually the molecule that NAD+ is broken down into once your body has used it. An advantage of niacinamide is that it does not cause a flush as niacin does.

The problem with using niacinamide to increase NAD+ levels, especially with higher doses, is that it is a direct inhibitor of the sirtuin Sirt1.[67] Since sirtuins require NAD+ to function, when niacinamide levels are high sirtuins tend to be inhibited and your longevity pathways become compromised. For this reason, many believe that niacinamide is not an ideal choice for a niacin precursor.

There are other NAD+ precursors, such as nicotinamide riboside (NR) and nicotinamide mononucleotide (NMN) and even the NAD+ molecule itself. But for most they are unnecessary at this time and beyond the scope of this book. Just understand that NAD+ augmentation support is one of the most important strategies you can use to stay healthy and these are the five best ways to do it.

Five Best Ways to Increase Your NAD+

- Limit your EMF exposure and sleep in a low-EMF bedroom

- Practice daily time-restricted eating where you only eat food in a 6- to 8-hour window or even less

- Engage in some type of daily exercise and seriously consider blood flow restriction training

- Supplement with molecular hydrogen

- Make sure you are getting about 25 mg of niacin a day and have regular magnesium supplementation to reach at least your RDA of 400 mg of elemental magnesium

Increasing NAD+ Indirectly Through NQO1

There is an elegant enzyme that will actually convert NADH back to NAD+. That enzyme has a heck of a long, complicated biochemical name—*NADPH dehydrogenase, quinone 1*. Thankfully, we can call it NQO1 for short.

NQO1 is really unusual in that it is one of the only enzymes that takes NADH and converts (oxidizes) it to NAD+.[68] This is helpful because what is important for your health and longevity may not be the actual concentration or level of NAD+ in your cells, but rather the NAD+/NADH ratio.

Also, it is well documented that NAD+ levels decrease with age due to a change in the balance between NAD creation and consumption.[69] So just about anything that increases NAD+ levels will help improve your health and also fuel PARP to help repair your DNA damage.

As a bonus, NQO1 plays a role in the direct removal of superoxide from your mitochondria.[70] Less superoxide means less formation of peroxynitrite.

You can increase NQO1 activity through heat exposure and photodynamic therapy, such as sitting in a near-infrared sauna. This is a great practice for a wide variety of other health reasons, such as energizing your mitochondria through photobiomodulation and helping to eliminate toxins through sweating. In my view a near-infrared (not far-infrared) sauna is one of the most valuable health tools out there.

But one of the other important ways to boost NQO1 is to activate a very important DNA transcription factor that you may not have heard of previously, the *Nrf2 pathway*, which I will describe next. This is also one of the pathways that molecular hydrogen activates.

NRF2 IS A KEY PATHWAY TO KEEP YOU HEALTHY

Nrf2 is an important biological pathway that emerged from obscurity in 1997 at the University of Tsukuba in Japan.[71] It's quite likely neither you nor your doctor have ever heard of it before.

This is unfortunate, because the Nrf2 pathway is the master regulator of responses to oxidative damage from free radicals, inflammation, and mitochondrial dysfunction. In addition to helping your body address the effects of EMFs, the Nrf2 pathway protects your cells from the damaging effects of ionizing radiation such as X-rays.[72,73]

Since its discovery, Nrf2 has become most known for its role in activating genes that have powerful antioxidant effects.[74] It does not indiscriminately suppress all free radicals; it is only called to action when your body needs to reduce free radical damage. At that point, it will trigger your DNA to activate up to 500 genes, including antioxidant proteins, and detoxifying enzymes.[75]

The Single Use of High Doses of Antioxidants Might Save Your Life

This is a tangent, but a potentially life-saving one. If you or someone you love ever comes down with a life-threatening sepsis infection, a relatively simple but highly effective cocktail of a massive IV dose of vitamin C, thiamine, and hydrocortisone could save your or your loved one's life.[76]

Septic shock from severe sepsis strikes more than a million Americans every year, and 15 to 30 percent of those people die.[77] That means 150,000 to 300,000 people die EVERY year in the United States from this problem; that's nearly 1,000 people every day. More than half of sepsis infections are acquired in the hospital.

If your doctor refuses to consider it, have him or her review the recent studies cited here that show this works.[78–81] All you need is to look up the references in the endnotes to the previous sentence and type the name of the article in your search engine. Alternatively, you can just go to PubMed (https://www.ncbi.nlm.nih.gov/pubmed) directly and type "vitamin C and sepsis" in the search field and you will get the list.

These articles are completely free to download. I hope you never need to access them, but if you do, you can print them and use the information to convince your medical team to use these simple life-saving strategies.

Nrf2 can activate the production of hundreds of antioxidant and stress-response genes. Some of these include the NQO1 gene we talked about earlier, glutathione peroxidase, thioredoxin, catalase, superoxide dismutase heme oxygenase-1, and many others.[82]

You will be pleased to know that Nrf2 also plays a major role in optimizing the entire family of NAD coenzymes. Not only does it increase NADPH, Nrf2 also activates NQO1.[83]

In addition, Nrf2 activates a total of 25 different detoxification genes, each of which produce an enzyme that acts in detoxification of various toxic chemicals.[84] This is very beneficial, because thanks to the industrialization of the 20th and 21st centuries, your exposure to chemical toxins has increased dramatically.

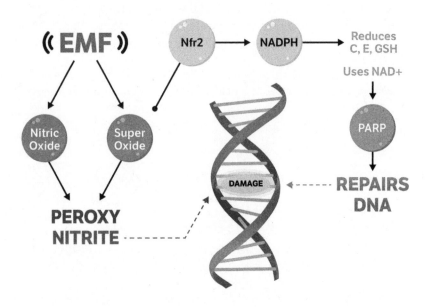

Figure 6.2: The complex ways you can damage and repair your DNA.

How Nrf2 Works

We believe that one of the general biologic strategies that enables Nrf2 to do its beneficial work is a process called *hormesis*.

If you haven't heard of hormesis before, it is best summed up by Friedrich Nietzsche's famous quote "That which does not kill us makes us stronger."

Another way of looking at hormesis is through one of the basic tenets of toxicology, which is "The dose makes the poison." Low doses of "toxin" may actually make you healthier. Many of the polyphenols (primarily micronutrient found in plants that are antioxidants) that activate Nrf2 are actually produced by plants to ward off predators. These chemicals can kill predators in large doses but, when used in smaller increments, are quite beneficial.

Moderate stress causes a response in your body that is protective against future insults: Exercise and calorie restriction are two other examples of this principle. To be effective, though, the stress must be pulsed; it cannot be continuous or chronic. This is why pulsing many Nrf2 activators is so important. It just isn't a wise strategy to take most of them continuously.

Exercise, for example, puts stress on muscles that cause your body to react in ways that increase muscle strength. Weight-bearing exercise puts stress on your bones, causing your body to react by increasing bone strength. And we all know that you need to have recovery periods after exercise. For example, if you exercise continuously without rest, it could be very damaging and counterproductive to your health.

In this same way, after an oxidative stress–inducing incident, your body requires time to clear out oxidation by-products and reestablish homeostasis. Your cells also likely require time to replenish their stocks of Nrf2.

Nrf2 and Health Span

Many researchers believe that Nrf2 is a master regulator of not only longevity, but also, more important, of health span.[85] Whereas life span refers to the oldest age you reach, health span is the oldest age at which you maintain all the aspects of being healthy. It is not a victory to live to an old age if you are crippled with arthritis and pain, immobile, frail, and lacking most of your mental capacity.

There are a number of genetic studies in mice and several other species that show that raising Nrf2 activity produces prolonged life spans and health spans, and that lowering Nrf2 produces the opposite.

Nrf2 may provide these benefits by facilitating the removal of senescent cells that have stopped reproducing and create silent inflammation.[86] Interestingly, when mice have their Nrf2 genes removed they develop premature cellular senescence.[87]

This makes perfect sense because one of the primary drivers for senescent cells is oxidative stress, and Nrf2 is magnificent for addressing this.[88] If you are older than 65, you will want to consider strategies to activate your Nrf2 pathways because you likely have diminished Nrf2 activation[89] in addition to lower NAD+ levels.

Also, it is well known that calorie restriction benefits your health primarily through activating *autophagy*, which comes from the Greek words for *self-eating*. It is a process that removes damaged and defective cellular parts, tags them for destruction, and then breaks down the cellular parts to their constituent elements so they can be recycled.

Nrf2 not only stimulates autophagy,[90] but it is also likely responsible for many of the health benefits afforded by calorie restriction.[91-95]

It just keeps on getting better with Nrf2 benefits, as researchers have found that this pathway also stimulates a process called *mitochondrial biogenesis*, which increases the number of your mitochondria and improves your mitochondrial function—essential for optimal health.[96,97]

An interesting side note on Nrf2 is that statins, the very popular drugs used to lower cholesterol levels in one in four Americans over the age of 40, appear to activate Nrf2, and this may explain some of their observed cardiovascular benefits.[98-100] That would make sense from my perspective, as in my view statins clearly don't benefit people by lowering their cholesterol levels. Fortunately, there are far less dangerous and less expensive strategies to raise Nrf2.

Natural Products Activate Nrf2

Many studies have shown that the consumption of fruits and vegetables is associated with reduced risk for cardiovascular disease and stroke. Experts used to believe that the protective effects of the phytochemicals, the protective chemicals that the plants produce, resulted from their direct antioxidant actions.

However, the understanding now is that the benefits conveyed by the phytonutrients in fruits and vegetables are likely largely related to their Nrf2-stimulating action and not their antioxidant action.

Fortunately, there are many natural products that will activate Nrf2 and not only stimulate NQO1 but also provide many other benefits. The scope of this book does not allow me to go deep into the details here, but I have provided references to the studies that go into more depth for you.

The Nrf2-boosting chemicals on the following list are mostly polyphenols. [101-108]

- Vitamin D[109]

- Molecular hydrogen[110-112]

- Sulforaphane[113] from broccoli

- Rutin from apples, black and green tea, and buckwheat[114-116]

- Quercetin, found in capers, red onions, berries, and broccoli[117-120]

- Curcumin[121-123] from turmeric

- Fisetin, which is found in strawberries, green tea, chamomile tea, and apples[124]

- Resveratrol, found in pistachios, grapes, blueberries, and dark chocolate[125-127]

- Green tea and its active ingredient epigallocatechin-3-gallate (EGCG)[128-130]

- Apple peel polyphenols[131,132]

- Pomegranate peel polyphenols[133-135]

- Delta- and gamma-tocopherols (vitamin E) and tocotrienols (not alpha, which has little activity), from rasperries, blackberries, soybeans (which you should only eat organic versions of to avoid genetically modified organisms), hazelnuts, and olive oil[136-139]

- Purple sweet potatoes[140-142]

- Astaxanthin[143-145] from microalgae and in some seafood, like krill

- Isothiocyanates from broccoli, cabbage, and other cruciferous foods[146,147]

- Triterpenoids and other terpenes, found in beans, apples, peppermint, oregano, and thyme[148,149]

- Sulfur compounds including allyl sulfides in garlic, onion, and allium foods such as chives and leeks[150,151]

- Carotenoids, particularly lycopene, which is found in tomatoes, watermelon, and guava [152,153]

- Fish oil (long-chain omega-3 fatty acids DHA and EPA)[154,155]

- Modest oxidative stress (hormesis), such as that induced by exercise[156]

- Melatonin[157]

While many consider daily consumption a useful protection strategy, I have some concerns that continuous use of the high-dose concentrated versions available in many supplements may be counterproductive. That's why I recommend you prioritize getting these polyphenols from whole foods.

I also suspect the use of these high-dose polyphenols is more appropriate when you have autophagy ("self-eating") activated through fasting or partial fasting of at least 40 hours. In this scenario the polyphenols would likely improve the level and benefits of autophagy.

THIS COMMON MINERAL CAN ALSO HELP

There is one more supplement strategy to address EMF damage that can be effective: to block excessive calcium channel activation. Magnesium can help with this. Magnesium is the fourth most abundant mineral in your body after calcium, potassium, and sodium. It activates more than 600 enzymes and is an important cofactor for the activation of a wide range of transporters and enzymes.[158]

Magnesium is essential for the stability of cell function, RNA and DNA synthesis, and cell repair. Interestingly, magnesium is also a natural calcium channel blocker.

Magnesium has been used for some time for lowering blood pressure because it acts like a natural calcium channel blocker.[159] If you can prevent activation of the calcium channels by EMFs then you could decrease the need for repairing peroxynitrite damage.

Magnesium is inexpensive and virtually free of side effects. Because it is also a natural laxative, it has a built-in safety mechanism. If you take too much oral magnesium you will simply eliminate it by having loose stools.

Additionally, it is well documented that more than half of Americans do not take enough magnesium. A baseline for "enough" is approximately 400 milligrams of *elemental* magnesium per day.[160] However, that is based on RDA (recommended daily allowance) values.

In my view, RDAs suggest a minimum amount, and not necessarily an optimal amount, especially to protect you against EMF. Taking this into account, it is likely that 80 percent or more of us have suboptimal levels of magnesium and could benefit from supplementation.

In addition to helping lessen the damage from EMF, magnesium supplementation can be helpful for improving your overall health. There are a wide variety of magnesium supplements available; whichever ones you choose, it is important to realize that you need to focus on the elemental magnesium in the supplement. This is the amount that is actually available for your body to use and it's what your requirements are based on.

It is easy to miss this important point, and many people do. You could take 400 milligrams of some magnesium supplements, but if they contain only 10 percent elemental magnesium, you would be getting only 40 milligrams and need to take 10 doses per day to get the advertised amount.

Another factor to consider is the type of magnesium used, as they each have different levels of absorbability. Magnesium oxide, for example, is commonly used as a supplement. Even though it has 50 percent elemental magnesium, which seems good, this form of magnesium is very poorly absorbed compared to other supplements, so I do not recommend taking it.

Here are some of my top choices for magnesium. Some products provide different forms of magnesium, but most don't. You can combine them to get some of the unique benefits each one offers. This is especially helpful since you will likely need to take more than one pill a day. We offer CannaCalm, which has citrate, threonate, and malate along with a very low dose of 5 mg of full spectrum non-psychoactive CBD.

- **Malate** is one of most bioavailable forms of magnesium, is well tolerated, and has a relatively high amount of elemental magnesium at 15.5 percent.

- **Citrate** is also highly bioavailable and has an elemental magnesium level of 11.4 percent. The benefit of using this form is that the citrate will help bind oxalates (naturally occurring molecules in many plants that can cause kidney stones and other biologic damage) and prevent them from absorbing the magnesium and also help dissolve existing oxalate crystals you have accumulated in your body.

- **Glycinate** has a high amount of elemental magnesium at 14 percent. In this form, the magnesium is attached to the amino acid glycine, which has additional benefits. It can help increase NADPH in your body and also contribute to connective tissue strength. Glycine is the primary amino acid in collagen and bone broth.

- **Threonate** has a low amount of elemental magnesium at 8 percent. Its claim to fame is that it's particularly good at passing the blood-brain barrier and increasing magnesium levels in your brain. Once it gets into the brain, it increases the density of synapses, which are the communication connections between brain cells.[161]

EVEN BETTER THAN REPAIRING DAMAGE

While the strategies I've covered here—to support your body's ability to repair the damage to your DNA and the oxidative stress that happens as a result of EMF exposure—are important, they aren't the most crucial for protecting your health. Instead of providing your body with the raw materials to build NAD+, you can increase your levels by not using as much of it in the first place.

It is clear that the first and most important strategy to keeping your DNA whole and your oxidative stress low is to avoid the things that cause damage. This is best done by optimizing your food choices (following the strategies I outlined in my books *Fat for Fuel* and *KetoFast)* and paying careful attention to your EMF exposures in order to limit DNA damage, which I cover at length in Chapter 7.

HOW TO PROTECT YOURSELF FROM EMFS

As helpful as it is to know how to remediate the damage that EMFs can inflict, the single most powerful way you have to protect yourself is to reduce your exposure to them in the first place.

Although most of this book does tend to paint a bleak picture, there are many practical ways to limit your EMF exposure and give yourself a chance to recover and repair from the pervasive and nearly continuous EMF exposure you've experienced already.

The tactics I outline in this chapter are beneficial for everyone. If you are challenged with a serious illness, it is imperative that you reduce your exposure as much as possible, as EMFs will only worsen your health challenges.

FOUR GUIDING PRINCIPLES TO REDUCE YOUR EMF EXPOSURE

The good news is that there are a wide variety of strategies to protect yourself from EMFs. The flip side of that is that it can be overwhelming to decide which strategies you'll implement and in what order. I want to help you prioritize your efforts and understand what you need to do, and why.

Because this is a book—which does not change once it's printed—and because technology evolves every day, there is a high likelihood that these recommendations will change in the future. For this reason I strongly recommend subscribing to my free newsletter at mercola.com to receive all the latest updates and strategies.

However, the framework for EMF remediation will not change, so I'll outline the basic principles here. Briefly, you want to seek to do the following four things, in this order:

- Avoid unnecessary exposure to EMFs, especially inside your own home and from your personal devices (such as your cell phone), where you have the most control.

- Put as much distance as you can between you and the EMFs you can't avoid.

- Decrease the amount of EMF exposure coming into your house from external sources.

- When all else fails, shield yourself.

I'll walk you through the various ways you can achieve all four of these goals in this chapter. But first, I want to make a case for why you should seriously consider purchasing a meter that measures EMFs, so that you can measure the effectiveness of each step you take. Seeing this evidence of progress will inspire you to continue to make changes and adopt a lower-EMF lifestyle.

Make the Invisible Visible

Part of the reason why EMFs are so dangerous is that, like X-rays, they are invisible, silent, and odorless. Unless you are EMF-hypersensitive, you won't see, feel, or hear your EMF exposures. This is why it's crucial to invest in devices that can locate and measure all hidden sources accurately.

Before you do anything to remediate your physical exposure to EMFs, it's vital for you to measure radiation levels already present. Measuring first provides you with a baseline and dramatically helps you fine-tune your mitigation efforts so they can be as effective as possible. The ability to see and hear current readings detected by EMF measuring devices will motivate you to take immediate action to address them.

Even if you are hyper-diligent and seek to address all the sources in the comprehensive list in this chapter, you can rest assured that some sources will escape your searches. The easiest, but most expensive, way to locate these stealth sources in your home and measure the fields they emit would be to hire a professional.

The most well-known professionals who offer this service are building biologists, trained and certified to analyze indoor environments and systematically seek to reduce chemical, mold, electric, magnetic, and radio-frequency irritants. They can also help you learn how to use your own meters, and add to your knowledge of how to determine, reduce, and eliminate EMFs that lurk in your home.

EMF professionals are particularly helpful in finding wiring errors in your home that can result in very high magnetic fields throughout your home, and they are relatively common. However, they are not easy to measure even if you have a meter of your own.

The more affordable approach is to purchase your own EMF meter and do the measuring yourself. Even if you hire a professional at the outset, it is best to purchase a few meters so you can measure your different EMF exposures yourself, as the exposures will change over time.

Professional-quality meters from Gigahertz Solutions, Geovital, and other companies cost thousands of dollars, but you don't
need to spend that much. Often a decent meter can be obtained
for somewhere between $200 and $400. There are different types
of meters to measure the following four types of EMFs:

- Radio frequency (RF) for cell phones, Wi-Fi, and
  smart meters

- Magnetic fields

- Electric fields

- Dirty electricity

Guidelines for Assessing EMF Readings in Your Home

Type of EMF Exposure	Maximum Safety Threshold
AC Electric Fields: Field strength with ground potential Field strength, potential-free Body voltage	 5 volts per meter 1.5 volts per meter 100 millivolts
AC Magnetic Fields	1 milligauss or 100 nanotesla
RF Radiation	10 microwatts per square meter
Dirty Electricity	Threshold varies depending on meter you use; check manual for guidelines

There are many inexpensive meters out there that measure
the first three, but some of these combination meters, particularly
older versions, may not be able to measure all the fields accurately.
It is likely that you'll need more than one meter to measure your
exposure to all the various forms.

I know that this is a technical topic with a load of details. Even so, it is possible to find the right combination of meters that are ideal for you. I have included a list of many of the best meters available on the market with their pros and cons in the Resources section at the back of this book.

Of course meters do cost money, and when you need to buy more than one, the investment can become significant. One cost-saving idea is to pool your resources with your neighbors or family members and purchase meters together that you'll share.

When I interviewed Magda Havas, Ph.D., who has studied the health effects of what some experts call "electrosmog" for decades and who researches and teaches courses on electromagnetic pollution at Trent University in Canada, here is how she described the process of measuring EMFs on your own:

> The more you play around with [using meters], the more comfortable you become with it. You'll find some real surprises when you have the meters, because things that you think might be turned off or aren't radiating may be and increasing your exposure. Doing your own testing is something I highly recommend.

Whatever meter you choose, you'll want to search YouTube for videos on how to use it properly. Lloyd Burrell became a dedicated researcher on how to reduce EMF exposure after experiencing dizziness and pain whenever he used his cell phone. He has made many videos on the topic; you can find them on his website, electricsense.com.

When it comes to selecting which meter to buy, it's important to know that there is no "best meter." Your choice of meters depends upon your answers to the following questions:

- What are your EMF concerns? The cell tower down the street? Your neighbor's Wi-Fi? The overhead power lines? Get clear on your concerns and then look at meters that can measure that type of EMF.

- How technically minded are you? Some meters are more novice-friendly than others. Make sure you consider your tolerance for learning to use new technology when selecting your model.

- Are you willing to invest in your health? If you buy cheap, you get cheap. This is particularly true with EMF meters. There are a few out there that are so insensitive and inaccurate they are a total waste of money. Your meter purchase is an investment. Do your research and invest wisely.

Once you have a meter and are familiar with how to use it, you are in an optimal position to start lessening your exposure. So let's go back to the four guiding principles and top priorities for EMF remediation.

PRIORITY NUMBER 1:
REDUCE EXPOSURE TO EMFS WITHIN YOUR HOME

Remediating your home from the EMFs that originate from inside it is the vital first step. If you shield your home from these outside sources without first remediating internal sources of EMFs, the strategy can backfire and increase EMF levels inside because the shielding will be reflecting EMFs from your home right back inside.

Reduce EMFs Emitted by Your Computer and Your Internet Connection

This is one of the two most important aspects of reducing EMF exposure in your home, because radio-frequency exposures are among the largest contributors to your EMF exposure load, especially Wi-Fi from your routers and other devices. What's more, Wi-Fi produces a modulated signal that is especially harmful to your body.

Your long-term goal should be to connect your home computer and printer to the Internet using a hard-wired Ethernet cable (local area network, or LAN) instead of wirelessly through a Wi-Fi enabled router.

Ideally, you'll be able to get a professional solution by hiring a low-voltage audio/video contractor or a home theater company to install Ethernet wires in your walls. As a money-saving alternative, you can do it yourself by running Ethernet wires from your modem and router along the walls at the baseboards of your home.

The less-expensive flat Ethernet cables, readily available at online retailers, work best in this scenario. Most new laptops do not have an Ethernet port, so you will need to purchase an inexpensive adaptor that fits into the USB-A, USB-C, or Thunderbolt port.

It's important to realize that your Ethernet connection will not be grounded, so if you have a laptop and you disable your Wi-Fi and plug in a standard Ethernet cable to get on the Internet, you will still have high electric fields when you put your hands on the laptop. You are essentially swapping one type of EMF for another.

You can avoid high electric fields by using a grounded Cat7 Ethernet cable (with metal ends) and an Ethernet grounding adapter kit (see Resources for recommendations).

Please understand that most cable and telephone company modems/routers are Wi-Fi enabled by default. Fortunately, the Wi-Fi can be turned off through the software. Contact your cable or telephone company to walk you through how to do this, or have them do it for you remotely over the phone. But be sure to check for yourself, as they may be giving you incorrect instructions. You will need to take out your RF meter and confirm that there is no wireless radiation coming from your device.

Additionally, your cable company may automatically update your modem's software and turn Wi-Fi back on without making you aware of it, which is why it is wise to check for this regularly with your RF meter. You can then easily confirm whether or not the wireless is truly disabled.

One solution is to purchase your own cable company-approved modem and your own separate router. Then you can avoid paying the monthly fee to rent the modem/router they install and avoid having Wi-Fi turned back on automatically with updates. The Arris Surfboard is one such cable company-approved modem. Choose a model that does not have Wi-Fi.

You will only have one Ethernet port, so if you have more than one computer in the house, you will need your own router. Purchase a router that doesn't come with Wi-Fi at all, or a router model that has switchable Wi-Fi—I suggest several models to choose from in the Resources section.

Also, realize that just because you are using a wired Ethernet connection doesn't mean your computer is not emitting a Wi-Fi signal. You will need to go to your settings and be sure to place your device in airplane mode. Most laptops have a wireless button or icon to switch it on and off. You can search for your model online to find out where it is or just look for an icon that looks like an antenna sending signals.

It is really important to remember and be sure to also disable Bluetooth on your PC or Mac, but only after replacing your wireless mouse and keyboard with a wired mouse and keyboard. You may need to actually unplug a Bluetooth dongle from a USB port to disable the Bluetooth on your computer.

If for whatever reason you are unable to disable the Wi-Fi on your router, the minimal first step is to use either an electronics timer to turn your Wi-Fi router off every night while sleeping, or a wireless switch that can turn it off and on when you need to. Just make sure it is always off when you are sleeping and place it far from a desk, couch, or anywhere people sit or stand in the daytime.

Another option—but not the one I recommend—is to keep your router but to cover it with an RF-shielding cloth or wire mesh box. Some examples are the Signal Tamer and the WaveCage, both available from LessEMF.com, and Router Guard, available from Smart Meter Guard. These do not eliminate the RF levels in the room altogether, they just reduce them.

Those in your family who insist on using their portable wireless devices will still get a signal but at least the RF signal from the router and other wireless devices will be reduced in the room. If you take this approach, at least try to locate routers far away from bedrooms and where people spend a lot of time in the daytime.

For any electric device that you put your hands on—especially a personal computer—make sure it has a grounded alternating current (AC) power cord with a three-pronged plug that is plugged into a properly grounded outlet. This is crucial for protecting against EMFs when using a laptop. If your PC computer doesn't have a power cord with a three-pronged plug, you can buy one that plugs into your USB port. (See Resources.)

For a Mac laptop, slide off and throw away the adapter on the transformer (the white brick in the power cord). The adapter is the piece with two blades that swing out and allow you to plug the transformer into an outlet or power strip—but that adapter is not grounded.

Instead, connect the transformer to the grounded AC power cord with the three-pronged plug that came in the box with older MacBooks. New MacBooks don't come with that grounded AC power cord. You can, however, purchase it online from Apple or other retailers. For added protection, purchase shielded AC power cords for your desktop computer, monitor, and printer. (See Resources for suggestions.)

Take Control of Your Phone

Your cell phone transmits radio-frequency radiation even when you are not on a call, because it is constantly updating its location and communicating with the nearest cell phone towers for updates, downloads, e-mails, and texts. Whenever you don't need to be making a call on your phone, switch it to airplane mode in order to avoid the continuous radiation it emits.

Also, put your mobile phone in airplane mode if you carry it on your body. This is the second most important strategy and for some the most important step you can take. Keeping this strong emitter of RF frequencies directly on your body is just asking for trouble.

Many women diagnosed with breast cancer carried their phone in their bra. Unless you have an emergency and need to be alert to incoming calls, it is best to avoid having your phone turned on when it is on your body.

Unfortunately, it's not as easy as it once was to disable the wireless antenna on your phone by simply selecting airplane mode in your phone's settings. Now you have to not only select airplane mode, but also turn off Wi-Fi, Bluetooth, and near-field communications (NFC).

Fortunately, you can do this by swiping up on an Apple phone and down on an Android; this will bring up a screen that shows you the icons for airplane mode, Wi-Fi, and Bluetooth so you can turn them all off in just a couple of taps. (You can also configure this page in the edit screen to put all the icons near each other to make it even easier.)

Avoid using your cell phone when the signal is weak, because when the phone has to work harder to establish a connection to a cell tower, it emits higher levels of radiation. In fact, a 2019 study found that phones emit up to 10,000 times more EMF radiation when the connectivity is low.[1] It's much better to wait until you're in a spot with full bars—and even then, to use speakerphone so that the phone is farther away from your body.

Beware of "Harmonizers"

Avoid the mistake that many make in believing that a "harmonizer" will protect you from EMFs. There are a wide variety of these devices out there; one example would be a sticker that enshrouds a polycarbonate disk that you place on your phone or laptop, which sellers claim emits a negative electrical field that counteracts, or "harmonizes," the radiation emitted by the phone—making it "safe" to use your phone.

I have met hundreds of people who have something attached to their phone that they believe makes them "protected." I have tested many of these devices and have never found any that actually reduce radiation exposure. If you don't trust me, then measure the radiation yourself with an RF meter. If your measurements are above the recommended biologically safe threshold of 1 milligauss, there's your proof.

I won't dispute that many find symptomatic improvement with some of these devices, but the danger is you get a false sense of security, thinking you are solving the problem and then go on using your devices, rather than taking the necessary measures to reduce your exposures.

Remember, EMF levels activate your calcium channels, which leads to peroxynitrite oxidative stress that damages your nuclear and mitochondrial DNA, cell membranes, mitochondria, stem cells, and proteins. The only way to prevent this process is through avoidance or actual shielding, not using a harmonizer.

I know this may sound challenging, but you also want to avoid using a cell phone in your car, or while you're on a bus or train, even when the connection to a cell tower is strong. Because you are in motion, the phone will need to work harder to stay in communication with the cell tower and again, will emit more radiation as a result.

Additionally, because you are encased in metal, all that extra radiation reflects off the inside surfaces of the vehicle, thereby intensifying the radiation. Better to keep your phone in airplane mode when you're in the car. If you commonly use it to listen to music or podcasts, download the content before you leave so that you can still enjoy it without being connected to a network.

Avoid sleeping with your cell phone in your bedroom unless it is in airplane mode or powered off completely. If possible, it is also wise to place it in a Faraday bag (which I discuss in more detail later in this chapter). While that may seem excessive, there's a possibility that you may have unknowingly downloaded spyware to your phone that will keep the device on even when you put it in airplane mode.

These programs can be difficult to find, so using a Faraday bag is a simple solution that offers additional protection and also guards against the more common scenario in which you forget to put your phone in airplane mode.

Sadly many people, including children, sleep with their phones on right under their pillow, with their head within inches of a device that transmits intermittent radio signals all night long. This is one of the worst things you can do for brain health; it is a virtual prescription for neurodegeneration and an increased risk of brain cancer.

Many people use their cell phones as alarm clocks. This is not a good idea either. If you choose to do this, the minimum precaution is to put your phone in airplane mode and in a Faraday bag. A better option is to use a talking clock that has no lights and will therefore not interfere with your sleep, even by disrupting melatonin. These clocks are available through online retailers.

Don't use wireless chargers for your cell phone, especially anywhere near your bed, as they too will increase EMFs throughout your home. Instead, use a standard plug-in charger and keep that charger and its cord well away from the bed. Wireless charging is also far less energy-efficient than using a dongle attached to a power plug, as it draws continuous power (and emits EMFs) whether you're using it or not.

For a way to use your cell phone *and* protect yourself from EMFs, you can copy a simple trick I use. When I'm home, I have a wired Ethernet connection on my desktop and I keep my phone in airplane mode so it doesn't emit any RF.

When someone calls my cell phone, it goes to my voicemail that I have configured using a service called YouMail, which will send me an e-mail with an audio attachment of any voice messages someone leaves for me. Best yet, the YouMail service is free and you can use it to report and block telemarketers.

You can also create a hardwired workaround that allows you to use your iPhone and iPad in airplane mode and still access the Internet. Use an Ethernet adapter power cord (see the Resources section for one that is shielded). Then use the same grounded, shielded Ethernet cable and Ethernet grounding adapter kit that I recommended for your computer.

This workaround allows you to access the Internet and other apps as you would on Wi-Fi without the radio-frequency EMFs from the device. You also won't have the electric fields you would if you did not use a grounded, shielded Ethernet cable.

You won't be able to make or receive phone calls, but that is what a corded landline telephone is for when you are home. Unfortunately this workaround is not yet doable with most Android cell phones and tablets, only iPhones and iPads.

Your Children and Cell Phones

Barring a life-threatening emergency, children should not use a cell phone or a wireless device of any type, for all the reasons I outlined in Chapter 4.

If your child wants to play a game on a tablet or phone, put the device in airplane mode. Restrict your child's total access to mobile devices to less than two hours a week. Hold out as long as you possibly can before giving your child a cell phone, especially a smartphone. There is a nationwide movement to Wait Until 8th (waituntil8th.org), a pledge that parents and kids take to say they won't get a smartphone until at least the eighth grade.

While the primary aim of the initiative is to "let kids be kids a little longer," the physical health benefits of subtracting years off your kids' lifetime exposure to cell phone radiation, especially when their bodies, brains, and skulls are still growing, is just as important as any social-emotional benefit, if not more so.

Once children are given cell phones, it is essential that they learn how to use them safely by keeping them in airplane mode at all times except when making a call, which should only be made using a speakerphone with the phone kept at least two feet away from the body during the call.

Reducing Common Indoor Sources of Magnetic Fields

If there are magnetic fields originating *inside* your house, it is due to internal wiring or grounding issues as well as devices that generate a high magnetic field (electric stove, hair dryer, etc.).

Sadly it is common for many homes to have wiring errors in which the magnetic fields created by current running on the hot and neutral wires of a circuit are unable to cancel each other out. This creates a dangerously high alternating current (AC) magnetic field when electric loads are turned on, such as overhead lights or appliances.

There are also areas near appliances with motors where you simply don't want to spend time when they are running. Some homes have the refrigerator against the wall in one room and, on the other side of the wall, a bedroom with a bed or living room with a chair or couch right up against the back of the fridge. The person sitting there or sleeping there will be exposed to high AC magnetic fields whenever the fridge motor is running.

A circuit breaker box and the large wires that connect it to the outside pole or meter are another area where magnetic fields can extend up to five feet out on both sides of the wall. Solar power inverters also have high AC magnetic fields.

Avoid these "point sources" of magnetic field exposure by measuring with your gauss meter and doing careful planning of where to put chairs, desks, couches, and beds relative to high magnetic field sources. Shielding, which you'll read more about later in this chapter, is often very difficult and expensive to achieve with magnetic fields.

Lower Dirty Electricity That Originates inside Your Home

As you'll remember from Chapter 1 and from earlier in this chapter, sources of dirty electricity include power lines, electrical wiring inside your home, compact fluorescent light bulbs, dimmer switches, pool pumps, heat pumps, air conditioners, power supplies for many electrical devices (such as TVs, monitors, and computers), and inverters on solar panels, all of which emit harmful EMFs.

Dirty electricity can also jump from one circuit to another within your house. It can even travel along power lines and enter your home from neighbors' homes through wiring, or even through the ground.

For these reasons, it's trickier to reduce your exposure to dirty electricity than it is to simply switch your Wi-Fi off, put your phone on airplane mode, or change the cords on your electrical devices. But addressing sources of dirty electricity within your home is still an important part of your EMF mitigation efforts.

The simplest way to remediate dirty electricity is by installing filters designed to reduce dirty electricity, which plug into a socket and use a specific electrical circuit to purge the dirty electricity pollution for the circuit it is plugged into.

Filters are portable, meaning you can move them from room to room—perhaps plugging one in near your desk if you work at home during the day and then moving it to your bedroom at night. Or you can bring it to work with you and then bring it home again at night.

In her research, Magda Havas of Trent University has found that dirty electricity filters could provide significant remediation of this invisible scourge and improvement of symptoms. In 2003, Havas designed and conducted an experiment at a school where one of the students was having health and attention challenges and was also electrohypersensitive.

She installed Stetzer Filters in the classrooms.[2] The teachers were not aware that the filters were being used. In an interview I conducted with her for my website, Havas recalled:

> I was very skeptical that you can put something in an electrical outlet and that would clean the electricity and everyone would be happy and healthy after that. . . . When I finally got to analyzing the data, I was absolutely shocked by what I found. . . .
>
> About 44 percent of the teachers improved while the filters were plugged in . . . and student behavior improved. Many of the symptoms that improved in the school were those we associate with attention-deficit hyperactivity disorder.

Of course, you could also buy multiple filters, but at about $40 each, it can be costly to place filters in every room of your house, as most homes will probably need at least 20, and a large home may need anywhere from 40 to 80 filters.

You can, however, get a discounted bulk rate if you call Stetzer Electric (608-989-2571). You won't find the discount online; you'll need to make a phone call to get the price down to around $25 per unit.

Ideally two to three filters should be installed in your bedroom (the most important), in rooms that have computers, and in the room close to your circuit breakers. It is imperative to use a dirty electricity meter (see Resources for suggestions) to help you place the filters properly, as some circuits will not need any while others may need a few filters. The only way to know is to measure with a dirty electricity meter.

An alternative approach to reducing dirty electricity that's generated in your own home is to use whole-house filters that are installed in your circuit breaker box. (See Resources for a specific product recommendation.) With a whole-house filter in use, the dirty electricity traveling on all circuits is cleaned before having the chance to infect other circuits. These filters also help with phase correction of the power before it reaches the fridge and other appliances, which will help them run more smoothly with less arcing and dirty power created.

When you use a whole-home system, there are many other benefits. This system causes less current (amps) to travel through your wires because the voltage is in line with the current. This is called *phase correction* and can also reduce magnetic fields. Less voltage traveling through all your electrical lines reduces voltage exposures, mitigates dirty electricity, and provides the added benefit of helping appliances run cooler, smoother, and more energy-efficient.

While that will help to filter out dirty electricity from coming into your home from neighbors, it will only marginally filter the dirty electricity that is created within your own home from switching power supplies and motors like your refrigerator.

That is why you should be careful to minimize the use of light bulbs and appliances that create dirty electricity in the first place and plug individual filters into outlets throughout your home based upon the readings on your plug-in microsurge meter.

Another increasingly common source of dirty electricity is the inverters that are used to convert the DC electricity that solar panels create to AC so your home and the grid can use the energy. There are special capacitors that can be installed in the solar inverter that take out dirty electricity frequencies in the 20 kHz range that are typically caused by inverters converting DC to AC electricity.

Other Strategies

- Replace all your wireless technology with wired alternatives. If you meet with resistance from other members of your household, then you'll need to educate
  everyone about the information in this book. At the
  very least, turning off all wireless devices in the house
  at night is the important first step and it's better than
  doing nothing.

  Use wired versions of keyboards, mice, and game
  controllers, and if these devices allow you to put them
  in airplane mode, please do so. Once you have replaced
  a wireless mouse and keyboard with wired versions,
  make sure to disable the Bluetooth on your computer.
  Otherwise, it will continue to emit radio frequencies.

  Connect your printer to your computer with a
  USB cable or networked through a hardwired router
  using an Ethernet cable (presuming your computer is
  also part of that hardwired network with an Ethernet
  cable). Then disable the Wi-Fi on the printer.

- Continue with your transition to wired technologies
  by rethinking your home phone. Ideally you will want
  to use a traditional landline or a Voice over Internet
  Protocol (VoIP) phone system at home or in the office,
  where you have a wired Internet connection. Plug in
  the term "free VoIP services" into your favorite search
  engine and you'll find a wide variety of options to use.
  One advantage is that all domestic calls will be free.

  Whichever type of phone connection you have,
  make sure not to use a cordless phone. They emit high
  levels of EMFs from their base at all times, even when
  the phone is not in use. If you have a cordless phone
  in your home, it should be at the top of your list of
  things to remove. Choose a phone with a handset

that is connected to the base by an old-fashioned cord and you will spare yourself a large amount of EMF exposure.

- Remove all the fluorescent bulbs and fixtures from your home. This is for three reasons. The primary one is that these fixtures produce dirty electricity, usually in the range of 62 kHz. The bulbs have toxic mercury inside, and if you happen to break one you'll have a toxic challenge to contend with. LED and fluorescent bulbs also flicker, which can impair your biology. The risks from flickering lights include seizures and less specific neurological symptoms, such as malaise and headaches.

  Seizures can also be triggered in individuals with no previous history or diagnosis of seizure disorder.[3] Lastly, they are a digital light source that can expose you to large amounts of blue light, which can disrupt your melatonin production and your sleep-wake cycles if you use them at night.

  It is best to have LEDs only in areas that you don't use very much. This is because if someone accidentally leaves them on, they will not consume as much energy as the healthier incandescent alternative. However, because most LEDs have the same digital blue light concern, it would be best to use the old clear incandescent bulbs in areas that you frequently have lit at night, like your kitchen, bathroom, and bedroom.

  Measure any light bulb you use for dirty electricity with a plug-in microsurge meter (see the Resources section for more information on specific meters) with lights on versus off. If the bulb raises the dirty electricity level above the baseline reading (with the bulb off), don't use it. Purchase "line voltage" LED bulbs that run straight off 120 volts and don't have a switched mode power supply in their base, which is what produces the dirty electricity.

However, be careful to avoid "smart" LED lights, which can be turned on and off with your cell phone or even have their color change. These bulbs emit radio-frequency signals similar to your Wi-Fi router or cell phone.

- Opt out of the Internet of Things (IoT) rage, which we discussed in Chapter 1, and avoid buying any smart appliances, thermostats, and digital assistants/smart speakers, as they are constantly seeking and receiving a Wi-Fi signal. Additionally, they are also invading your privacy and constantly listening to your conversations—particularly smart TVs[4] and digital assistants/smart speakers such as Alexa[5] and Google Home.[6]

The other challenge with virtually every new smart TV is that it is impossible to disable the Wi-Fi. This means it will be regularly blasting you with Wi-Fi even when you don't have any Wi-Fi enabled on your router in your home.

Consider using a large high-resolution computer monitor as your TV instead, as it won't have this issue. They also typically have less flicker than a TV. The other benefit of watching your video on a computer monitor is that you can use software from a company like Iris (https://iristech.co/) that allow you to filter out blue light when you watch TV at night.

Sony brand smart TVs do allow you to disable the Wi-Fi. Plug an Ethernet cable into the Ethernet jack that all smart TVs have on the back. On other brands of smart TVs, plug the TV's power cord into a power strip and flip off the power to the TV when you're not watching it.

That kills the Wi-Fi in the room (which can emit upstairs into nearby bedrooms at night). Measure the RF in the room with your meter with your non-Sony smart TV on and sit far enough back that the RF level where you sit is as close to, or less than, 10 microwatts per meter square (uW/m^2) (or less than 0.01 Watts per meter square(W/m^2)) as possible.

- If you still use a microwave oven, consider replacing it with a steam convection oven, which will heat your food as quickly and far more safely. When they are on, microwave ovens are among the largest radio-frequency EMF polluters in your home and they also emit a very high magnetic field several feet into the kitchen (when running).

  You really don't want to be within 100 feet of a microwave that is running, so it's best to remove it from your home. Remember though, that cumulatively your cell phone and wireless router are the biggest sources of EMF exposure in your home.

- Plug a grounded Ethernet cable into the back of your Roku or Apple TV device. This will automatically shut off the Wi-Fi on the Roku, but it will take several minutes.

  You will then need to purchase an infrared (IR) remote control from Roku to shut off the wireless connect, a separate transmitter in the Roku device that allows you to control it from your smartphone. The wireless connect feature does not shut off by simply plugging in an Ethernet cable.

  On Apple TV devices, the Wi-Fi does not shut off at all when you plug in an Ethernet cable, but you can place the device inside a Signal Tamer to reduce the RF in the room when you watch TV, and plug it into a power strip that you flip off when you are done watching. That kills the Wi-Fi on the Apple TV device.

- Avoid wearing metal-framed glasses. Researchers have found that metal frames can, in certain cases, cause an increase in field levels by up to approximately 20 decibels (dB), which is about a tenfold increase over that seen without them.[7] It would be best to switch to plastic frames for any glasses that you wear.

- Replace your dimmer switches with regular on-off light switches, as the dimmer switches produce dirty electricity. If you want to control the level of lighting, look for incandescent light bulbs with multiple levels of intensity.

- Choose alarm systems carefully. Make sure you are using a system that does not require a Wi-Fi router. Ideally, wire as many of the sensors as you can. If you have a few wireless sensors, that should be fine, as typically they do emit a continuous wireless signal but only go on for a few seconds a day.

  Tell your security system contractor that you want to avoid a system that "polls" the sensors every 30 seconds or several times a day. This is done with radio frequencies, where the central control unit asks all the sensors to check back in with a radio signal of their own to make sure the system is working.

- Toss out your baby monitor. In a cruel irony, most baby monitors are a major source of RF radiation.[8] Moving your baby's crib into your bedroom so that you can do away with the baby monitor altogether is the best way to avoid the radiation emitted by these devices. If you must use an existing monitor, keep it as far away from your baby's crib and mom's bedside or kitchen countertop as possible.

  For baby monitors that are either hardwired or emit low levels of EMFs, see the Resources section. You still want to keep all these monitors as far away from baby's crib, as well as mom's bed and the kitchen counter, as possible, like across the room.

Remember, parents raised children for thousands of years without baby monitors; you too can do without one.

- Refuse a smart utility meter on your home as long as you can. If your utility does not offer an opt-out program, put a smart meter guard over your smart electric, water, and gas meter. They are available from smartmetercovers.com and smartmeterguard.com.

- Avoid purchasing smart appliances like thermostats and refrigerators.

- Hire an EMF-experienced electrician, plumber, or EMF expert to fix wiring errors that can cause spikes in magnetic field exposures. Sources of magnetic fields from appliances, such as a refrigerator motor or the back of a breaker panel, can be shielded with special materials ordered from Europe, but they need to be assessed and installed professionally.

- Avoid electrical radiant floor heating systems, which emit both high magnetic and electric EMFs that can be measured even at waist height, unless you use a brand that neutralizes EMFs (see Resources). Ideally it is best to consider another heating solution.

- Keep unnecessary EMFs out of the bedroom by using a battery-operated alarm clock instead of one that plugs into the wall, and don't use electric blankets. If you have a bed that has components with electric cords that plug into a wall outlet, you are sleeping in a huge electric field that does not allow for deep, rejuvenating sleep.

Some electric beds, like hospital beds, also have a transformer mounted right up under the mattress, putting high magnetic fields into the middle part of your body all night long. This is potentially very harmful. Make sure the cord is plugged into a power strip and that you shut off the switch on the power strip when you sleep. This eliminates both the electric and magnetic field at the same time.

Ideally, it's best to turn off the electricity to your bedroom altogether when you sleep. While this may seem like a challenge, there are relatively simple devices at emfkillswitch.com that, once installed, will allow you to easily turn off all the power in the bedroom by pressing one button.

- Unplug chargers and appliances from the wall outlet when not in use. Keep them away from your bed at night. Use battery-operated power banks to charge your phones and devices at night. In combination with a shutoff switch, these power banks can be kept plugged into a wall and they will charge during the day and charge your phone at night. Just remember to keep your phone in airplane mode.

- For electrical devices that you don't use all that often, plug them into a grounded power cord, available at any hardware store, and then switch the power cord off any time you aren't using those devices. A shielded power strip is available from ElectraHealth.com. You can also use manual plug-in switches, such as one called a tap cube with on-off switch, available from online retailers or a local hardware store.

- If you have a sauna in your home, choose one that has shielded wires in the walls to heating elements as well as the AC power cord to the wall outlet. Many, but certainly not all, saunas are designed to keep magnetic fields low, and they have certifications to prove that.

These certifying labs, however, focus only on magnetic fields, the "M" of EMFs, and not also on electric fields, the "E" of EMFs. As a result, EMF experts have measured high electric fields in saunas that tout their low EMF levels, and certain electrically sensitive clients who cannot tolerate electric fields, which is most of them, are not comfortable in saunas with high electric fields.

For recommendations of sauna companies that have converted their wiring to shielded wiring and have documented low electric *and* magnetic fields inside them, see the Resources section.

Turn Your Bedroom into an EMF Sanctuary

One final, but no less important, touch to remediate your home is to make your bedroom as EMF-free as you possibly can. I've already mentioned a few precautions that apply to the bedroom; in this section, I'll explain in detail why reducing EMFs in this part of your home is so important and how to do it effectively.

Your body does an enormous amount of repair and regeneration at night. If you have high EMF exposures and secondary oxidative stress, it will be nearly impossible to optimally activate these repair and regeneration programs so that you can recover from the EMF exposures that you have no control over during the day when you are outside your home. This is why it is so important to create an EMF-free zone in your home—especially in the room where you sleep.

Even with the lights off in your bedroom and everything unplugged, there are still large amounts of AC electric pressure, known as voltage, coming off the hot wire in circuits inside the walls.

Electric fields from this voltage extend out six to eight feet into your living and sleeping space from the walls and floor and from cords plugged in near the bed. These electric fields jostle back and forth in the air, ready to resonate with charged ions and subatomic protons and electrons in every cell in your body and cause biologic havoc. This is easily verified with a body voltage meter.

These fields don't stay confined within the wires of your wall. They disperse outward and onto anything conductive, alternating between positive and negative polarity 60 times per second. They energize metal bed frames, springs in your mattresses, and ultimately your body as you lie on the mattress. This is one of the reasons I sleep on a bed that doesn't have any metal parts (even screws) and on a mattress without springs.

Electrical engineers have made it clear that electrons don't actually flow out of circuits into the air around them. Instead, it is the invisible electric field that emanates out from the hot wire, jostling the electrons in the air, your body, and the metal objects you are near that causes the problem.

Even seemingly nonconductive objects in your room that are near walls can be energized and bring AC electric fields toward your body. Prior to the 20th century your AC body voltage was zero. Now EMF remediation experts are finding that the average body voltage is anywhere between 500 and 3,000 millivolts, or 0.5 and 3 volts. In homes wired with knob and tube wiring in the 1920s and '30s, it can be as high as 12,000 millivolts.

So what happens when you are surrounded by electricity at night and your body voltage is upward of 3,000 millivolts? This energy causes muscle microcontractions that can deplete your mineral stores and increase your cortisol, which in turn lowers your melatonin at night while you're sleeping. Electric fields essentially rob you of a good night's sleep. You don't spend enough time in deep sleep every 90-minute cycle, and you wake up tired.

Deep sleep occurs in the final stage of non-REM sleep. Deep sleep is also referred to as "slow wave sleep" (SWS), or delta sleep. This is your recovery and regeneration stage of sleep where your heartbeat and breathing become their slowest as your muscles relax. Insufficient deep sleep can contribute to many health problems.

You can reduce AC electric field levels where you sleep by applying shielding paint to the walls, ceiling, and, if possible, the floor and having an electrician properly ground these painted surfaces.

If your bedroom is properly shielded, you don't have to shut off the electricity at night before you go to sleep. If your bedroom is not properly shielded, then shutting off the bedroom electricity at night is a helpful step to lower your electric field exposures.

This is why I strongly recommend, if your bedroom is not properly shielded, getting an EMF Kill Switch installed next to your circuit breaker panel and turning off the electricity in all your bedrooms with a remote switch at night while you are sleeping, as shutting off power in homes with old fuse boxes can be dangerous.

Be sure to employ the help of an EMF expert to determine precisely which circuits to shut off for each bedroom. These will be the circuits that pass within six to eight feet of each bed. All the other circuits in the house can stay on at night.

Have lamps rewired with shielded cords at a lamp repair shop, or slide a plastic, conductive tube over the existing cord and use what's known as a plug-to-gator groundpatch cord to ground it (both available at LessEMF.com).

If you use the plastic tubing, you should still move the lamp so that it is as far away from you as possible, as the electric wire inside the lamp that the cord attaches to will not be shielded and the metal of the lamp will amplify that field, and these are the parts of the lamp that are closest to you. It is far better to have the lamp professionally rewired with shielded cord.

For whatever cords you can't or don't shield, move them as far away from you as possible to minimize the electric fields. It would be helpful to use an electrical body voltage meter to see how various plug-in devices and lamps are affecting your body voltage. It's easy to tell if something is or isn't a problem if you just test it yourself or have a professional test it for you.

If so, you can have an electrician run new, dedicated circuits to those appliances using flexible metal-clad cable. That way they can remain on when you sleep without raising electric field levels.

Clients of EMF experts who turn off their breakers at night notice a significant improvement in health, including more energy, vitality, and mental clarity. They report dreaming again. Many nagging health symptoms drop away and health treatments provided by health-care practitioners just work better. Identifying and reducing electric fields is a vastly overlooked part of EMF mitigation strategies, often cited by clients as the missing link for them when they did everything else right up to that point.

PRIORITY NUMBER 2: INCREASE THE DISTANCE BETWEEN YOU AND THE EMFS YOU CAN'T AVOID

When it comes to EMFs, distance is your friend. The strength of an electromagnetic field is subject to Newton's inverse-square law, which states that the strength of a force is inversely proportional to the square or cube of the distance from that force, depending upon the source.

So if you're one foot away from an EMF, you're exposed to only one-fourth to one-eighth of the radiation you would experience if you were in contact with the source. If you're two feet away, the strength of the field that reaches you is one-sixteenth of the full strength.

Magnetic fields drop off even more quickly as you move away from them, often as much as 90 percent within one to two feet, depending upon the source.

So when you can't avoid a radiation-emitting device, find ways to put more distance between it and your body. This one little step can radically reduce your exposure. Here are some ways to do just that:

- When on a cell phone call in a private place, use the speakerphone while placing the phone at least three feet away from you. If you need privacy, your best bet is an air-tube headset, which uses hollow plastic tubes to transmit sound between you and your phone. These headsets don't allow EMFs to travel along with the sound, unlike headsets that use only metal wires, which can conduct EMFs all the way to your ear.

  Avoid all Bluetooth headsets including AirPods or their clones. You might think that using a Bluetooth headset would be good, but it isn't.

  Most people using them still have their phone on their body. But even if you had your phone 30 feet away, though you would limit your cell phone exposure, the Bluetooth signal would eradicate any benefit. Bluetooth devices generate significant EMF signals and broadcast them directly into your brain.

- If you can't make the transition away from a Wi-Fi router, at least move it as far from your living and sleeping areas as possible. Use a Signal Tamer, WaveCage, or Router Guard to further reduce the signal.

- Keep extension cords away from your desks, couches, and beds—or any location where you spend long periods of time—as they emit electric fields unless you are using a shielded electrical cable. For devices that have the option of plugging the AC cord directly into them without a switched mode power supply, such as desktop computers, monitors, and some printers, purchase shielded AC power cables that will help lower your electric field exposure. (See Resources section for where to buy these cables.)

- Avoid carrying your cell phone on your body unless it is in airplane mode. Of course, there are circumstances when you will need to be available and have to have your phone on, but it is best not to put it on your body.

    It is better to put it in your purse or backpack and remember to return it to airplane mode as soon as you can. If you must carry it on your body, or in your purse or backpack, use a Faraday bag (which I discuss on page 216), which will radically decrease if not completely eliminate the RF fields.

- Have your bedroom tested for electric fields by an EMF expert and have them show you which circuits to shut off at night. If that is not possible, you could paint your wall and floor with shielding, grounded paint. Moving your bed and desk one foot away from the walls will only slightly reduce electrical field exposure emanating from wiring in the walls.

    If you live in a commercial building, however, shutting off breakers is not necessary as the building codes for commercial buildings and residences in many large cities like New York and Chicago require electrical wires to be encased in metal conduit. This was done for fire protection, but the side effect is that it also eliminates electric fields.

    However, it would still be wise to use manual or remote plug-in switches to eliminate electric fields from unshielded AC power cords plugged into the wall that are within six to eight feet of the bed when you sleep. Alternatively, you could change all the wires plugged into your bedroom and have a lamp repair shop rewire bedside lamps with shielded cords, as discussed earlier (see Resources for a retailer that sells these).

- Train yourself and your child to keep as much distance as possible between your body and your wireless device. If you need to use a laptop, use it on a table instead of on your lap. If you must use it on your lap, put a large pillow between the device and your lap.

  Remember to turn off the Wi-Fi and Bluetooth on your laptop, use a grounded power cord (instead of the battery), and connect to the Internet using a grounded Ethernet cable plugged into an Ethernet grounding adapter kit (see Resources for a retailer that sells these).

PRIORITY NUMBER 3: REDUCE OUTSIDE SOURCES OF EMF

Although remediating the above sources is of primary importance, some remediators say the sources outside the home can be just as pervasive—if they turn off all the wireless devices inside the home they can still measure high EMF readings from the surrounding cell phone towers in many homes tested.

Much of the EMF radiation coming from outside your home originates from mobile phone towers, radio/TV stations, neighboring Wi-Fi, power lines, and smart meters. These are invariably bombarding you 24/7 and they can't be turned off. This will only get worse when 4G/5G small cell transmitters go up outside homes in residential neighborhoods, particularly in large cities.

Even though they are pervasive, there is still a lot you can do to protect yourself from these external sources.

A Few Words about 5G

I talked at length at the beginning of this book about the dangers of fifth generation cellular technology, or 5G. I also mentioned that some small cell stations will have always-on 4G LTE transmitters emitting constant RF into your home at high intensities because they will be so close to your home. That 4G signal will geolocate mobile and fixed devices. The 5G antenna will then send in data at high speeds when a 5G device requests it.

I also made the point that engineers say that 5G beamformed signals are on demand, not always on like 4G signals. These 5G signals will be narrow, roughly 15 degrees wide compared to the broader 120 degrees of width for always-on 4G signals. Engineers have made it clear that to save electricity, small cell stations will send out 5G signals primarily when users' mobile handsets request a connection along with a much weaker but frequent reference signal looking for 5G-enabled cell phones.

All 4G cell phones are programmed to prefer Wi-Fi by default when given the choice. However, when a visitor, resident, or passerby with a 5G-enabled cell phone does initiate a connection to the small cell 5G antenna outside, that signal will come into your home with a relatively narrow and focused beam.

That means that electrically hypersensitive people who want to avoid 5G from coming into their homes can be partially protected by avoiding the purchase and use of 5G-enabled cell phones, smart speakers, routers, and other devices, which started coming on the market in 2019. Shielding strategies that we review below should block most of the weak 5G reference signal.

The important point to remember is that the somewhat narrow 5G beamformed signals will be beamed into your neighbor's homes, but not so much into yours *unless* you or a family member invites that signal in by buying and using these devices yourselves. Finally, certain shielding materials will be effective against beamformed 5G signals and accompanying 4G signals. For more details on shielding, see the section that starts on page 212.

Protecting Yourself from the EMFs Emitted by Power Lines

Magnetic fields from outside overhead power lines or power lines that are buried in the ground alongside or under your house can penetrate throughout the house.

The magnetic field is a function of current flowing through the line, and this will fluctuate with time of day. (The electric field, on the other hand, is a function of the line voltage and will remain stable.)

As a result, magnetic fields from external power lines are usually only a factor when there are high current levels, such as in the evening when lights and other appliances are on, and during hot summer weather when air-conditioning use is high.

Not all power lines have high magnetic fields. You cannot tell by just looking at them. You always need to measure with your gauss meter, preferably a three-axis model (see more about specific EMF meters in the Resources section).

All overhead electric power lines will have some magnetic fields because they are uninsulated and thus must be kept separate from one another in order to prevent them from knocking together in the wind and shorting out. The farther the distance between these two lines, the higher the magnetic fields will be.

If you measure an elevated magnetic field in a room and it does not change wherever you go in the room, and only increases as you walk toward the front or back of the house, chances are you will look out the window and see power lines.

Walk out the door and the field will continue to increase. If you don't see power lines but the reading still increases, you are dealing with leakage from underground lines. Remember that magnetic fields will extend out farther in hot weather. Always measure with your gauss meter several times throughout the day, evening, and night.

Magnetic fields come from current, not voltage. That means that lower-voltage neighborhood distribution lines can have more magnetic fields than high-voltage transmission lines, even though the voltage is often much lower.

You can, however, still have seriously high magnetic fields coming up out of the ground onto your property and into your house from buried power lines. This might be due to a broken neutral wire at someone's house, or on the utility power lines, which the utility provider will fix once informed of the problem.

It can also happen because utilities ground their transformers to the earth, allowing current to bleed into soil, resulting in high amounts of dirty electricity. This is a practice they refuse to change because it costs more for the company to do it the correct way, as it's done on most every continent other than North America.

Neighborhood power lines are generally not a problem as there will usually not be a magnetic field extending beyond 20 to 30 feet as long as current loads are relatively balanced. Additionally, magnetic fields are only dangerous to your body when you are physically in their field. Normally they only radiate a few inches to a few feet from the source.

Just because you have a magnetic field somewhere in a corner in your home or apartment doesn't mean it is dangerous. The only way a magnetic field can affect your body biologically is if you measure the field where it meets your body and it is above the recommended threshold of 1 milligauss.

EMF experts typically find hot spots of magnetic field exposure somewhere in most apartments and condos. Often they simply advise clients to avoid that spot and sit or sleep elsewhere. Unfortunately, there is not a practical way to block magnetic fields from power lines, although they have been shown to have a negative health impact even at very low levels of 1 milligauss in multiple studies.

Reducing Dirty Electricity Begins Outside Your Home

Earlier in this chapter, I touched on the topic of dirty electricity and how to eliminate it within your home. It's worth repeating here. To reduce dirty electricity flowing into your home from neighbors, you should consider plugging four filters into two double outlets, one on each wire, installed by an electrician in a metal box mounted next to the circuit breaker panel.

Measure EMFs Before You Buy or Rent a Home

That being said, you do not want to choose a home with magnetic fields over 1 milligauss. And that's why it's important to measure the electric and magnetic fields of a home *before* you move in. (And one more reason to have your own meters.)

Apartments and condos can be particularly problematic because you only have control over the wiring coming out of the subpanel in your unit. There can be and often are unbalanced current loads on feeder cables to neighbors' subpanels that run through your walls and floor, or there may be current that runs along the grounding system.

One thing to be very vigilant about is avoiding electric radiant heat in your ceiling, or, even worse, in your floor—or in the ceiling of the apartment or condo below you. Avoid renting or buying a unit with an in-ceiling electric heating system, and if you live in one now, seriously consider moving (unless you live on the first floor of the building).

When the heat is turned on, magnetic fields measured from your own ceiling heat can be 5–10 milligauss at your bed or chair, and higher at head level when you stand.

If your downstairs neighbor's ceiling heat is on, you may measure 25 milligauss and higher at your feet and bed. This is far too high and will nearly guarantee health complications. Magnetic fields can cause fatigue, insomnia, depression, and even cancer. They strongly suppress your immune system and vitality.

These same radiant heating systems also usually cause very high and potentially unhealthy AC electric fields because of their design, even if the thermostat on the wall is turned off. EMF experts have measured electric field levels in the thousands of millivolts with the body voltage meter, which is far too high for good health.

These are only some of the reasons you must always measure magnetic fields before buying or renting a house or apartment to see what your potential exposure may be. Understand that magnetic fields coming in from outdoors (or from in-ceiling electric radiant heat) is usually a problem that cannot be fixed, whereas indoor sources—like wiring errors, current on metal grounding paths, and point sources—can, in most cases, be remedied.

If you live near power lines and magnetic fields are penetrating your home, usually the recommendation is to move. Unfortunately, shielding has not been proven to be effective for magnetic fields from outside power lines. This should be a deal-breaker when purchasing a new home, and many people have chosen to move from their existing homes when magnetic fields are shown to be above 1 to 2 milligauss from outside sources.

When you measure the levels of magnetic fields in a prospective home, keep in mind that magnetic field levels will be highest in the evening, when everyone is home and many appliances are turned on, and lowest at night, when loads are off while people are sleeping. Summertime is also a time of high electricity use because of air-conditioning. If at all possible, measure at various different times before you buy a new house.

PRIORITY NUMBER 4: SHIELD YOURSELF AND YOUR HOME FROM EMFS YOU CAN'T OTHERWISE REMEDIATE

The term *shielding* refers to enveloping either the source of the EMFs or yourself so that the radiation reaching you is blocked, or at least reduced. Shielding is never the first step to lowering your

EMF exposure. Rather, it is the step you take when you have done everything else you can do to limit your exposure to EMFs.

Not all EMFs are amenable to shielding and no one type of shielding blocks all types of EMFs. You need to learn the specifics and solicit the help of an EMF expert for the best results. Shielding your bedroom is definitely the most important step to see an actual impact on your health.

People turn off their Wi-Fi and remove all the wireless devices from their homes, but more often than not it's not until they shield their bedrooms that heart palpitations, insomnia, tinnitus, night terrors, and night sweats disappear. This is because cell tower, smart meter, and radio broadcast tower exposures are especially damaging to your physiology, as the waveforms are designed to collect on conductive surfaces like your body.

The golden rule is to have an RF meter available to take readings before and after shielding to ensure its effectiveness. If you start blindly shielding without taking readings, not only could you be wasting your money, but you also might make matters worse. For example, using a bed canopy made of non-groundable shielding fabric does block RF, but it also amplifies AC electric fields from circuits in nearby walls.

This is one of the reasons I have developed the Silver Shield EMF Sleeping Tent. I travel quite a bit and want to make sure I sleep in a shielded room. The only practical way for me to do this was to create a lightweight, easily collapsible tent out of RF shielding fabric that can be grounded.

The tent has zippers so you can easily get in and out of it from either side and it can also be grounded by plugging it into a properly grounded outlet. In effect you're creating a grounded Faraday cage for yourself.

This way, not only are you shielded from the typically very high RF fields in most hotels, but you are also able to ground out the electrical fields that would normally go into your body, especially from sleeping on a mattress that has metal springs in it.

For those who are unable to remediate their bedroom, using a tent could be a simple and economical way to introduce shielding. Keep in mind that you will need one tent for every person in your home. I hope that by the time you read this, tents will be available on my website, mercola.com.

I feel the best recommendation is to have an EMF expert help guide you through proper shielding. The expert should know about the other types of EMFs that are also present in the bedroom and know the right way to use shielding materials. The problem is that not all EMF experts know how to guide people through the process and don't follow up. Ask people you're considering hiring if they do have these skills, which the profession is teaching to its students. Shielding is a rather complex skill to master.

Here are some other supplies that can help you shield yourself and your home from EMFs. For more specific recommendations, refer to the Resources section:

- EMF-shielding paint. This is an effective shielding solution for blocking RF from entering your bedroom, but you will need to paint the ceiling, walls, floor, and door and window frames, and also have shielding fabric, film, and/or a metal mesh screen for your windows.

  This is typically a far better, and likely less expensive, strategy than sleeping in an EMF shielding canopy which you have to go into and out of every night, which collects dust and typically can't be washed due to the silver particles shedding off. (See Resources for my recommendation.)

  When shielding paint does not work, the reason is often that people apply it wrong; they don't understand the pitfalls of grounding, and they treat it like normal paint. Just type in "Geovital shielding paint" on YouTube and you will find a series of videos that provide detailed instruction on how to apply the shielding paint.

These are generic instructions that also apply to other brands of paint and metallic grounding tape. Just keep in mind that shielding paint and shielding cloth only protect from electric fields and wireless radiation—not magnetic fields.

Also, it's a shame for some people to paint their walls when they have wiring errors that sometimes require them to tear apart the walls to fix the errors. I have trouble simply selling the shielding paint on my website because of this.

Remember that you will need to check your bedroom for magnetic fields first before you apply shielding paint, as the shielding paint will not block magnetic fields.

- Supplies to protect against small cell signals. Remember, small cell antennas will include 4G LTE transmitters that are always on, spraying your home with constant RF exposure, as well as 5G antennas that will send beamformed data signals, but on demand in a relatively narrow beam (along with constant but much weaker reference signals).

    EMF experts and engineers believe that YShield and other RF-shielding paints as well as thicker building-grade aluminum foil will both be effective at blocking RF frequencies from 600 MHz through the part of the GHz millimeter wave (MMW) band that will be used for 5G.

    Remember, 4G will continue to use 600 MHz through 6 GHz, and new 5G technology will use the entire range from 600 MHz to 39 GHz, and eventually beyond 39 GHz. A good shielding paint and aluminum building foil will effectively block this entire range. While you could rely on a shielded tent, most current shielding fabrics are not known to be as effective above about 12 GHz.

Windows will have to be shielded against 4G and 5G frequencies with a combination of transparent window film, standard aluminum or steel metal-mesh insect screen, and RF-shielding fabric sewn onto the back of curtains.

Use your RF meter to at least measure the 4G LTE component before and after shielding. (5G RF meters that measure frequencies above 20 GHz are under development.)

- Faraday bags. They come in different sizes to fit cell phones, laptops, and tablets, and while they are commonly used to protect against remote access of your devices by hackers, Faraday bags are just as effective at keeping EMFs in as they are at keeping hackers out. Of course, you can't use your device when it's in a bag. But since cell phones emit EMFs even when they're on standby and off, it's a good idea to use the bags whenever you aren't actively using your phone.

Many online retailers offer a wide selection of bags for purchase. Whichever one you choose, please be sure to do before and after measurements with your RF meter to confirm the bag is indeed shielding you effectively.

They are inexpensive at about $5, and are highly effective at eliminating any signal from coming from your mobile phone. I use these all the time so that I'm covered in case I forget to put my phone in airplane mode.

Please remember, though, that Faraday bags do not protect you from keeping your phone on your body when it's not in airplane mode or off.

- EMF-protective clothing. It is possible to purchase hats, T-shirts, underwear, and even full burkas and hoodies made out of materials that are designed to shield EMFs.

- Smart meter guards. This is a simple enclosure that slips over your smart electric, gas, or water meter, and you can probably install it yourself easily. The guard blocks up to 99 percent of the radiation emanating out of the front and sides of the meter.[9] Yet your utility will still be able to get their signal (which indicates just how overpowered these transmitters are).

  You will still need to cover the back of the meter; metal plates can be used for this, either directly on the back of the meter if you can access it, or on the interior side of the wall where the meter is mounted. The metal of the smart meter base in the wall does afford some RF shielding itself.

REMEMBER YOUR PRIORITIES

I know that I have given you many things to consider in this chapter and you may be feeling overwhelmed. Remember to work on your EMF-remediation strategies following the order of priorities I outlined in the beginning of this chapter. They will help you tackle the most important things first and keep you on track.

Once you start taking some of these high-priority measures—like replacing as many wireless devices as you can with wired options, changing the way you use your cell phone, and making your bedroom as low-EMF as you can—you'll start to feel so much more energized and vital that it will be that much easier to keep going.

CHAPTER 8

THE PATH FROM HERE

I hope it is clear from the facts about EMFs I've revealed in this book that the rapid technological advancements of the 21st century have created a health challenge like no previous generation has been forced to face.

Ironically, it may be these very challenges—and the healthcare costs that accompany them—that provide a ray of hope that the economic forces that are responsible for our planet being deluged by EMFs will also play a role in reducing them.

INSURANCE COMPANIES TO THE RESCUE?

As the wireless industry unceasingly marches forward to blanket the Earth in an ever-growing intensity of EMFs, it may come to pass that insurance companies do the work of derailing, or at least slowing, the progression of EMFs. I hope this happens, as I don't have much faith that the government and its captured federal regulatory agencies will step in to protect us from the dangers of EMFs.

Insurance companies are in the business of making money, and they can't afford to blindly accept the misleading claims of the telecommunication industry that its products pose no threat to human health. Over the past several years, commercial insurance companies have begun refusing to cover cell phone manufacturers and wireless service providers for product liability health-related claims.

A 2018 article in *The Nation* titled "How Big Wireless Made Us Think That Cell Phones Are Safe: A Special Investigation" reported:

> One key player has not been swayed by all this wireless-friendly research: the insurance industry. In our reporting for this story, we found not a single insurance company that would sell a product-liability policy that covered mobile phone radiation.
>
> "Why would we want to do that?" one executive asked with a chuckle before pointing to more than two dozen lawsuits outstanding against wireless companies, demanding a total of $1.9 billion in damages.[1]

This isn't a new development, either. An underwriter of the insurer Lloyd's of London has refused to cover cell phone manufacturers against customer claims of health harms since 1999.[2]

Lloyd's of London itself kept a close eye on the advancements in EMF research, even issuing a white paper in 2010 that compared EMFs to asbestos, although it concluded that the links between EMFs and cancer weren't yet well established enough to warrant a change in strategy.[3]

Then, in 2015, it quietly updated its policies to include electromagnetic radiation in its list of general insurance exclusions, with the language:

We will not a) make any payment on your behalf for any claim, or b) incur any costs and expenses, or c) reimburse you for any loss, damage, legal expenses, fees or costs sustained by you, or d) pay any medical expenses [from any claims] . . . directly or indirectly arising out of, resulting from or contributed to by electromagnetic fields, electromagnetic radiation, electromagnetism, radio waves or noise.[4]

Because Lloyd's of London is such a prominent player in the insurance industry—and one that is considered to be fairly risk-tolerant—its adoption of this stance has made it a standard practice throughout the industry, to the point that the wireless companies themselves are now clear to warn investors about their inability to procure insurance.

As evidence, Crown Castle, which describes itself on its website as America's "largest provider of communications infrastructure," included this language on pages 12 and 13 of its 2016 annual report:

If radio frequency emissions from wireless handsets or equipment on our wireless infrastructure are demonstrated to cause negative health effects, potential future claims could adversely affect our operations, costs or revenues. . . . We currently do not maintain any significant insurance with respect to these matters.[5]

It's not difficult to envision a future in which telecommunications companies are forced to pay huge fines and watch their stock prices plummet as a result—something that has already happened to tobacco companies, as I detailed in Chapter 3.

Another way insurance companies may impact the unchecked proliferation of EMFs is from the costs they pay for health care. Because EMFs contribute to chronic health conditions and inflammation, it is likely that a good portion in the rise in health-care spending is related to the accumulating effects of EMF.

It is reasonable to assume that insurance costs will need to keep rising past the point that consumers and employers will want to pay, and something in the system will have to give. I'm hoping that something will, at long last, be limits on EMFs.

In the meantime, it's up to you to protect yourself and your family. It's up to all of us to become advocates and activists for better legislative policies regarding EMF-exposing products and infrastructures that permeate our world.

Now is the time to consider not just the health of yourself and your family, but the impact that it will have on future generations and to do everything you can to minimize these threats.

Exposure to EMFs should be treated like exposure to any of the well-known damaging effects to your health, such as eating nonorganic and processed food, inactivity, and poor sleeping habits. It is vital to avoid them whenever possible. I hope this book has provided you with the basic tools and resources to prevent harm from this growing problem and given you solid evidence to educate others.

Here are some general strategies to consider to help move us forward.

ADVOCATE FOR THE PRECAUTIONARY PRINCIPLE

The Precautionary Principle calls for wide-ranging policies developed by governments and other regulatory bodies to use discretion regarding environmental decisions that have a plausible possibility of leading to harm of people and/or nature, especially when scientific consensus is lacking and our understanding is incomplete.

There is more than sufficient peer-reviewed research documenting the clear biologic damage that results from EMF exposure to implement this policy, especially in light of progressively increasing exposures like 5G and satellite internet.

Specifically, the Precautionary Principle counsels that an estimation of the cost of immediate action needs to be compared to the potential cost of inaction. If the potential cost of inaction is plausible, significant, and irreversible, then immediate action should be taken to prevent the potential effects of inaction. In other words, it's better to be safe than sorry.

It was first endorsed as a principle in 1982 when the United Nations General Assembly adopted the World Charter for Nature. Since then, it has been baked into the Montreal Protocol, the Rio Declaration, the Kyoto Protocol, and the Paris Agreement. Leaders at every level need to be reminded that this is a global guideline that has been widely adopted yet is being neglected.

DISREGARD CURRENT SAFETY LEVELS

Remember, the current levels of wireless exposure that the FCC has deemed "safe" are based only on the short-term thermal effects they cause. Now you know that there are long-term, non-thermal reactions initiated by exposure to nonionizing radiation, and that you can't trust the safety guidelines to truly keep you safe.

There are no two ways about it: It is in our race's and our Earth's best interests to lower the levels of exposure that are currently deemed safe, and to do it by factors of 100 to 1,000.

PUSH BACK AGAINST THE ADOPTION OF "SMART" TECHNOLOGIES

Do you truly need these smart televisions, utility meters, plant waterers, and fitness trackers, simply because they are available? Consumer electronics companies can't exist without customers; use your voice and your dollars to send a message about how much radiation exposure and data mining you will and won't accept.

Ask your utility company for an old analog meter—and stay strong when your efforts are met with resistance. Show up to the parent-teacher organization at your local school and start to build awareness of the risks of Wi-Fi on kids.

BRING BACK THE CORDS

Much of our exposure can be reduced by returning to using corded phones at home, corded headsets instead of Bluetooth, and Ethernet cables to connect computers, printers, televisions, and other devices to the Internet.

PUSH YOUR COMMUNITY TO ADOPT A FIBER-OPTIC ALTERNATIVE TO 5G

There is no disagreement or controversy that we would benefit from faster Internet connections. The central issue is how these connections are delivered. We need to push our communities for more wired connections. Dr. Timothy Schoechle, an expert on communications technology and a senior research fellow of the National Institute for Science, Law, and Public Policy, wrote a 156-page report for that institution in 2018, which states:

> Wired infrastructure is *inherently more* future-proof, more reliable, more sustainable, more energy efficient, and more essential to many other services. Wireless networks and services are inherently more complex, more costly, more unstable, and more constrained.[6]

GET INVOLVED IN THE FIGHT

As Elizabeth "Libby" Kelley, M.A., a director of the International EMF Scientist Appeal Campaign to the U.N., has stated:

> Solutions must be found that place the highest priority on protecting people and the planet over the powerful economic

forces driving new technologies without thought for biology. We can have both innovation and public safety if there is political will.

The way to build political will is to get engaged. Many of the safeguards will have to come from the government, and for that to happen we need to have politicians in office who are aware of the risks of wireless technology and who know they have the support of their constituents to push for greater regulation of wireless companies.

Probably one of the most important strategies is to get involved in schools. Remember children are among the groups most susceptible to EMF exposures. We need to band together and convince schools to convert their wireless routers to Ethernet wired connections.

Working to create societal change is unglamorous, tedious, sometimes difficult work. But every time a person speaks out about the risks, it is like a drip of water that may not seem consequential in the moment but over time can cut through the stone of our current laws and norms.

It will certainly be a long road. It may at times feel like an unwinnable fight. But humans have stood up to dark forces in the past and have prevailed. We can, and will, do it again. This is your chance—our collective chance—to be on the right side of history. If we don't start speaking up and taking different actions, there may not be much more history left to write.

YOUR CLOSING TO-DO LISTS

I wrote this book to not only inform you why you are being lied to about EMFs and the very real threat they present to your biology, but also to inspire you to take action. It is not enough to realize there is danger. You must take action to protect yourself and those you love from this pernicious and pervasive exposure.

So let me highlight some of my strongest recommendations for you in these quick checklists.

Your To-Do List for Reducing Your EMF Exposure

☐ **Get a Meter** EMFs are an invisible threat. You can't typically see, hear, or feel them, yet they are able to cause enormous damage. A meter will present visible evidence to you and help you understand the sea of frequencies you are swimming in. There are a number of very good meters out there that I detail in the Resources section. I recommend you purchase an RF and a magnetic meter.

☐ **Remove W-Fi from Your Home** While turning off your Wi-Fi at night is a good first step, it is only putting your toe in the water. It is important to create an EMF sanctuary in your home where you can recover from the enormous exposures you will have when out in public, especially with the introduction of 5G. A Wi-Fi router is like having a cell phone tower in your home, and it is simply impossible to create an EMF sanctuary with your Wi-Fi on. This will involve installing Ethernet cables and getting Ethernet adapters for your computers.

☐ **Minimize EMFs in Your Bedroom** If you are committed to being healthy, you know that restorative sleep is an absolute essential. It is vital for you to remediate your bedroom as described in Chapter 7, applying the specific strategies discussed to make your bedroom a sanctuary where you can heal and repair.

☐ **Bring Back the Cords** Much of your EMF exposure can be reduced by returning to using corded phones at home, corded headsets instead of Bluetooth, and Ethernet cables to connect computers, printers, televisions, and other devices to the Internet.

☐ **Take Control of Your Cell Phone** This is one of the most important steps you can take. I encourage you to reread the section that begins on page 186. Keep your cell phone in airplane mode whenever possible and while carrying it on your body. Ideally you will want to conduct as many of your calls as possible through an Internet connection or traditional landline, not wirelessly on your cell phone.

☐ **Help Your Body Repair the Damage from Exposure to EMFs** Thankfully your body has the capacity to repair this damage. Remember to take your magnesium. Nearly everyone is deficient in this important mineral, and one of its functions is to help block some of the calcium channels that EMFs stimulate.

Keeping your NAD+ levels optimized is key to your DNA repair, and the older you are the more important this is as NAD+ levels drop very dramatically as you age. I have provided some background and basic recommendations, but there is an enormous amount of research going on and it is challenging to make solid recommendations at this time.

I plan on offering some breakthrough strategies for NAD+ replacement that are relatively inexpensive and effective. It is best to subscribe to my newsletter at mercola.com so you can be informed when they are available.

Until then, the best ways to optimize your NAD+ levels and remediate the physiological damage triggered by EMFs are:

☐ Practice daily time restricted eating where you only eat food in a 6- to 8-hour window or even less.

☐ Engage in some type of daily exercise and seriously consider blood flow restriction training.

☐ Supplement with molecular hydrogen.

☐ Make sure you are getting about 25 mg of niacin a day and have regular magnesium supplementation to reach at least your RDA of 400 mg of elemental magnesium.

DON'T TAKE AS LONG AS I DID TO MAKE CHANGES

Health has been my passion and full-time profession for more than four decades, and tech is another one of my primary passions. I was an early and enthusiastic adopter of the Internet. I took my first programming class in high school. It was 1968 and I learned Fortran and Cobol.

I was online in the 1970s, well before the introduction of the World Wide Web in the mid-'90s. A few years after the Web was launched and before there was Google, I started my website, mercola.com, which has been the most visited natural-health site since 2003.

It was easy for me to be complacent about EMFs when public health authorities and the media made a strong case that the research proved that there is minimal to no danger from prudent exposure to EMFs.

Even though I regularly wrote about the seriousness of EMFs in my daily online newsletter, and have interviewed many experts on the topic on my website, I believed that EMFs posed little to no threat to me personally. I believed that living a healthy lifestyle and following a healthy diet, exercise, and supplement program would be more than enough to safeguard anyone from EMF-related danger.

Boy, did I have that one confused. After a serious, objective, and detailed analysis I realized that it is virtually impossible to achieve high levels of health in the 21st century unless you are addressing your EMF exposure and giving your body what it needs to remediate the damage this exposure causes.

Now I rarely use my cell phone unless I am traveling and then mostly for getting a ride to where I am going. My home has no Wi-Fi as all my Internet connections are through an Ethernet cable.

I shielded my bedroom from RF with EMF shielding paint and I now turn off the electricity in the room at night to keep electric fields low. I have also installed filters for dirty electricity throughout my house and at the main circuit breakers, and I have installed capacitors in all my solar panel inverters.

In other words, I now take EMFs seriously. I wrote this book to help you do the same. Now you have the basic tools and resources to prevent further harm, as well as solid evidence that you can use to educate others.

As you have learned from reading this book, the research that shows the impact of EMFs on your biology is being suppressed. It is my sincere wish that what you have learned has led you to the conclusion that you must take steps to protect yourself, your family, and the planet from these harmful frequencies. I hope that your eyes are now open and you are inspired to take action.

RESOURCES

EMF METERS

The EMF-measuring meters I recommend include:

- **The Acousticom 2.** This RF-only meter is about the size of a deck of cards and very portable as it easily fits into your pocket. I bring it with me when I travel. This meter does not give you a digital display of the actual measurement; it merely blinks LED lights at different levels. But I have found this more than adequate to guide my RF debugging strategies.

    The Acousticom 2 is easy to use and has great sensitivity. It measures RF sources between 200 MHz and 8 GHz and emits an audio sound for each wireless source that gets louder as you get closer to the signal. This feature makes the Acousticom 2 very intuitive to understand your RF exposure levels and to locate sources.

    The Acousticom 2 displays a graduated progression of lights that indicate the intensity of the RF level in Volts/meter present for the peak value, which is the measurement I recommend you focus on (not the average value).
    Cost: Under $200.

- **Safe and Sound Pro.** This RF-only meter is comparable to the Acousticom 2, although it has a larger frequency range, from 200 MHz to 12 GHz, and somewhat more sensitivity than the Acousticom 2 at measuring Wi-Fi and cordless telephones in the 5.8 GHz range (Wi-Fi transmits at both 2.4 and 5.8 GHz). The Safe and Sound Pro can also measure the quick RF micro pulses from smart electric meters.

  The Safe and Sound Pro measures peak RF readings in microWatts/meter squared (uW/m²) at power densities up to 2 million uW/m². The speaker emits a sound in the presence of wireless EMFs, with a volume control and headphone jack.
  Cost: Under $400.

- **Safe and Sound Classic.** This RF-only meter is comparable to the Acousticom 2, although it also has more sensitivity when measuring 5.8 GHz signals. The Classic model has the same RF sensitivity, range and sound capability as its more expensive cousin, the Safe, and Sound Pro.

  The primary difference is that the Classic has a row of LEDs without a numeric display to keep the cost down. Use the handy guide to see how many uW/m2 each LED setting compares to.
  Cost: Under $200.

- **The Cornet ED88T Plus** also measures RF, but because it is a combination EMF meter, it also measures electric fields and magnetic fields. Please understand that its user manual is particularly bad, but thankfully there are great YouTube video manuals to show you how to properly use it.

  The single most important feature is its tri-mode functionality. This means it can measure RFs, electric fields, and magnetic fields. It offers good RF mode functionality with a slightly broader frequency range than the Acousticom 2; it measures down to 100 MHz as opposed to 200 MHz for the Acousticom 2.

One difference between the two meters is that the lowest the Cornet will measure is .0147 volts/meter or .005 microwatts/meter. These are very low, safe readings but you will not be able to measure below them with this meter. The Acousticom 2's lower limit is .01 volts/meter.

Beware, this meter gives a lot of information. For example, it also has a frequency display function (100 MHz to 2.7 GHz), meaning it tells you what the frequency is of the strongest RF source that it is measuring at a particular location. If you want easy "point and play" this meter is not for you, but if you're willing to play around with it, you won't be disappointed. Also includes a USB socket for data logging.

Like the Acousticom 2, the Cornet has an audio function that can help you not only identify the strength of the RF signal but also tell you the device that is transmitting that signal.

Use a headset to best hear the sound. (To access an audio clip that lets you hear the varying sounds that the different microwave sources generate, visit http://www.slt.co/Education/EMFSounds.aspx.)
Cost: Under $200

- **The Electrosmog Indicator ESI-24.** This meter has a triple-axis gauss meter, which means it measures in all three planes and the RF has a sound setting that's a bit louder and more sensitive than the Acousticom 2.

    The default setting measures Magnetic, Electric, and RF simultaneously so you can start to understand the difference between the different frequencies right away. There is a higher sensitivity RF setting as well.

This meter does not give you a digital display of the actual measurement. It merely blinks LED lights at different levels, but this is more than adequate to guide EMF debugging strategies.

Convert the magnetic field reading, given in nanotesla (nT), into milligauss by dividing the number of nT by 100 (there are 100 nanoteslas in one milligauss). Then compare that reading with building biology safe levels.

Cost: $300

- **Trifield TF2 Meter.** The older Trifield meters were popular because they did a good job of measuring magnetic fields, but weren't nearly as good on the RF and the electric field measurements. All that's changed with the new Trifield TF2 meter.

  Only use the magnetic field nonweighted setting on this meter. Ideal numbers for magnetic fields in homes are below 0.5 milligauss (50 nanotesla) in daytime areas and below 0.3 milligauss (30 nanotesla) in sleeping areas.

  Although the new Trifield TF2 has RF measurement capability comparable with the Cornet and Acousticom2, many EMF professionals have found the new Trifield 2 to be inferior when RF and electric fields measure.

  This is likely a result of the fact that for electric field setting to be accurate one needs to use the meter only when the body is grounded. All the best meters that measure electric fields are grounded themselves to get a real indication of what the true electric field reading is.

  Pay attention to the peak value in the upper left corner on the TF2 when measuring RF. This number holds the highest RF reading measured by the meter in the previous three seconds. Hold the bottom of the meter when measuring RF to avoid covering the RF antenna inside with your hand.

The Trifield TF2 has similar sensitivity to the Cornet in magnetic field mode but the TF2 trumps the Cornet because it measures magnetic fields in 3-axis (you need to rotate the Cornet to get the best reading).

This means you get the same magnetic field reading at a given location with the TF2, no matter what orientation you hold it in. With a single-axis Gauss meter, on the other hand, like the Cornet ED88T, you have to hold it in all three positions (X, Y, and Z axes) wherever you are measuring to find the highest value. Otherwise, you may miss the true magnetic field reading. (Once you get the hang of using a single-axis Gauss meter, it is just as useful as a three-axis Gauss meter.)

Cost: Under $200

- **ENV RD-10.** The ENV RD-10 offers tri-mode functionality as it can measure three distinct types of EMFs—so it's like having three meters in one. It offers good sensitivity for the price, and compares very well with other more expensive meters (Acousticom2, Cornet ED88TPlus, and Trifield TF2).

  The ENV RD-10 offers Windows and Android connectivity for data logging. That means by connecting to a cell phone (on airplane mode) or computer you can get actual readings as opposed to relying on interpreting the LEDs. It has a compact and handy size; it's so small you can almost fit it in your wallet. It is much smaller than any similar meters on the market.

  The downside is that the EMF mode selector switch is a bit awkward to use, particular care is required to get on the magnetic field setting and not confuse it with the other settings. It does not have a digital display to give you an actual reading. Also, it is a single-axis magnetic field meter.

Its size might make you think that it's not a meter you can take seriously. But you can use it as a detector, or by using the USB cable to connect to your cell phone or computer, you can get precise readings, which effectively makes it into an EMF meter.

Cost: Under $200.

- **AlphaLabs UHS2 3-Axis Gaussmeter.** If you want to measure magnetic field EMFs with a very accurate, three-axis Gaussmeter, this is the one to buy. It measures magnetic fields from 13 Hz to 75,000 Hz (75 kHz), which include many dirty electricity frequencies. (Remember, dirty electricity is defined as the electric and magnetic field components of any harmonic frequency above 60 Hz, which is the frequency of AC electricity in North America.)

  Cost: Just over $300

- **Dirty Electricity Meters.** There's a tendency for many to overlook measuring dirty electricity. One of the reasons might be because you do need a separate meter to measure this form of EMF. But dirty electricity shouldn't be overlooked. It's certainly not any less harmful than any of the other types of EMF exposures, and for some, it can be the principle source of illness.

  Fortunately, it's easy to measure. Dr. Martin Graham and Dave Stetzer, who did some of the earliest research on dirty electricity, devised the Stetzerizer® Microsurge Meter, which you just plug into your wall outlet and it gives you a number in Graham-Stetzer, or GS, units.

  According to the manufacturers, the reading should ideally be below 50 GS units. If it's not, you should seek to eliminate devices that are causing this high reading and/or install filters to reduce your exposure. Greenwave also makes a popular alternative to the Stetzerizer meters. Some people prefer the Greenwave to Stetzerizer and vice versa. This really seems to be a personal thing.

Cost: Stetzer and Greenwave Microsurge Meters each retail for around $100.

A note about measuring the RF of MMW (millimeter wave) 5G signals: The band used by true 5G devices, above 20 GHz, will not be measured with any RF meter on this list. Such meters do not yet exist. There are spectrum analyzers that can measure above 20 GHz. They are very expensive and focus on average rather than peak readings, and are not considered sensitive enough by engineers who know about the health effects of 5G for our purposes.

Several companies and engineers are hard at work perfecting an affordable RF detector for frequencies above 20 GHz. I expect that those meters will be on the market shortly after this book is published in 2020.

Remember that some small cell antennas will have 4G transmitters and some will have 5G transmitters, so all of the RF meters mentioned on this list will adequately detect any 4G LTE RF signal from a small cell antenna with a 4G transmitter if you are unfortunate enough to have one go up in your neighborhood. New 5G signals from any updated 4G LTE small cell transmitter below 6 GHz will also be picked up by all RF meters on this list, as most of these meters go up to 8 GHz and even higher.

Two last tips:

- Each EMF meter is different. For instance, most of the meters mentioned above are single-axis meters, so you would need to orient them in different directions to get the highest reading—read the manufacturer's instructions on how to use them.

- Be methodical when using an EMF meter. Have a note-pad on hand where you note your readings in precise locations so you can keep track of them and refer back to them when you take subsequent readings later that day and in a few weeks or months.

RF and Magnetic Field Conversion Chart

As you can see from the list of recommended meters in this section, there are a wide variety of instruments, and each provides measurements in one specific unit. Use the charts on pages 246 and 247 to convert the measurement used by any meter to the units you are interested in.

OTHER PRODUCT RECOMMENDATIONS

Dirty electricity filters

Stetzer and Greenwave each make dirty electricity filters. Sometimes people report feeling unwell after they've installed filters. In order to avoid this possibility for yourself, check your electrical wiring for so-called wiring errors (as I discussed in Chapter 7) before you install these filters.

If you have wiring errors, this could cause your filters to create abnormally high magnetic fields in your house or apartment while they drop the dirty electricity levels. Fortunately, wiring errors can be repaired. Then use your filters without worrying about increasing magnetic fields. (Just don't put them right next to a bed or chair, as filters have a one- to two-foot magnetic field of their own.)

These filters do change the quality of your electricity, so after installing them you should give yourself a couple of weeks to "break them in" before you come to a conclusion about how effective they are.

Cost: $25-35 each; they are typically less expensive if purchased in volume.

Whole-house dirty electricity filters

There are also whole-house dirty electricity-reduction technologies. The one I recommend is the Super Power Perfect Box.

They need to be installed by an electrician at your circuit breaker. You still may need some of the Stetzer or Greenwave filters, but far fewer than you would otherwise require.

Cost: $1495, at shieldedhealing.com

Shielded power cables and power strips

You can use shielded power cables to power your electronic devices, and shielded power strips to plug those devices into the wall.

Cost: From $7-$15 for extension and device cords and $75-$85 for power strips; all available from Electrahealth.com

Grounded power cords for laptops

To insure that your laptop is grounded, get a grounded power cord that plugs into a USB port.

Cost: $8.95 at LessEMF.com.

Shielded wiring

Use MµCord™ to re-wire your lamps, particularly in the bedroom. (I suggest having a licensed electrician do this for you.)

Cost: $1.75 a foot, available from LessEMF.com.

Ethernet grounding adapter kit

In order for your Ethernet cable to be grounded (and thus, not producing dirty electricity), you'll need an Ethernet grounding adapter kit.

Cost: $29.97 from Electrahealth.com

Grounded Ethernet-to-USB adapters

If you need an adapter to plug an Ethernet cable into your computer, that needs to be grounded as well. Thunderbolt-to-Ethernet adapters from Apple are grounded. For the newest MacBooks, you'll need a USB-C-to-Ethernet adapter that is also grounded (the AmazonBasics USB 3.1 Type-C to 3 Port USB Hub is one such model).
Cost: About $20

Corded router with no Wi-Fi, or a feature that allows you to turn Wi-Fi off

The Trendnet 4-Port Broadband Router has no Wi-Fi at all. The Netgear N750 (Model WND4300), N900 (Model WNDR4500), or AC1200 (Model R6230) are routers with switchable Wi-Fi.

Corded modem

The Arris Surfboard is a cable company-approved modem that you can use with a wired router, or a router where you can switch the Wi-Fi off.
Cost: Ranges from $49.99 to $159.99, depending on model

RF-shielding wire mesh box (for covering a router)

Signal Tamer and the Wave Cage, both available from LessEMF; and Router Guard, available from Smart Meter Guard.
Cost: $34.95 (for Signal Tamer), $12.95 - $24.95 (for Wave Cage), $62.95 or $82.50, depending on size (for Router Guard)

Flicker-free monitors

Flicker-free monitors from Asus have Eye Care Technology.
Cost: About $125, depending on size and retailer

Smart electric, gas, and water meter covers

Wire mesh covers intended to shield the RFs emitted by smart utility meters can be found at smartmetercovers.com and smartmeterguard.com. Smartmeterguard.com also sells RF-shielding cloth covers for smart gas and water meters.
Cost: $59.95 to $159.95, depending on size needed

Manual plug-in switches

You can also use manual plug-in switches, called a cube tap with switch, available from online retailers or a local hardware store.
Cost: $5–$10

EMF protective clothing

My favorite source for clothing that protects your body from EMFs—everything from hats to T-shirts to gloves to full-on burquas—is LessEMF.com.
Cost: Varies depending on item

Shielding paint

The best shielding paint I have found to date is YShield, which can be purchased at LessEMF.com.
Cost: $29.95 for a four-ounce can

Dirty electricity filters for solar panel inverters

Among the photovoltaic inverters that are on the market for solar panel systems, SMA Sunny Boy is designed to keep dirty electricity to a minimum. But even these filters will create dirty electricity.

The capacitor/filter can be purchased from Sager Electronics. The part number for a 5KW inverter (the most common size) is

50FC10. Unfortunately, this is a business to business to company and very consumer unfriendly.

It is a painful process to work with Sager and get the filters so you can have an electrician install them in your inverter(s), but it is the only option I know of. If your inverters are different than 5KW, you will need to talk to their technical staff and give them the part number for the 5KW part and they can recommend the part number you need.

Cost: Less than $150 for Sager capacitor/filter

Baby monitors

Instead of a typical wireless video baby monitor, use a camera and microphone that can be hardwired, such as the D-Link HD Wi-Fi Camera with Remote Viewing, available from online retailers. The Wi-Fi on that camera shuts off when you plug in an Ethernet cable. Verify that with your RF meter.

If you are searching for a new wireless baby monitor with low RF levels, seek out the SmartNOVA Baby Monitor, which emits 97 percent less radiation than standard baby monitors (a newly designed model is under development).

Several other low-RF options are listed on The Gentle Nursery website, at https://www.gentlenursery.com/natural-baby-registry-guide/low-emission-baby-monitors/. In Europe, the Nuk-Babyphone is a good option.

Radiant heating floor units

Manufacturers of safer heaters include Schluter Ditra-Heat E-HK, Warmzone ComfortTile, and ThermoTile by Thermosoft. These products have very low magnetic and electric fields because of how they are designed.

Dimmer switches

Lutron and other high-end manufacturers make cleaner dimmer switches than other manufacturers, and central lighting control systems by Lutron, Crestron, and Control4 tend to have clean, expensive dimming modules.

This is done to keep electronic noise out of home theater speaker systems, but they also help keep dirty electricity off electric circuits and plastic AC power cords that you leave plugged in around the house.

Infrared saunas

The lowest and best saunas are near infrared and the best of these are from SaunaSpace (saunaspace.com), which makes a completely EMF-free sauna that is grounded and shielded and uses special full spectrum near infrared bulbs.

EDUCATIONAL RESOURCES

For pregnant women or women who plan to become pregnant

Visit the website babysafeproject.org for specific guidelines on protecting your baby from EMFs.

5g support groups

- Ban All 5G Technology: https://petitions.moveon.org/sign/ban-all-5g-technology

- International Appeal to Stop 5G on Earth and in Space: https://www.5gspaceappeal.org/

- Stop Hazardous 5G Small Cell Units from Being Installed: http://stop5g.whynotnews.eu/?page_id=580

- Take Action by Writing, Emailing, or Calling: http://www.parentsforsafetechnology.org/stop-5g-spectrum-frontiers.html

- How to File an ADA Accommodations Request for Electrosensitivity to Avoid Small Cells and Wi-Fi:

  - http://www.electrosmogprevention.org/ada-accommodations-for-rf-exposures/ada-for-es-to-avoid-small-cells-and-wifi/

  - http://keepyourpower.org/

  - https://www.5gcrisis.com/ (To find a 5G group near you)

- Urging City Council to Halt 5G in Charlotte: https://www.change.org/p/charlotte-area-residents-urging-city-council-to-halt-5g-in-charlotte

- Ireland:

  - Galway Public Awareness Meeting on Wireless Technologies and 5G: https://www.facebook.com/events/2190209274396632/

  - Dublin Meeting to Stop 5G: https://www.facebook.com/events/673336026446726/

- England:

  - 5G Awareness Topsham Event: https://www.facebook.com/events/444897969609210/

  - Stop 5G!: https://www.facebook.com/events/601831420318009/

  - 5G World 2019 Protest: https://www.facebook.com/events/341771203144683/

  - Stop 5G Demonstration: https://docs.google.com/document/d/1wLFv3wlWDtc9kW81dOAa7j9ejqCQVfO0H2xtXv5zNvA

/edit?fbclid=IwAR28cEvFLeJngAcdyqmJCbkt2gdUA
Jgh2YYeagjBBWHc1K5TPJ5UtuBHjcA

- Stop the Trial of 5G on the Isles of Scilly and Corn-wall: https://you.38degrees.org.uk/petitions/stop-the-trial-of-5g-on-the-isles-of-scilly-and-cornwall

- Australia:

  - 5G Rollout in Australia: https://www.communi tyrun.org/petitions/5g-roll-out-in-australia

  - 5G Tower Locations around Australia:

  - https://tottnews.com/2019/05/16/5g-tower-loca tions-australia/?fbclid=IwAR2G3fiL1oVthsltKMVc c1vM8kGU7e_rLpJu4TxM5yXV6xjByUmhmmOata8

  - No 5G in the Blue Mountains:

  - https://www.no5gbluemountains.org/what-you-can-do.html

- New Zealand

  - Petition of Terri Takau: Stop 5G: https://www.par liament.nz/en/pb/petitions/document/PET_87686/ petition-of-terri-takau-stop-5g

MAGNETIC FIELD CONVERSION CHART

Gauss	milliGauss	microGauss	Tesla	milliTesla	microTesla	nanoTesla
0.000,000,01 G	0.000,01 mG	0.01 µG	0.000,000,000,001 T	0.000,000,001 mT	0.000,001 µT	0.001 nT
0.000,000,1 G	0.0001 mG	0.1 µG	0.000,000,000,01 T	0.000,000,01 mT	0.000,01 µT	0.01 nT
0.000,001 G	0.001 mG	1 µG	0.000,000,000,1 T	0.000,000,1 mT	0.0001 µT	0.1 nT
0.000,01 G	0.01 mG	10 µG	0.000,000,001 T	0.000,001 mT	0.001 µT	1 nT
0.0001 G	0.1 mG	100 µG	0.000,000,01 T	0.000,01 mT	0.01 µT	10 nT
0.001 G	1 mG	1,000 µG	0.000,000,1 T	0.0001 mT	0.1 µT	100 nT
0.01 G	10 mG	10,000 µG	0.000,001 T	0.001 mT	1 µT	1,000 nT
0.1 G	100 mG	100,000 µG	0.000,01 T	0.01 mT	10 µT	10,000 nT
1 G	1,000 mG	1,000,000 µG	0.0001 T	0.1 mT	100 µT	100,000 nT
10 G	10,000 mG	10,000,000 µG	0.001 T	1 mT	1,000 µT	1,000,000 nT
100 G	100,000 mG	100,000,00 µG	0.01 T	10 mT	10,000 µT	10,000,000 nT

Radio Frequency "RF" Power Density to Volts Per Meter Unit Conversion Chart

milliVolts Per Meter	Volts Per Meter	Watts/Sq Meter	milliWatts/sq Meter	microWatts/sq Meter	Watts/Sq Centimeter	milliWatts/Sq Centimeter	microWatts/Sq Centimeter
0.001,94 mV/m	0.000,001,94 V/m	0.000,000,000,000,01 W/m²	0.000,000,000,01 mW/m²	0.000,000,01 µW/m²	0.000,000,000,000,000,001 W/cm²	0.000,000,000,000,001 mW/cm²	0.000,000,000,001 µW/cm²
0.006,14 mV/m	0.000,006,14 V/m	0.000,000,000,000,1 W/m²	0.000,000,000,1 mW/m²	0.000,000,1 µW/m²	0.000,000,000,000,000,01 W/cm²	0.000,000,000,000,01 mW/cm²	0.000,000,000,01 µW/cm²
0.019,4 mV/m	0.000,019,4 V/m	0.000,000,000,001 W/m²	0.000,000,001 mW/m²	0.000,001 µW/m²	0.000,000,000,000,000,1 W/cm²	0.000,000,000,000,1 mW/cm²	0.000,000,000,1 µW/cm²
0.0614 mV/m	0.000,061,4 V/m	0.000,000,000,01 W/m²	0.000,000,01 mW/m²	0.000,01 µW/m²	0.000,000,000,000,001 W/cm²	0.000,000,000,01 mW/cm²	0.000,000,001 µW/cm²
0.194 mV/m	0.000,194 V/m	0.000,000,000,1 W/m²	0.000,000,1 mW/m²	0.000,1 µW/m²	0.000,000,000,000,01 W/cm²	0.000,000,000,1 mW/cm²	0.000,000,01 µW/cm²
0.614 mV/m	0.000,614 V/m	0.000,000,001 W/m²	0.000,001 mW/m²	0.001 µW/m²	0.000,000,000,000,1 W/cm²	0.000,000,000,1 mW/cm²	0.000,000,1 µW/cm²
1.94 mV/m	0.001,94 V/m	0.000,000,01 W/m²	0.000,01 mW/m²	0.01 µW/m²	0.000,000,000,001 W/cm²	0.000,000,01 mW/cm²	0.000,001 µW/cm²
6.14 mV/m	0.006,14 V/m	0.000,000,1 W/m²	0.000,1 mW/m²	0.1 µW/m²	0.000,000,000,01 W/cm²	0.000,000,1 mW/cm²	0.000,01 µW/cm²
19.4 mV/m	0.019,4 V/m	0.000,001 W/m²	0.001 mW/m²	1 µW/m²	0.000,000,000,1 W/cm²	0.000,001 mW/cm²	0.000,1 µW/cm²
61.4 mV/m	0.061,4 V/m	0.000,01 W/m²	0.01 mW/m²	10 µW/m²	0.000,000,001 W/cm²	0.000,01 mW/cm²	0.001 µW/cm²
194 mV/m	0.194 V/m	0.000,1 W/m²	0.1 mW/m²	100 µW/m²	0.000,000,01 W/cm²	0.000,1 mW/cm²	0.01 µW/cm²
614 mV/m	0.614 V/m	0.001 W/m²	1 mW/m²	1,000 µW/m²	0.000,000,1 W/cm²	0.001 mW/cm²	0.1 µW/cm²
1,942 mV/m	1.94 V/m	0.01 W/m²	10 mW/m²	10,000 µW/m²	0.000,001 W/cm²	0.01 mW/cm²	1 µW/cm²
6,140 mV/m	6.14 V/m	0.1 W/m²	100 mW/m²	100,000 µW/m²	0.000,01 W/cm²	0.1 mW/cm²	10 µW/cm²
19,415 mV/m	19.4 V/m	1 W/m²	1,000 mW/m²	1,000,000 µW/m²	0.000,1 W/cm²	1 mW/cm²	100 µW/cm²
61,400 mV/m	61.4 V/m	10 W/m²	10,000 mW/m²	10,000,000 µW/m²	0.001 W/cm²	10 mW/cm²	1,000 µW/cm²
194,164 mV/m	194 V/m	100 W/m²	100,000 mW/m²	100,000,000 µW/m²	0.01 W/cm²	100 mW/cm²	10,000 µW/cm²
614,003 mV/m	614 V/m	1,000 W/m²	1,000,000 mW/m²	1,000,000,000 µW/m²	0.1 W/cm²	1,000 mW/cm²	100,000 µW/cm²
1,941,648 mV/m	1942 V/m	10,000 W/m²	10,000,000 mW/m²	10,000,000,000 µW/m²	1 W/cm²	10,000 mW/cm²	1,000,000 µW/cm²
6,140,032 mV/m	6140 V/m	100,000 W/m²	100,000,000 mW/m²	100,000,000,000 µW/m²	10 W/cm²	10,000 mW/cm²	10,000,000 µW/cm²

Formulas: V/m = √ (W/m² x 377) Volts per meter = the square root of the product of Watts per square meter times 337
Note: V/m and mV/m are rounded

APPENDIX A

Damaging Effects of Excessive Peroxynitrite

- Damages DNA, and when PARP repairs the damage it reduces cellular NAD+ stores. Once the level of cellular damage inflicted by peroxynitrite supersedes any possibility of repair, the cell eventually dies via one of the two main pathways of cell demise, necrosis or apoptosis.[1]

- Depletes antioxidant reserves, especially glutathione.[2]

- Creates a self-reinforcing vicious cycle of chronic inflammation.[3]

- Triggers lipid peroxidation in membranes, liposomes, and lipoproteins by abstracting a hydrogen atom from polyunsaturated fatty acids, generating lipid radicals that propagate free radical reactions, thereby degrading membrane lipids and increasing risk of cardiovascular diseases.[4]

- Represents the major species responsible for DNA mutations linking NO overproduction with cancer.[5]

- Exacerbates oxidative damage to mitochondrial proteins.[6]

- Alters protein structure and function.[7]

- Inhibits most components of the mitochondrial electron transport chain, thus decreasing ATP.[8]

- Inhibits superoxide dismutase, thereby preventing the breakdown of locally produced superoxide, which further fuels the formation of peroxynitrite.[9]

- Initiates peroxidation of myelin lipids leading to demyelination and plays a critical role in inflammatory diseases of the nervous system.[10]

- Causes endothelial dysfunction by inactivating prostacyclin synthase (PGI2 synthase) and limiting endothelial NO production by inactivating eNOS through oxidation of its zinc thiolate center.[11]

- Causes tyrosine nitration in proteins, which is consistently observed in cardiovascular diseases and neurodegeneration.[12]

- PARP-dependent reduction of cellular NAD may also suppress NO formation by depleting endothelial stores of NADPH, an essential cofactor of NOS.[13]

- As one ages, it activates NFκB, a redox-sensitive transcription factor involved in the induction of the transcription of a large range of genes implicated in inflammation, including cytokines (e.g., TNF-α, IL-6, and IL-1β).[14]

- Oxidizes and depletes tetrahydrobiopterin (BH4), which is known to produce a partial uncoupling of the NO synthases (eNOS, nNOS and iNOS). When these NOSs are uncoupled, they produce superoxide in place of NO.[15]

- Causes cardiolipin, the inner membrane of the mitochondrion, peroxidation, which leads to lowered activity of some of the enzymes in the electron transport chain and impaired ATP synthesis.[16]

- Inactivates Mn-SOD and makes mitochondria more vulnerable in neurodegeneration.[17]

APPENDIX B

Studies That Demonstrate
Harmful Effects of EMFs

Cellular DNA damage: single strand and double strand breaks in cellular DNA and oxidized bases in cellular DNA, leading to chromosomal and other mutational changes:

1. Glaser ZR, PhD. "Naval Medical Research Institute Research Report." Bibliography of Reported Biological Phenomena ("Effects") and Clinical Manifestations Attributed to Microwave and Radio-Frequency Radiation. Report No. 2, revised. (June 1971). https://apps.dtic.mil/dtic/tr/fulltext/u2/750271.pdf. Accessed September 9, 2017.

2. Goldsmith JR. "Epidemiologic Evidence Relevant to Radar (Microwave) Effects." *Environmental Health Perspectives*. Vol. 105, supplement 6. (December 1997): 1579-1587. doi: 10.1289/ehp.97105s61579.

3. Yakymenko IL, Sidorik EP, Tsybulin AS. "Metabolic Changes in Cells Under Electromagnetic Radiation of Mobile Communication Systems." [Article in Russian] *Ukrainskii Biokhimicheskii Zhurnal* (1999). Vol. 83, no. 2. (March-April 2011): 20-28.

4. Aitken RJ, De Iuliis GN. "Origins and Consequences of DNA Damage in Male Germ Cells." *Reproductive BioMedicine Online*. Vol. 14, no. 6. (June 2007): 727-733. doi: 10.1016/S1472-6483(10)60676-1.

5. Hardell L, Sage C. "Biological Effects from Electromagnetic Field Exposure and Public Exposure Standards." *Biomedicine & Pharmacotherapy*. Vol. 62, no. 2. (February 2008): 104-109. doi: 10.1016/j.biopha.2007.12.004.

6. Hazout A, Menezo Y, Madelenat P, Yazbeck C, Selva J, Cohen-Bacrie P. "Causes and Clinical Implications of Sperm DNA Damages." [Article in French] *Gynécologie Obstétrique & Fertilité*. Vol. 36, no. 11. (November 2008): 1109- 1117. doi: 10.1016/j.gyobfe.2008.07.017.

7. Phillips JL, Singh NP, Lai H. "Electromagnetic Fields and DNA Damage." *Pathophysiology.* Vol. 16, no. 2-3. (August 2009): 79-88. doi: 10.1016/j.pathophys.2008.11.005.

8. Ruediger HW. "Genotoxic Effects of Radiofrequency Electromagnetic Fields." *Pathophysiology.* Vol. 16, no. 2-3. (August 2009): 89-102. doi: 10.1016/j.pathophys.2008.11.004.

9. Makker K, Varghese A, Desai NR, Mouradi R, Agarwal A. "Cell Phones: Modern Man's Nemesis?" *Reproductive BioMedicine Online.* Vol. 18, no 1. (January 2009): 148-157. doi: 10.1016/S1472-6483(10)60437-3.

10. Yakymenko I, Sidorik E. "Risks of Carcinogenesis from Electromagnetic Radiation and Mobile Telephony Devices." *Experimental Oncology.* Vol. 32, no. 2. (June 2010): 54-60.

11. Yakymenko IL, Sidorik EP, Tsybulin AS. "Metabolic Changes in Cells Under Electromagnetic Radiation of Mobile Communication Systems." [Article in Russian] *Ukrainskii Biokhimicheskii Zhurnal* (1999). Vol. 83, no. 2. (March-April 2011): 20-28.

12. Gye MC, Park CJ. "Effect of Electromagnetic Field Exposure on the Reproductive System." *Clinical and Experimental Reproductive Medicine.* Vol. 39, no. 1. (March 2012): 1-9. doi: 10.5653/cerm.2012.39.1.1.

13. Pall ML. "Electromagnetic Fields Act via Activation of Voltage-Gated Calcium Channels to Produce Beneficial or Adverse Effects." *Journal of Cellular and Molecular Medicine.* Vol. 17, no. 8. (August 2013): 958-965. doi: 10.1111/jcmm.12088.

14. Pall ML. "Scientific Evidence Contradicts Findings and Assumptions of Canadian Safety Panel 6: Microwaves Act Through Voltage-Gated Calcium Channel Activation to Induce Biological Impacts at Non-Thermal Levels, Supporting a Paradigm Shift for Microwave/Lower Frequency Electromagnetic Field Action." *Reviews on Environmental Health.* Vol. 30, no. 2. (May 2015): 99-116. doi: 10.1515/reveh-2015-0001.

15. Hensinger P, Wilke E. "Mobilfunk-Studienergebnisse bestätigen Risiken Studienrecherche 2016-4 veröffentlicht." *Umwelt Medizin Gesellschaft.* Vol. 29, no. 3. (2016).

16. Houston BJ, Nixon B, King BV, De Iuliis GN, Aitken RJ. "The Effects of Radiofrequency Electromagnetic Radiation on Sperm Function." *Reproduction.* Vol. 152, no. 6. (December 2016): R263-R276. doi: 10.1530/REP-16-0126.

17. Batista Napotnik T, Reberšek M, Vernier PT, Mali B, Miklavčič D. "Effects of High Voltage Nanosecond Electric Pulses on Eukaryotic Cells (In Vitro): A Systematic Review." *Bioelectrochemistry.* Vol. 110. (August 2016): 1-12. doi: 10.1016/j.bioelechem.2016.02.011.

18. Asghari A, Khaki AA, Rajabzadeh A, Khaki A. "A Review on Electromagnetic Fields (EMFs) and the Reproductive System." *Electronic Physician.* Vol. 8, no. 7. (July 2016): 2655-2662. doi: 10.19082/2655.

19. Pall ML. "Chapter 7: How Cancer Can Be Caused by Microwave Frequency Electromagnetic Field (EMF) Exposures: EMF Activation of Voltage-Gated Calcium Channels (VGCCs) Can Cause Cancer Including Tumor Promotion, Tissue Invasion and Metastasis via 15 Mechanisms." In Markov M (Ed). *Mobile Communications and Public Health* (pp 163-184). New York, CRC Press, 2018.

20. Pall ML. "Wi-Fi Is an Important Threat to Human Health." *Environmental Research.* Vol. 164. (July 2018): 405-416. doi: 10.1016/j.envres.2018.01.035.

21. Wilke I. "Biological and Pathological Effects of 2.45 GHz Radiation on Cells, Fertility, Brain and Behavior." *Umwelt Medizin Gesellschaft.* Vol. 31, supplement 1. (2018): 1-32.

Lowered fertility, including tissue remodeling changes in the testis, lowered sperm count and sperm quality, lowered female fertility including ovarian remodeling, oocyte (follicle) loss, lowered estrogen, progesterone, and testosterone levels (that is sex hormone levels), increased spontaneous abortion incidence, lowered libido:

1. Glaser ZR, PhD. "Naval Medical Research Institute Research Report." *Bibliography of Reported Biological Phenomena ("Effects") and Clinical Manifestations Attributed to Microwave and Radio-Frequency Radiation. Report No. 2, revised.* (June 1971). https://apps.dtic.mil/dtic/tr/fulltext/u2/750271.pdf. Accessed September 9, 2017.

2. Tolgskaya MS, Gordon ZV. *Pathological Effects of Radio Waves,* translated by B Haigh. New York/London, Consultants Bureau, 1973, 146 pages. doi: 10.1007/978-1-4684-8419-9.

3. Goldsmith JR. "Epidemiologic Evidence Relevant to Radar (Microwave) Effects." *Environmental Health Perspectives.* Vol. 105, supplement 6. (December 1997): 1579-1587. doi: 10.1289/ehp.97105s61579.

4. Aitken RJ, De Iuliis GN. "Origins and Consequences of DNA Damage in Male Germ Cells." *Reproductive BioMedicine Online.* Vol. 14, no. 6. (June 2007): 727-733. doi: 10.1016/S1472-6483(10)60676-1.

5. Hazout A, Menezo Y, Madelenat P, Yazbeck C, Selva J, Cohen-Bacrie P. "Causes and Clinical Implications of Sperm DNA Damages." [Article in French] *Gynécologie Obstétrique & Fertilité.* Vol. 36, no. 11. (November 2008): 1109- 1117. doi: 10.1016/j.gyobfe.2008.07.017.

6. Makker K, Varghese A, Desai NR, Mouradi R, Agarwal A. "Cell Phones: Modern Man's Nemesis?" *Reproductive BioMedicine Online.* Vol. 18, no 1. (January 2009): 148-157. doi: 10.1016/S1472-6483(10)60437-3.

7. Kang N, Shang XJ, Huang YF. "Impact of Cell Phone Radiation on Male Reproduction." [Article in Chinese] *Zhonghua Nan Ke Xue.* Vol. 16, no. 11. (November 2010): 1027-1030.

8. Gye MC, Park CJ. "Effect of Electromagnetic Field Exposure on the Reproductive System." *Clinical and Experimental Reproductive Medicine.* Vol. 39, no. 1. (March 2012): 1-9. doi: 10.5653/cerm.2012.39.1.1.

9. La Vignera S, Condorelli RA, Vicari E, D'Agata R, Calogero AE. "Effects of the Exposure to Mobile Phones on Male Reproduction: A Review of the Literature." *Journal of Andrology.* Vol. 33, no. 3. (May-June 2012): 350-356. doi: 10.2164/ jandrol.111.014373.

10. Carpenter DO. "Human Disease Resulting from Exposure to Electromagnetic Fields." *Reviews on Environmental Health.* Vol. 28, no. 4. (2013): 159-172. doi: 10.1515/reveh-2013-0016.

11. Nazıroğlu M, Yüksel M, Köse SA, Özkaya MO. "Recent Reports of Wi-Fi and Mobile Phone-Induced Radiation on Oxidative Stress and Reproductive Signaling Pathways in Females and Males." *The Journal of Membrane Biology.* Vol. 246, no. 12. (December 2013): 869-875. doi: 10.1007/s00232-013-9597-9.

12. Adams JA, Galloway TS, Mondal D, Esteves SC, Mathews F. "Effect of Mobile Telephones on Sperm Quality: A Systematic Review and Meta-Analysis." *Environment International.* Vol. 70. (September 2014): 106-112. doi: 10.1016/j.envint.2014.04.015.

13. Liu K, Li Y, Zhang G, Liu J, Cao J, Ao L, Zhang S. "Association Between Mobile Phone Use and Semen Quality: A Systematic Review and Meta-Analysis." *Andrology.* Vol 2, no. 4. (July 2014): 491-501. doi: 10.1111/j.2047-2927.2014.00205.x.

14. K Sri N. "Mobile Phone Radiation: Physiological & Pathophysiological Considerations. *Indian Journal of Physiology and Pharmacology.* Vol. 59, no. 2. (April 2015): 125-135.

15. Hensinger P, Wilke E. "Mobilfunk-Studienergebnisse bestätigen Risiken Studienrecherche 2016-4 veröffentlicht." *Umwelt Medizin Gesellshaft.* Vol. 29, no. 3. (2016).

16. Houston BJ, Nixon B, King BV, De Iuliis GN, Aitken RJ. "The Effects of Radiofrequency Electromagnetic Radiation on Sperm Function." *Reproduction.* Vol. 152, no. 6. (December 2016): R263-R276. doi: 10.1530/REP-16-0126.

17. Pall ML. "Wi-Fi Is an Important Threat to Human Health." *Environmental Research.* Vol. 164. (July 2018): 405-416. doi: 10.1016/j.envres.2018.01.035.

18. Wilke I. "Biological and Pathological Effects of 2.45 GHz Radiation on Cells, Fertility, Brain and Behavior." *Umwelt Medizin Gesellschaft.* Vol. 31, supplement 1. (2018): 1-32.

Neurological/neuropsychiatric effects:

1. Marha K. "ATD Report 66-92." *Biological Effects of High-Frequency Electromagnetic Fields (Translation).* ATD Work Assignment. No. 78, task 11. (July 13, 1966). http://www.dtic.mil/docs/citations/AD0642029. Accessed March 12, 2018.

2. Glaser ZR, PhD. "Naval Medical Research Institute Research Report." *Bibliography of Reported Biological Phenomena ("Effects") and Clinical Manifestations Attributed to Microwave and Radio-Frequency Radiation. Report No. 2, revised.* (June 1971). https://apps.dtic.mil/dtic/tr/fulltext/u2/750271.pdf. Accessed September 9, 2017.

3. Tolgskaya MS, Gordon ZV. *Pathological Effects of Radio Waves,* translated by B Haigh. New York/London, Consultants Bureau, 1973, 146 pages. doi: 10.1007/978-1-4684-8419-9.

4. Bise W. "Low Power Radio-Frequency and Microwave Effects on Human Electroencephalogram and Behavior." *Physiological Chemistry and Physics.* Vol. 10, no. 5. (1978): 387-398.

5. Raines, JK. "National Aeronautics and Space Administration Report." *Electromagnetic Field Interactions with the Human Body: Observed Effects and Theories.* (April 1981): 116 pages.

6. Frey AH. "Electromagnetic Field Interactions with Biological Systems." *The FASEB Journal.* Vol. 7, no. 2. (February 1, 1993): 272-281. doi: 10.1096/fasebj.7.2.8440406.

7. Lai H. "Neurological Effects of Radiofrequency Electromagnetic Radiation." In JC Lin (Ed). *Advances in Electromagnetic Fields in Living Systems, Vol. 1* (pp 27-88). New York, Plenum Press, 1994.

8. Grigor'ev IuG. "Role of Modulation in Biological Effects of Electromagnetic Radiation." [Article in Russian] *Radiatsionnaia Biologiia Radioecologiia.* Vol. 36, no. 5. (September-October 1996): 659-670.

9. Lai, H. "Mobile Phone and Health Symposium Workshop Paper." *Neurological Effects of Radiofrequency Electromagnetic Radiation.* (1998). http://www.mapcruzin.com/radiofrequency/henry_lai2.htm.

10. Aitken RJ, De Iuliis GN. "Origins and Consequences of DNA Damage in Male Germ Cells." *Reproductive BioMedicine Online.* Vol. 14, no. 6. (June 2007): 727-733. doi: 10.1016/S1472-6483(10)60676-1.

11. Hardell L, Sage C. "Biological Effects from Electromagnetic Field Exposure and Public Exposure Standards." *Biomedicine & Pharmacotherapy.* Vol. 62, no. 2. (February 2008): 104-109. doi: 10.1016/j.biopha.2007.12.004.

12. Makker K, Varghese A, Desai NR, Mouradi R, Agarwal A. "Cell Phones: Modern Man's Nemesis?" *Reproductive BioMedicine Online.* Vol. 18, no 1. (January 2009): 148-157. doi: 10.1016/S1472-6483(10)60437-3.

13. Khurana VG, Hardell L, Everaert J, Bortkiewicz A, Carlberg M, Ahonen M. "Epidemiological Evidence for a Health Risk from Mobile Phone Base Stations." *International Journal of Occupational and Environmental Health.* Vol. 16, no. 3. (July-September 2010): 263-267. doi: 10.1179/107735210799160192.

14. Levitt BB, Lai H. "Biological Effects from Exposure to Electromagnetic Radiation Emitted by Cell Tower Base Stations and Other Antenna Arrays." *Environmental Reviews.* Vol. 18, no. 1. (2010): 369-395. doi.org/10.1139/A10-018.

15. Carpenter DO. "Human Disease Resulting from Exposure to Electromagnetic Fields." *Reviews on Environmental Health.* Vol. 28, no. 4. (2013): 159-172. doi: 10.1515/reveh-2013-0016.

16. Politański P, Bortkiewicz A, Zmyślony M. "Effects of Radio- and Microwaves Emitted by Wireless Communication Devices on the Functions of the Nervous System Selected Elements." [Article in Polish] *Medycyna Pracy.* Vol. 67, no. 3. (2016): 411-421. doi: 10.13075/mp.5893.00343.

17. Hensinger P, Wilke E. "Mobilfunk-Studienergebnisse bestätigen Risiken Studienrecherche 2016-4 veröffentlicht." *Umwelt Medizin Gesellshaft.* Vol. 29, no. 3. (2016).

18. Pall ML. "Microwave Frequency Electromagnetic Fields (EMFs) Produce Widespread Neuropsychiatric Effects Including Depression." *Journal of Chemical Neuroanatomy*. Vol. 75, part B. (September 2016): 43-51. doi:10.1016/j.jchemneu.2015.08.001.

19. Hecht, K. "Brochure 6: Brochure Series of the Competence Initiative for the Protection of Humanity, the Environment and Democracy." *Health Implications of Long-Term Exposures to Electrosmog*. (2016). http://kompetenzinitiative.net/KIT/wp-content/uploads/2016/07/KI_Brochure-6_K_Hecht_web.pdf. Accessed February 11, 2018.

20. Sangün Ö, Dündar B, Çömlekçi S, Büyükgebiz A. "The Effects of Electromagnetic Field on the Endocrine System in Children and Adolescents." *Pediatric Endocrinology Reviews*. Vol. 13, no. 2. (December 2015): 531-545.

21. Belyaev I, Dean A, Eger H, Hubmann G, Jandrisovits R, Kern M, Kundi M, Moshammer H, Lercher P, Müller K, Oberfeld G, Ohnsorge P, Pelzmann P, Scheingraber C, Thill R. "EUROPAEM EMF Guideline 2016 for the Prevention, Diagnosis and Treatment of EMF-Related Health Problems and Illnesses." *Reviews on Environmental Health*. Vol. 31, no. 3. (September 2016): 363-397. doi: 10.1515/reveh-2016-0011.

22. Zhang J, Sumich A, Wang GY. "Acute Effects of Radiofrequency Electromagnetic Field Emitted by Mobile Phone on Brain Function." *Bioelectromagnetics*. Vol. 38, no 5. (July 2017): 329-338. doi: 10.1002/bem.22052.

23. Lai H. "Chapter 8: A Summary of Recent Literature (2007–2017) on Neurological Effects of Radio Frequency Radiation." In Markov M (Ed). *Mobile Communications and Public Health* (pp 185-220). New York, CRC Press, 2018.

24. Pall ML. "Wi-Fi Is an Important Threat to Human Health." *Environmental Research*. Vol. 164. (July 2018): 405-416. doi: 10.1016/j.envres.2018.01.035.

25. Wilke I. "Biological and Pathological Effects of 2.45 GHz Radiation on Cells, Fertility, Brain and Behavior." *Umwelt Medizin Gesellschaft*. Vol. 31, supplement 1. (2018): 1-32.

Apoptosis/cell death (an important process in production of neurodegenerative diseases that is also important in producing infertility responses):

1. Glaser ZR, PhD. "Naval Medical Research Institute Research Report." Bibliography of Reported Biological Phenomena ("Effects") and Clinical Manifestations Attributed to Microwave and Radio-Frequency Radiation. Report No. 2, revised. (June 1971). https://apps.dtic.mil/dtic/tr/fulltext/u2/750271.pdf. Accessed September 9, 2017.

2. Tolgskaya MS, Gordon ZV. Pathological Effects of Radio Waves, translated by B Haigh. New York/London, Consultants Bureau, 1973, 146 pages. doi: 10.1007/978-1-4684-8419-9.

3. Raines, JK. "National Aeronautics and Space Administration Report." *Electromagnetic Field Interactions with the Human Body: Observed Effects and Theories*. (April 1981): 116 pages.

4. Hardell L, Sage C. "Biological Effects from Electromagnetic Field Exposure and Public Exposure Standards." *Biomedicine & Pharmacotherapy.* Vol. 62, no. 2. (February 2008): 104-109. doi: 10.1016/j.biopha.2007.12.004.

5. Makker K, Varghese A, Desai NR, Mouradi R, Agarwal A. "Cell Phones: Modern Man's Nemesis?" *Reproductive BioMedicine Online.* Vol. 18, no 1. (January 2009): 148-157. doi: 10.1016/S1472-6483(10)60437-3.

6. Levitt BB, Lai H. "Biological Effects from Exposure to Electromagnetic Radiation Emitted by Cell Tower Base Stations and Other Antenna Arrays." *Environmental Reviews.* Vol. 18, no. 1. (2010): 369-395. doi.org/10.1139/A10-018.

7. Yakymenko I, Sidorik E. "Risks of Carcinogenesis from Electromagnetic Radiation and Mobile Telephony Devices." *Experimental Oncology.* Vol. 32, no. 2. (June 2010): 54-60.

8. Yakymenko IL, Sidorik EP, Tsybulin AS. "Metabolic Changes in Cells Under Electromagnetic Radiation of Mobile Communication Systems." [Article in Russian] *Ukrainskii Biokhimicheskii Zhurnal* (1999). Vol 83, no. 2. (March-April 2011): 20-28.

9. Pall ML. "Electromagnetic Fields Act via Activation of Voltage-Gated Calcium Channels to Produce Beneficial or Adverse Effects." *Journal of Cellular and Molecular Medicine.* Vol. 17, no. 8. (August 2013): 958-965. doi: 10.1111/jcmm.12088.

10. Pall ML. "Microwave Frequency Electromagnetic Fields (EMFs) Produce Widespread Neuropsychiatric Effects Including Depression." *Journal of Chemical Neuroanatomy.* Vol. 75, part B. (September 2016): 43-51. doi:10.1016/j.jchemneu.2015.08.001.

11. Batista Napotnik T, Reberšek M, Vernier PT, Mali B, Miklavčič D. "Effects of High Voltage Nanosecond Electric Pulses on Eukaryotic Cells (In Vitro): A Systematic Review." *Bioelectrochemistry.* Vol. 110. (August 2016): 1-12. doi: 10.1016/j.bioelechem.2016.02.011.

12. Asghari A, Khaki AA, Rajabzadeh A, Khaki A. "A Review on Electromagnetic Fields (EMFs) and the Reproductive System." *Electronic Physician.* Vol. 8, no. 7. (July 2016): 2655-2662. doi: 10.19082/2655.

13. Pall ML. "Wi-Fi Is an Important Threat to Human Health." *Environmental Research.* Vol. 164. (July 2018): 405-416. doi: 10.1016/j.envres.2018.01.035.

Oxidative stress/free radical damage (important mechanisms involved in almost all chronic diseases; direct cause of cellular DNA damage):

1. Raines, JK. "National Aeronautics and Space Administration Report." *Electromagnetic Field Interactions with the Human Body: Observed Effects and Theories.* (April 1981): 116 pages.

2. Hardell L, Sage C. "Biological Effects from Electromagnetic Field Exposure and Public Exposure Standards." *Biomedicine & Pharmacotherapy.* Vol. 62, no. 2. (February 2008): 104-109. doi: 10.1016/j.biopha.2007.12.004.

3. Hazout A, Menezo Y, Madelenat P, Yazbeck C, Selva J, Cohen-Bacrie P. "Causes and Clinical Implications of Sperm DNA Damages." [Article in French] *Gynécologie Obstétrique & Fertilité*. Vol. 36, no. 11. (November 2008): 1109- 1117. doi: 10.1016/j.gyobfe.2008.07.017.

4. Makker K, Varghese A, Desai NR, Mouradi R, Agarwal A. "Cell Phones: Modern Man's Nemesis?" *Reproductive BioMedicine Online*. Vol. 18, no 1. (January 2009): 148-157. doi: 10.1016/S1472-6483(10)60437-3.

5. Desai NR, Kesari KK, Agarwal A. "Pathophysiology of Cell Phone Radiation: Oxidative Stress and Carcinogenesis with Focus on Male Reproductive System." *Reproductive Biology and Endocrinology*. Vol. 7. (October 22, 2009): 114. doi: 10.1186/1477-7827-7-114.

6. Yakymenko I, Sidorik E. "Risks of Carcinogenesis from Electromagnetic Radiation and Mobile Telephony Devices." *Experimental Oncology*. Vol. 32, no. 2. (June 2010): 54-60.

7. Yakymenko IL, Sidorik EP, Tsybulin AS. "Metabolic Changes in Cells Under Electromagnetic Radiation of Mobile Communication Systems." [Article in Russian] *Ukrainskii Biokhimicheskii Zhurnal* (1999). Vol 83, no. 2. (March-April 2011): 20-28.

8. Consales C, Merla C, Marino C, Benassi B. "Electromagnetic Fields, Oxidative Stress, and Neurodegeneration." *International Journal of Cell Biology*. Vol. 2012. (2012): 683897. doi: 10.1155/2012/683897.

9. La Vignera S, Condorelli RA, Vicari E, D'Agata R, Calogero AE. "Effects of the Exposure to Mobile Phones on Male Reproduction: A Review of the Literature." *Journal of Andrology*. Vol. 33, no. 3. (May-June 2012): 350-356. doi: 10.2164/jandrol.111.014373.

10. Pall ML. "Electromagnetic Fields Act via Activation of Voltage-Gated Calcium Channels to Produce Beneficial or Adverse Effects." *Journal of Cellular and Molecular Medicine*. Vol. 17, no. 8. (August 2013): 958-965. doi: 10.1111/jcmm.12088.

11. Nazıroğlu M, Yüksel M, Köse SA, Özkaya MO. "Recent Reports of Wi-Fi and Mobile Phone-Induced Radiation on Oxidative Stress and Reproductive Signaling Pathways in Females and Males." *The Journal of Membrane Biology*. Vol. 246, no. 12. (December 2013): 869-875. doi: 10.1007/s00232-013-9597-9.

12. Pall ML. "Scientific Evidence Contradicts Findings and Assumptions of Canadian Safety Panel 6: Microwaves Act Through Voltage-Gated Calcium Channel Activation to Induce Biological Impacts at Non-Thermal Levels, Supporting a Paradigm Shift for Microwave/Lower Frequency Electromagnetic Field Action." *Reviews on Environmental Health*. Vol. 30, no. 2. (May 2015): 99- 116. doi: 10.1515/reveh-2015-0001.

13. Yakymenko I, Tsybulin O, Sidorik E, Henshel D, Kyrylenko O, Kysylenko S. "Oxidative Mechanisms of Biological Activity of Low-Intensity Radiofrequency Radiation." *Electromagnetic Biology and Medicine*. Vol. 35, no. 2. (2016): 186-202. doi: 10.3109/15368378.2015.1043557.

14. Hensinger P, Wilke E. "Mobilfunk-Studienergebnisse bestätigen Risiken Studienrecherche 2016-4 veröffentlicht." *Umwelt Medizin Gesellshaft*. Vol. 29, no. 3. (2016).

15. Houston BJ, Nixon B, King BV, De Iuliis GN, Aitken RJ. "The Effects of Radiofrequency Electromagnetic Radiation on Sperm Function." *Reproduction*. Vol. 152, no. 6. (December 2016): R263-R276. doi: 10.1530/REP-16-0126.

16. Dasdag S, Akdag MZ. "The Link Between Radiofrequencies Emitted from Wireless Technologies and Oxidative Stress." *Journal of Chemical Neuroanatomy*. Vol. 75, part B. (September 2016): 85-93. doi: 10.1016/j.jchemneu.2015.09.001.

17. Wang H, Zhang X. "Magnetic Fields and Reactive Oxygen Species." *International Journal of Molecular Sciences*. Vol. 18, no. 10. (October 2017): 2175. doi: 10.3390/ijms18102175.

18. Pall ML. "Wi-Fi Is an Important Threat to Human Health." *Environmental Research*. Vol. 164. (July 2018): 405-416. doi: 10.1016/j.envres.2018.01.035.

19. Wilke I. "Biological and Pathological Effects of 2.45 GHz Radiation on Cells, Fertility, Brain and Behavior." *Umwelt Medizin Gesellschaft*. Vol. 31, supplement 1. (2018): 1-32.

Endocrine/hormonal effects:

1. Glaser ZR, PhD. "Naval Medical Research Institute Research Report." Bibliography of Reported Biological Phenomena ("Effects") and Clinical Manifestations Attributed to Microwave and Radio-Frequency Radiation. Report No. 2, revised. (June 1971). https://apps.dtic.mil/dtic/tr/fulltext/u2/750271.pdf. Accessed September 9, 2017.

2. Tolgskaya MS, Gordon ZV. *Pathological Effects of Radio Waves*, translated by B Haigh. New York/London, Consultants Bureau, 1973, 146 pages. doi: 10.1007/978-1-4684-8419-9.

3. Raines, JK. "National Aeronautics and Space Administration Report." *Electromagnetic Field Interactions with the Human Body: Observed Effects and Theories*. (April 1981): 116 pages.

4. Hardell L, Sage C. "Biological Effects from Electromagnetic Field Exposure and Public Exposure Standards." *Biomedicine & Pharmacotherapy*. Vol. 62, no. 2. (February 2008): 104-109. doi: 10.1016/j.biopha.2007.12.004.

5. Makker K, Varghese A, Desai NR, Mouradi R, Agarwal A. "Cell Phones: Modern Man's Nemesis?" *Reproductive BioMedicine Online*. Vol. 18, no 1. (January 2009): 148-157. doi: 10.1016/S1472-6483(10)60437-3.

6. Gye MC, Park CJ. "Effect of Electromagnetic Field Exposure on the Reproductive System." *Clinical and Experimental Reproductive Medicine*. Vol. 39, no. 1. (March 2012): 1-9. doi: 10.5653/cerm.2012.39.1.1.

7. Pall ML. "Scientific Evidence Contradicts Findings and Assumptions of Canadian Safety Panel 6: Microwaves Act Through Voltage-Gated Calcium Channel Activation to Induce Biological Impacts at Non-Thermal Levels, Supporting a Paradigm Shift for Microwave/Lower Frequency Electromagnetic Field Action." *Reviews on Environmental Health*. Vol. 30, no. 2. (May 2015): 99-116. doi: 10.1515/reveh-2015-0001.

8. Sangün Ö, Dündar B, Çömlekçi S, Büyükgebiz A. "The Effects of Electromagnetic Field on the Endocrine System in Children and Adolescents." *Pediatric Endocrinology Reviews*. Vol. 13, no. 2. (December 2015): 531-545.

9. Hecht, K. "Brochure 6: Brochure Series of the Competence Initiative for the Protection of Humanity, the Environment and Democracy." *Health Implications of Long-Term Exposures to Electrosmog*. (2016). http://kompetenzinitiative.net/ KIT/wp-content/uploads/2016/07/KI_Brochure -6_K_Hecht_web.pdf. Accessed February 11, 2018.

10. Asghari A, Khaki AA, Rajabzadeh A, Khaki A. "A Review on Electromagnetic Fields (EMFs) and the Reproductive System." *Electronic Physician*. Vol. 8, no. 7. (July 2016): 2655-2662. doi: 10.19082/2655.

11. Pall ML. "Wi-Fi Is an Important Threat to Human Health." *Environmental Research*. Vol. 164. (July 2018): 405-416. doi: 10.1016/j.envres.2018.01.035.

12. Wilke I. "Biological and Pathological Effects of 2.45 GHz Radiation on Cells, Fertility, Brain and Behavior." *Umwelt Medizin Gesellschaft*. Vol. 31, supplement 1. (2018): 1-32.

Increased intracellular calcium: intracellular calcium is maintained at very low levels (typically about 2 X 10-9 M) except for brief increases used to produce regulatory responses, such that sustained elevation of intracellular calcium levels produces many pathophysiological (that is disease-causing) responses):

1. Adey WR. "Cell Membranes: The Electromagnetic Environment and Cancer Promotion." *Neurochemical Research*. Vol. 13, no. 7. (July 1988): 671-677. doi: 10.1007/bf00973286.

2. Walleczek, J. "Electromagnetic Field Effects on Cells of the Immune System: The Role of Calcium Signaling." *The FASEB Journal*. Vol. 6, no. 13. (October 1992): 3177-3185. doi: 10.1096/fasebj.6.13.1397839.

3. Adey, WR. "Biological Effects of Electromagnetic Fields." *Journal of Cellular Biochemistry*. Vol. 51, no. 4. (April 1993): 410-416.

4. Frey AH. "Electromagnetic Field Interactions with Biological Systems." *The FASEB Journal*. Vol. 7, no. 2. (February 1, 1993): 272-281. doi: 10.1096 /fasebj.7.2.8440406.

5. Funk RHW, Monsees T, Özkucur N. "Electromagnetic Effects—From Cell Biology to Medicine." *Progress in Histochemistry and Cytochemistry*. Vol. 43, no. 4. (2009): 177-264. doi: 10.1016/j.proghi.2008.07.001.

6. Yakymenko IL, Sidorik EP, Tsybulin AS. "Metabolic Changes in Cells Under Electromagnetic Radiation of Mobile Communication Systems." [Article in Russian] *Ukrainskii Biokhimicheskii Zhurnal* (1999). Vol 83, no. 2. (March-April 2011): 20-28.

7. Gye MC, Park CJ. "Effect of Electromagnetic Field Exposure on the Reproductive System." *Clinical and Experimental Reproductive Medicine.* Vol. 39, no. 1. (March 2012): 1-9. doi: 10.5653/cerm.2012.39.1.1.

8. Pall ML. "Electromagnetic Fields Act via Activation of Voltage-Gated Calcium Channels to Produce Beneficial or Adverse Effects." *Journal of Cellular and Molecular Medicine.* Vol. 17, no. 8. (August 2013): 958-965. doi: 10.1111 /jcmm.12088.

9. Pall ML. "Electromagnetic Field Activation of Voltage-Gated Calcium Channels: Role in Therapeutic Effects." *Electromagnetic Biology and Medicine.* Vol. 33, no. 4. (December 2014): 251. doi: 10.3109/15368378.2014.906447.

10. Pall ML. "How to Approach the Challenge of Minimizing Non-Thermal Health Effects of Microwave Radiation from Electrical Devices." *International Journal of Innovative Research in Engineering & Management.* Vol. 2, no. 5. (September 2015): 71-76.

11. Pall ML. "Scientific Evidence Contradicts Findings and Assumptions of Canadian Safety Panel 6: Microwaves Act Through Voltage-Gated Calcium Channel Activation to Induce Biological Impacts at Non-Thermal Levels, Supporting a Paradigm Shift for Microwave/Lower Frequency Electromagnetic Field Action." *Reviews on Environmental Health.* Vol. 30, no. 2. (May 2015): 99-116. doi: 10.1515/reveh-2015-0001.

12. Pall ML. "Electromagnetic Fields Act Similarly in Plants as in Animals: Probable Activation of Calcium Channels via Their Voltage Sensor." *Current Chemical Biology.* Vol. 10, no. 1. (July 2016): 74-82. doi: 10.2174/22127968106661 60419160433.

13. Pall ML. "Microwave Frequency Electromagnetic Fields (EMFs) Produce Widespread Neuropsychiatric Effects Including Depression." *Journal of Chemical Neuroanatomy.* Vol. 75, part B. (September 2016): 43-51. doi:10.1016/j .jchemneu.2015.08.001.

14. Batista Napotnik T, Reberšek M, Vernier PT, Mali B, Miklavčič D. "Effects of High Voltage Nanosecond Electric Pulses on Eukaryotic Cells (In Vitro): A Systematic Review." *Bioelectrochemistry.* Vol. 110. (August 2016): 1-12. doi: 10.1016/j.bioelechem.2016.02.011.

15. Asghari A, Khaki AA, Rajabzadeh A, Khaki A. "A Review on Electromagnetic Fields (EMFs) and the Reproductive System." *Electronic Physician.* Vol. 8, no. 7. (July 2016): 2655-2662. doi: 10.19082/2655.

Pulsed EMFs are, in most cases, much more biologically active than are non-pulsed EMFs. This is important because all wireless communication devices communicate via pulsations, and the "smarter" the devices are, the more they pulse, because the pulsations convey the information. What should be obvious is that you could not study such pulsation roles if there were no biological effects produced by such EMFs. The pulsation studies alone tell us that there are many such EMF effects:

1. Osipov YuA. Labor Hygiene and the Effect of Radiofrequency Electromagnetic Fields on Workers. Leningrad Meditsina Publishing House, 1965, 220 pages.

2. Pollack H, Healer J. "Review of Information on Hazards to Personnel from High-Frequency Electromagnetic Radiation. Institute for Defense Analyses; Research and Engineering Support Division." IDA/HQ 67-6211, Series B, May 1967.

3. Frey AH. "Differential Biologic Effects of Pulsed and Continuous Electromagnetic Fields and Mechanisms of Effect." *Annals of the New York Academy of Sciences.* Vol. 238. (1974): 273-279. doi: 10.1111/j.1749-6632.1974 .tb26796.x.

4. Creighton MO, Larsen LE, Stewart-DeHaan PJ, Jacobi JH, Sanwal M, Baskerville JC, Bassen HE, Brown DO, Trevithick JR. "In Vitro Studies of Microwave-Induced Cataract. II. Comparison of Damage Observed for Continuous Wave and Pulsed Microwaves." *Experimental Eye Research.* Vol. 45, no. 3. (1987): 357-373. doi: 10.1016/s0014-4835(87)80123-9.

5. Grigor'ev IuG. "Role of Modulation in Biological Effects of Electromagnetic Radiation." [Article in Russian] *Radiatsionnaia Biologiia Radioecologiia.* Vol. 36, no. 5. (September-October 1996): 659-670.

6. Belyaev I. "Non-Thermal Biological Effects of Microwaves." *Microwave Review.* Vol. 11, no. 2. (November 2005): 13-29.

7. Belyaev I. "Non-Thermal Biological Effects of Microwaves: Current Knowledge, Further Perspective and Urgent Needs." *Electromagnetic Biology and Medicine.* Vol. 24, no. 3. (2005): 375-403. doi.org/10.1080/15368370500381844.

8. Markov MS. "Pulsed Electromagnetic Field Therapy: History, State of the Art and Future." *The Environmentalist.* Vol. 27, no. 4. (December 2007): 465-475. doi: 10.1007/s10669-007-9128-2.

9. Van Boxem K, Huntoon M, Van Zundert J, Patijn J, van Kleef M, Joosten EA. "Pulsed Radiofrequency: A Review of the Basic Science as Applied to the Pathophysiology of Radicular Pain: A Call for Clinical Translation." *Regional Anesthesia & Pain Medicine.* Vol. 39, no. 2. (March-April 2014): 149-159. doi: 10.1097/AAP.0000000000000063.

10. Belyaev, I. "Biophysical Mechanisms for Nonthermal Microwave Effects." In Markov M (Ed). *Electromagnetic Fields in Biology and Medicine* (pp 49-67). New York, CRC Press, 2015.

11. Pall ML. "Scientific Evidence Contradicts Findings and Assumptions of Canadian Safety Panel 6: Microwaves Act Through Voltage-Gated Calcium Channel Activation to Induce Biological Impacts at Non-Thermal Levels, Supporting a Paradigm Shift for Microwave/Lower Frequency Electromagnetic Field Action." *Reviews on Environmental Health.* Vol. 30, no. 2. (May 2015): 99-116. doi: 10.1515/reveh-2015-0001.

12. Panagopoulos DJ, Johansson O, Carlo GL. "Real Versus Simulated Mobile Phone Exposures in Experimental Studies." *BioMed Research International.* Vol. 2015, no. 4. (2015): 607053. doi: 10.1155/2015/607053.

13. Batista Napotnik T, Reberšek M, Vernier PT, Mali B, Miklavčič D. "Effects of High Voltage Nanosecond Electric Pulses on Eukaryotic Cells (In Vitro): A Systematic Review." *Bioelectrochemistry.* Vol. 110. (August 2016): 1-12. doi: 10.1016/j.bioelechem.2016.02.011.

Cancer causation by EMF exposures:

1. Dwyer MJ, Leeper DB. "DHEW Publication (NIOSH)." *A Current Literature Report on the Carcinogenic Properties of Ionizing and Nonionizing Radiation.* No. 78-134. (March 1978).

2. Marino AA, Morris DH. "Chronic Electromagnetic Stressors in the Environment. A Risk Factor in Human Cancer." *Journal of Environmental Science and Health. Part C: Environmental Carcinogenesis Reviews.* Vol. 3, no. 2. (1985): 189-219. doi.org/10.1080/10590508509373333.

3. Adey WR. "Cell Membranes: The Electromagnetic Environment and Cancer Promotion." *Neurochemical Research.* Vol. 13, no. 7. (July 1988): 671-677. doi: 10.1007/bf00973286.

4. Adey WR. "Joint Actions of Environmental Nonionizing Electromagnetic Fields and Chemical Pollution in Cancer Promotion." *Environmental Health Perspectives.* Vol. 86. (June 1990): 297-305. doi: 10.1289/ehp.9086297.

5. Frey AH. "Electromagnetic Field Interactions with Biological Systems." *The FASEB Journal.* Vol. 7, no. 2. (February 1, 1993): 272-281. doi: 10.1096/fasebj.7.2.8440406.

6. Goldsmith JR. "Epidemiological Evidence of Radiofrequency Radiation (Microwave) Effects on Health in Military, Broadcasting and Occupational Settings." *International Journal of Occupational and Environmental Health.* Vol. 1, no. 1. (January 1995): 47-57. doi: 10.1179/oeh.1995.1.1.47.

7. Goldsmith JR. "Epidemiologic Evidence Relevant to Radar (Microwave) Effects." *Environmental Health Perspectives.* Vol. 105, supplement 6. (December 1997): 1579-1587. doi: 10.1289/ehp.97105s61579.

8. Kundi M, Mild K, Hardell L, Mattsson M. "Mobile Telephones and Cancer—A Review of the Epidemiological Evidence." *Journal of Toxicology and Environmental Health, Part B.* Vol. 7, no. 5. (September-October 2004): 351-384. doi: 10.1080/10937400490486258.

9. Kundi M. "Mobile Phone Use and Cancer." *Occupational & Environmental Medicine.* Vol. 61, no. 6. (2004): 560-570. doi: 10.1136/oem.2003.007724.

10. Behari J, Paulraj R. "Biomarkers of Induced Electromagnetic Field and Cancer." *Indian Journal of Experimental Biology.* Vol. 45, no. 1. (January 2007): 77-85.

11. Hardell L, Carlberg M, Soderqvist F, Hansson Mild K. "Meta-Analysis of Long-Term Mobile Phone Use and the Association with Brain Tumors." *International Journal of Oncology.* Vol. 32, no. 5. (May 2008): 1097-1103.

12. Khurana VG, Teo C, Kundi M, Hardell L, Carlberg M. "Cell Phones and Brain Tumors: A Review Including the Long-Term Epidemiologic Data." *Surgical Neurology.* Vol. 72, no. 3. (September 2009): 205-214. doi: 10.1016/j.surneu.2009.01.019.

13. Desai NR, Kesari KK, Agarwal A. "Pathophysiology of Cell Phone Radiation: Oxidative Stress and Carcinogenesis with Focus on Male Reproductive System." *Reproductive Biology and Endocrinology.* Vol. 7. (October 22, 2009): 114. doi: 10.1186/1477-7827-7-114.

14. Davanipour Z, Sobel E. "Long-Term Exposure to Magnetic Fields and the Risks of Alzheimer's Disease and Breast Cancer: Further Biological Research." *Pathophysiology.* Vol. 16, no. 2-3. (August 2009): 149-156. doi: 10.1016/j.pathophys.2009.01.005.

15. Yakymenko I, Sidorik E. "Risks of Carcinogenesis from Electromagnetic Radiation and Mobile Telephony Devices." *Experimental Oncology.* Vol. 32, no. 2. (June 2010): 54-60.

16. Carpenter DO. "Electromagnetic Fields and Cancer: The Cost of Doing Nothing." *Reviews on Environmental Health.* Vol. 25, no. 1. (January-March 2010): 75-80.

17. Giuliani L, Soffriti M (Eds). "Non-Thermal Effects and Mechanisms of Interaction Between Electromagnetic Fields and Living Matter. An ICEMS Monograph." *European Journal of Oncology.* Vol. 5. National Institute for the Study and Control of Cancer and Environmental Diseases "Bernardino Ramazzini." Bologna, Italy. (2010).

18. Khurana VG, Hardell L, Everaert J, Bortkiewicz A, Carlberg M, Ahonen M. "Epidemiological Evidence for a Health Risk from Mobile Phone Base Stations." *International Journal of Occupational and Environmental Health.* Vol. 16, no. 3. (July-September 2010): 263-267. doi: 10.1179/107735210799160192.

19. Yakymenko I, Sidorik E, Kyrylenko S, Chekhun V. "Long-Term Exposure to Microwave Radiation Provokes Cancer Growth: Evidences from Radars and Mobile Communication Systems." *Experimental Oncology.* Vol. 33, no. 2. (June 2011): 62-70.

20. BioInitiative Working Group: Carpenter D, Sage C (Eds). "BioInitiative 2012: A Rationale for Biologically-Based Exposure Standards for Low-Intensity Electromagnetic Radiation." *The BioInitiative Report 2012.* https://bioinitiative.org/table-of-contents.

21. Ledoigt G, Belpomme D. "Cancer Induction Molecular Pathways and HF-EMF Irradiation." *Advances in Biological Chemistry.* Vol. 3. (2013): 177-186. doi.org/10.4236/abc.2013.32023.

22. Hardell L, Carlberg M. "Using the Hill Viewpoints from 1965 for Evaluating Strengths of Evidence of the Risk for Brain Tumors Associated with Use of Mobile and Cordless Phones." *Reviews on Environmental Health.* Vol. 28, no. 2-3. (2013): 97-106. doi: 10.1515/reveh-2013-0006.

23. Hardell L, Carlberg M, Hansson Mild K. "Use of Mobile Phones and Cordless Phones Is Associated with Increased Risk for Glioma and Acoustic Neuroma." *Pathophysiology.* Vol. 20, no. 2. (2013): 85-110. doi: 10.1016/j.pathophys.2012.11.001.

24. Carpenter DO. "Human Disease Resulting from Exposure to Electromagnetic Fields." *Reviews on Environmental Health.* Vol. 28, no. 4. (2013): 159-172. doi: 10.1515/reveh-2013-0016.

25. Davis DL, Kesari S, Soskolne CL, Miller AB, Stein Y. "Swedish Review Strengthens Grounds for Concluding that Radiation from Cellular and Cordless Phones Is a Probable Human Carcinogen." *Pathophysiology.* Vol. 20, no. 2. (April 2013): 123-129. doi: 10.1016/j.pathophys.2013.03.001.

26. Morgan LL, Miller AB, Sasco A, Davis DL. "Mobile Phone Radiation Causes Brain Tumors and Should Be Classified as a Probable Human Carcinogen (2A) (Review)." *International Journal of Oncology*. Vol. 46, no. 5. (May 2015): 1865-1871. doi: 10.3892/ijo.2015.2908.

27. Mahdavi M, Yekta R, Tackallou SH. "Positive Correlation Between ELF and RF Electromagnetic Fields on Cancer Risk." *Journal of Paramedical Sciences*. Vol. 6, no. 3. (2015). ISSN 2008-4978.

28. Carlberg M, Hardell L. "Evaluation of Mobile Phone and Cordless Phone Use and Glioma Risk Using the Bradford Hill Viewpoints from 1965 on Association or Causation." *BioMed Research International*. Vol. 2017. (2017): 9218486. doi: 10.1155/2017/9218486.

29. Bortkiewicz A, Gadzicka E, Szymczak W. "Mobile Phone Use and Risk for Intracranial Tumors and Salivary Gland Tumors—A Meta-Analysis." *International Journal of Occupational Medicine and Environmental Health*. Vol. 30, no. 1. (February 2017): 27-43. doi: 10.13075/ijomeh.1896.00802.

30. Bielsa-Fernández P, Rodríguez-Martín B. "Association Between Radiation from Mobile Phones and Tumour Risk in Adults." [Article in Spanish] *Gaceta Sanitaria*. Vol. 32, no. 1. (January-February 2018): 81-91. doi: 10.1016/j .gaceta.2016.10.014.

31. Alegría-Loyola MA, Galnares-Olalde JA, Mercado M. "Tumors of the Central Nervous System." [Article in Spanish] *Revista Medica del Instituto Mexicano del Seguro Social*. Vol. 55, no. 3. (2017): 330-340.

32. Prasad M, Kathuria P, Nair P, Kumar A, Prasad K. "Mobile Phone Use and Risk of Brain Tumours: A Systematic Review of Association Between Study Quality, Source of Funding, and Research Outcomes." *Neurological Sciences*. Vol. 38, no. 5. (May 2017): 797-810. doi: 10.1007/s10072-017- 2850-8.

33. Miller A. "References on Cell Phone Radiation and Cancer." (2017). https:// ehtrust.org/references-cell-phone-radio-frequency-radiation-cancer. Accessed September 9, 2017.

34. Hardell L. "World Health Organization, Radiofrequency Radiation and Health—A Hard Nut to Crack (Review)." *International Journal of Oncology*. Vol. 51, no. 2. (August 2017): 405-413. doi: 10.3892/ijo.2017.4046.

35. Pall ML. "Chapter 7: How Cancer Can Be Caused by Microwave Frequency Electromagnetic Field (EMF) Exposures: EMF Activation of Voltage-Gated Calcium Channels (VGCCs) Can Cause Cancer Including Tumor Promotion, Tissue Invasion and Metastasis via 15 Mechanisms." In Markov M (Ed). *Mobile Communications and Public Health* (pp 163-184). New York, CRC Press, 2018.

ENDNOTES

Introduction

1. Kılıç AO, Sari E, Yucel H, Oğuz MM, Polat E, Acoglu EA, Senel S. "Exposure to and Use of Mobile Devices in Children Aged 1–60 Months." *European Journal of Pediatrics*. Vol. 178, no. 2. (2019): 221-227. doi: 10.1007/s00431-018-3284-x.

Chapter 1: Understanding EMFs

1. Lawrence T, editor; and Rosenberg S, editor. *Cancer: Principles and Practice of Oncology*. Lippincott Williams and Wilkins, Philadelphia, PA. 2008.

2. Reisz JA, Bansai N, Qian J, Zhao W, Furdui CM. "Effects of Ionizing Radiation on Biological Molecules—Mechanisms of Damage and Emerging Methods of Detection." *Antioxidants & Redox Signaling*. Vol. 21, no. 2. (July 10, 2014): 260–292. doi: 10.1089/ars.2013.5489.

3. United States Nuclear Regulatory Commission. "Doses in Our Daily Lives." October 2, 2017. https://www.nrc.gov/about-nrc/radiation/around-us/doses-daily-lives .html.

4. International Commission on Non-Ionizing Radiation Protection. "ICNIRP Guidelines for Limiting Exposure to Time-Varying Electric, Magnetic and Electromagnetic Fields (Up to 300 Ghz)." *Health Physics*. Vol. 74, no. 4. (1998): 494–522. https://www.icnirp.org/cms/upload/publications/ICNIRPemfgdl.pdf.

5. Investigate Europe. "How Much Is Safe?" March 14, 2019. https://www.investigate -europe.eu/publications/how-much-is-safe/.

6. Pressman AS. *Electromagnetic Fields and Life*. Plenum Press, New York. 1977.

7. Dubrov AP. *The Geomagnetic Field and Life: Geomagnetobiology*. Plenum Press, New York. 1978.

8. Panagopoulos DJ, Johansson O, Carlo GL. "Real versus Simulated Mobile Phone Exposures in Experimental Studies." *BioMed Research International*. (2015): 607053. doi: 10.1155/2015/607053.

9. Frei M, Jauchem J, Heinmets F. "Physiological Effects of 2.8 GHz Radio-Frequency Radiation: A Comparison of Pulsed and Continuous-Wave Radiation." *Journal of Microwave Power and Electromagnetic Energy.* Vol. 23, no. 2. (1988): 88. https://www.ncbi.nlm.nih.gov/pubmed/3193341.

10. Huber R, Treyer V, Borbély AA, Schuderer J, Gottselig JM, Landolt HP, Werth E, Berthold T, Kuster N, Buck A, Achermann P. "Electromagnetic Fields, Such as Those from Mobile Phones, Alter Regional Cerebral Blood Flow and Sleep and Waking EEG." *Journal of Sleep Research.* Vol. 11, no. 4. (2002): 289–295. https://www.ncbi.nlm.nih.gov/pubmed/12464096.

11. Campisi A, Gulino M, Acquaviva R, Bellia P, Raciti G, Grasso R, Musumeci F, Vanella A, Triglia A. "Reactive Oxygen Species Levels and DNA Fragmentation on Astrocytes in Primary Culture after Acute Exposure to Low Intensity Microwave Electromagnetic Field." *Neuroscience Letters.* Vol. 473, no. 1. (2010): 52–5. doi: 10.1016/j.neulet.2010.02.018.

12. Höytö A, Luukkonen J, Juutilainen J, Naarala J. "Proliferation, Oxidative Stress and Cell Death in Cells Exposed to 872 MHz Radiofrequency Radiation and Oxidants." *Radiation Research.* Vol. 170, no. 2. (2008): 235–243. doi: 10.1667/RR1322.1.

13. Goodman EM, Greenebaum B, Marron MT. "Effects of Electromagnetic Fields on Molecules and Cells." *International Review of Cytology.* Vol. 158. (1995): 279–338. https://www.ncbi.nlm.nih.gov/pubmed/7721540.

14. Panagopoulos DJ, Karabarbounis A, Lioliousis C. "ELF Alternating Magnetic Field Decreases Reproduction by DNA Damage Induction." *Cell Biochemistry and Biophysics.* Vol. 67, no. 2. (2013): 703–716. doi: 10.1007/s12013-013-9560-5.

15. Franzellitti S, Valbonesi P, Ciancaglini N, Biondi C, Contin A, Bersani F, Fabbri E, "Transient DNA Damage Induced by High-Frequency Electromagnetic Fields (GSM 1.8 GHz) in the Human Trophoblast HTR-8/SVneo Cell Line Evaluated with the Alkaline Comet Assay." *Mutation Research.* Vol. 683, no. 1-2. (2010): 35–42. doi: 10.1016/j.mrfmmm.2009.10.004.

16. Zhao L, Liu X, Wang C, Yan K, Lin X, Li S, Bao H, LiuX. "Magnetic Fields Exposure and Childhood Leukemia Risk: A Meta-Analysis Based on 11,699 Cases and 13,194 Controls." *Leukemia Research.* Vol.38, no. 3. (2014): 269-274. doi: 10.1016/j.leukres.2013.12.008.

17. Wertheimer N, Leeper E. "Electrical Wiring Configurations and Childhood Cancer." *American Journal of Epidemiology.* Vol. 109, no. 3. (March 1979): 273–284. doi: 10.1093/oxfordjournals.aje.a112681.

18. Wartenberg D. "Residential Magnetic Fields and Childhood Leukemia: a Meta-Analysis." *American Journal of Public Health.* Vol. 88, no. 12. (1998): 1787–1794. doi:10.2105/ajph.88.12.1787.

19. Li D-K, Odouli R, Wi S, Janevic T, Golditch I, Bracken TD, Senior R, Rankin R, Iriye R. "A Population-Based Prospective Cohort Study of Personal Exposure to Magnetic Fields During Pregnancy and the Risk of Miscarriage." *Epidemiology.* Vol. 13, no. 1. (January 2002): 9–20.

20. Lee GM, Neutra RR, Hristova L, Yost M, Hiatt RA. "A Nested Case-Control Study of Residential and Personal Magnetic Field Measures and Miscarriages." *Epidemiology.* Vol. 13, no. 1. (January 2002): 21–31

21. "Dirty Electricity—Stealth Trigger of Disease Epidemics and Lowered Life Expectancy," Mercola.com, May 28, 2017.

22. United Nations Department of Economic and Social Affairs. "High-Level Political Forum Goals in Focus. Goal 7: Ensure Access to Affordable, Reliable, Sustainable and Modern Energy for All." Accessed July 23, 2019. https://unstats.un.org/sdgs /report/2018/goal-07/.

23. International Energy Agency. "Sustainable Development Goal 7: Ensure Access to Affordable, Reliable, Sustainable and Modern Energy for All." Accessed July 23, 2019. https://www.iea.org/sdg/electricity/.

24. The International Energy Agency. "World Energy Outlook 2017." 2017. https:// www.iea.org/weo2017/.

25. Anonymous, "Is the X Ray a Curative Agent?" *Chicago Daily Tribune*. April 14, 1896.

26. "Operated on 72 Times." *New York Times*. March 12, 1926, page 22.

27. Bavley, H. "Shoe-Fitting with X-Ray." *National Safety News*. Vol. 62, no. 3. (1950): 107–111.

28. "City Sets Control of X-Ray Devices; Health Board Restricts Use and Sale to Professionals to Cut Radiation Peril." *New York Times*. January 23, 1958, page 29.

29. Van Allen WW, Van Allen WW. "Hazards of Shoe-Fitting Fluoroscopes." *Public Health Reports*. Vol. 66, no. 12. (1951): 375-378. doi: 10.2307/4587674.

30. "X Ray Shoe Fitters a Peril, Ewing Says." *New York Times*. March 29, 1950, page 38.

31. Miller RW. "Some Potential Hazards of the Use of Roentgen Rays." *Pediatrics*. Vol. 11, no. 3. (March 1953): 294–303.

32. Wheatley GM. "Shoe-Fitting Fluoroscopes." *Pediatrics*. Vol. 11, no. 2. (February 1953): 189–90.

33. ICRP. "Recommendations of the International Commission on Radiological Protection." *British Journal of Radiology*. Supplement 6. 1955.

34. "X-Rays for Shoes Barred." *New York Times*. January 27, 1957, page 65.

35. "Shoe X-Rays Scored; Health Service Urges States to Curb the Fluoroscopes." *New York Times*. August 19, 1960, page 10.

36. "The Hazards of Shoe Fitting." *Canadian Medical Association Journal*. Vol. 74, no. 3. (February 1, 1956): 234.

37. "U.S. Census Bureau History: Did You Know?" October 2015. https://www.census .gov/history/www/homepage_archive/2015/october_2015.html.

38. Peter Kerr. "Cordless Phones Catching On." *New York Times*. February 16, 1983.

39. Eric Mack. "The First Commercial Cell Call Was Made 30 Years Ago on a $9,000 Phone." *Forbes*. October 13, 2013.

40. Mercola.com.

41. Telecommunication Development Bureau. "ICT Facts & Figures: The World in 2015." International Telecommunications Union. May 2015. https://www.itu.int /en/ITU-D/Statistics/Documents/facts/ICTFactsFigures2015.pdf.

42. Mercola.com.

43. World Bank, TCdata360. "Mobile Network Coverage, % Population." Accessed July 25, 2019. https://tcdata360.worldbank.org/indicators/entrp.mob .cov?country=USA&indicator=3403&viz=line_chart&years=2012,2016.

44. Mercola.com.

45. Aaron Smith. "Record Shares of Americans Now Own Smartphones, Have Home Broadband." *Factank*, Pew Research Center. January 12, 2017.

46. Statista Research Department. "Number of Tablet Users in the United States from 2014 to 2020 (in Millions)." Edited March 2, 2016.

47. Jeffrey I. Cole, Ph.D., Michael Suman, Ph.D., Phoebe Schramm, Ph.D., Liuning Zhou, Ph.D. "The 2017 Digital Future Report: Surveying the Digital Future." Center for the Digital Future. University of Southern California. 2017.

48. Statista Research Department. "Internet of Things (IoT) Connected Devices Installed Base Worldwide from 2015 to 2025 (in Billions)." Edited November 27, 2016.

49. Johansson O, Flydal E. "Health Risk from Wireless? The Debate Is Over." ElectromagneticHealth.org (blog). 2014. http://electromagnetichealth.org /electromagnetic-health-blog/article-by-professor-olle-johansson-health-risk-from-wireless-the-debate-is-over/.

Chapter 2: 5G: The Single Biggest Health Experiment Ever

1. Burrell L. "5G Radiation Dangers: 11 Reasons to Be Concerned." ElectricSense. Last modified April 24, 2019. https://www.electricsense.com/5g-radiation-dangers/.

2. "Gartner Says 8.4 Billion Connected 'Things' Will Be in Use in 2017, up 31 Percent from 2016." Gartner press release. Egham, U.K. February 7, 2017. https://www .gartner.com/en/newsroom/press-releases/2017-02-07-gartner-says-8-billion-connected-things-will-be-in-use-in-2017-up-31-percent-from-2016.

3. Selena Larson. "Verizon to Test 5G in 11 Cities." CNN Business. February 22, 2017. https://money.cnn.com/2017/02/22/technology/verizon-5g-testing/index.html.

4. "AT&T Bringing 5G to More U.S. Cities in 2018." AT&T.com. July 20, 2018. https:// about.att.com/story/5g_to_launch_in_more_us_cities_in_2018.html.

5. "Mobile 5G Becoming a Reality in 12 Cities with Rapid Enhancements to Follow as the Ecosystem Evolves." AT&T.com. December 18, 2018. https://about.att.com /story/2018/att_brings_5g_service_to_us.html.

6. James Temperton, "A 'Fourth Industrial Revolution' Is about to Begin (In Germany)." *Wired*. May 21, 2015. https://www.wired.co.uk/article/factory-of-the-future.

7. IHS Economics and IHS Technology. "The 5G Economy: How 5G Technology Will Contribute to the Global Economy." IHS.com. January, 2017. https://www .qualcomm.com/media/documents/files/ihs-5g-economic-impact-study.pdf.

8. Allan Holmes. "5G Cell Service Is Coming. Who Decides Where It Goes?" *New York Times*. March 2, 2018. https://www.nytimes.com/2018/03/02/technology/5g -cellular-service.html.

9. CSPAN. "FCC Chair Tom Wheeler Delivers Remarks on 5G Networks." June 25, 2016. https://archive.org/details/CSPAN_20160625_230000_FCC_Chair_Tom _Wheeler_Delivers_Remarks_on_5G_Networks.

10. John P. Thomas. "5G from Space: 20,000 Satellites to Blanket the Earth." Technocracy. January 8, 2019. http://www.technocracy.news/5g-from-space -20000-satellites-to-blanket-the-earth/.
Jeanine Marie Russaw. "SpaceX Looks to Add 30,000 New Satellites to Starlink Mission." *Newsweek.* October 19, 2019. https://www.newsweek.com/spacex -satellites-starlink-mission-1466480.

11. Eric Ralph. "SpaceX's First Dedicated Starlink Launch Announced as Mass Production Begins." Teslarati. April 8, 2019. https://www.teslarati.com/spacex -starlink-first-launch-date.

12. Global Union Against Radiation Deployment from Space. "Planned Global WiFi from Space Will Destroy Ozone Layer, Worsen Climate Change, and Threaten Life on Earth." Accessed April 14, 2019. http://www.stopglobalwifi.org.

13. ISPreview. "London Scientists Prep 10 Gbps Home Wireless Network Using Li-Fi and 5G." September 14, 2017. https://www.ispreview.co.uk/index.php/2017/09 /london-scientists-prep-10gbps-home-wireless-network-using-li-fi-5g.html.

14. Electronic Products. "5G in a Light Bulb? Scientists Explore LED-Based 10-Gbps Li-Fi Network." September 21, 2017. https://www.electronicproducts.com/ Optoelectronics/LEDs/5G_in_a_light_bulb_Scientists_explore_LED_based_10 _Gbps_Li_Fi_network.aspx.

15. EMFields Solutions. "5G Update." August 15, 2017. http://www.lessemf.com/5G .pdf.

16. Lebedeva NN. "Sensor and Subsensor Reactions of a Healthy Man to Peripheral Effects of Low-Intensity Millimeter Waves." (In Russian.) *Millimetrovie Volni v Biologii i Meditcine.* Vol. 2 (1993): 5–23.

17. Lebedeva NN. "Neurophysiological Mechanisms of Biological Effects of Peripheral Action of Low-Intensity Nonionizing Electromagnetic Fields in Humans." (In Russian.) 10th Russian Symposium "Millimeter Waves in Medicine and Biology," Moscow, Russia. (April 1995): 138–140.

18. Golovacheva TV. "EHF Therapy in Complex Treatment of Cardiovascular Diseases." (In Russian.) 10th Russian Symposium "Millimeter Waves in Medicine and Biology," Moscow, Russia. (April 1995): 29–31.

19. Afanas'eva TN, Golovacheva TV. "Side Effects of the EHF-therapy for Essential Hypertension." (In Russian.) 11th Russian Symposium "Millimeter Waves in Medicine and Biology," Zvenigorod, Russia. (April 1997): 26–28.

20. Zalyubovskaya NP. "Biological Effect of Millimeter Radiowaves." (In Russian.) *Vracheboyne Delo.* No. 3. (1977): 116–119. https://drive.google.com/file/d/1mX1fSrT zvWIxJBOC0Q8POLD0XhBQSpDv/view.
Joel Moskowitz. "5G Wireless Technology: Millimeter Wave Health Effects." Electromagnetic Radiation Safety. November 14, 2018 (updated February 22, 2019). https://www.saferemr.com/2017/08/5g-wireless-technology-millimeter-wave.html.

21. EMFields Solutions. "5G Update." August 15, 2017. http://www.lessemf.com/5G.pdf.

22. Jody McCutcheon. "Frightening Frequencies: The Dangers of 5G." *Eluxe Magazine.* Accessed on April 15, 2019. https://eluxemagazine.com/magazine/dangers-of-5g/.

23. ElectricSense. "The Dangers of 5G—11 Reasons to Be Concerned." May 30, 2018. https://ecfsapi.fcc.gov/file/1053072081009/5G%20Radiation%20Dangers%20 -%2011%20Reasons%20To%20Be%20Concerned%20_%20ElectricSense.pdf.

24. Dr. Cindy Russell. "A 5G Wireless Future: Will It Give Us a Smart Nation or Contribute to an Unhealthy One?" *The Bulletin.* January–February 2017. https:// ecfsapi.fcc.gov/file/10308361407065/5%20G%20Wireless%20Future-SCCMA%20 Bulletin_FEb%202017_pdf.pdf.

25. References for "A 5G Wireless Future" by Dr. Cindy Russell (PDF). http:// www.sccma-mcms.org/Portals/19/assets/docs/References5garticle. pdf?ver=2017-03-10-112153-967.

26. Prost M, Olchowik G, Hautz W, Gaweda R. "Experimental Studies on the Influence of Millimeter Radiation on Light Transmission through the Lens." *Klin Oczna.* Vol. 96, no. 8-9 (August–September 1994): 257–9. https://www.ncbi.nlm .nih.gov/pubmed/7897988.

27. Kojima M, Hanazawa M, Yamashiro Y, Sasaki H, Watanabe S, Taki M, Suzuki Y, Hirata A, Kamimura Y, Sasaki K. "Acute Ocular Injuries Caused by 60-Ghz Millimeter-Wave Exposure." *Health Physics.* Vol. 97, no. 3. (September, 2009): 212–8. doi: 10.1097/HP.0b013e3181abaa57.

28. Wang KJ, Yao K, Lu DQ, Jiang H, Tan J, Xu W. "Effect of Low-Intensity Microwave Radiation on Proliferation of Cultured Epithelial Cells of Rabbit Lens." *Zhonghua Lao Dong Wei Sheng Zhi Ye Bing Za Zhi (Chinese Journal of Industrial Hygiene and Occupational Diseases).* Vol. 21, no. 5. (October 2003): 346–9.

29. Potekhina IL, Akoev GN, Enin LD, Oleiner VD. "The Effect of Low-Intensity Millimeter-Range Electromagnetic Radiation on the Cardiovascular System of the White Rat." (In Russian.) *Fiziol Zh SSSR Im I M Sechenova (Sechenov Physiological Journal of the USSR).* Vol. 78, no. 1. (January 1992): 35–41.

30. Dr. Cindy Russell. "A 5G Wireless Future: Will It Give Us a Smart Nation or Contribute to an Unhealthy One?" *The Bulletin.* January–February 2017. https:// ecfsapi.fcc.gov/file/10308361407065/5%20G%20Wireless%20Future-SCCMA%20 Bulletin_FEb%202017_pdf.pdf.

31. References for "A 5G Wireless Future" by Dr. Cindy Russell (PDF). http://www. sccma-mcms.org/Portals/19/assets/docs/References5garticle .pdf?ver=2017-03-10-112153-967.

32. Dr. Cindy Russell. "A 5G Wireless Future: Will It Give Us a Smart Nation or Contribute to an Unhealthy One?" *The Bulletin.* January–February 2017. https://ecfsapi.fcc.gov/file/10308361407065/5%20G%20Wireless%20Future -SCCMA%20Bulletin_FEb%202017_pdf.pdf.

33. References for "A 5G Wireless Future" by Dr. Cindy Russell (PDF). http:// www.sccma-mcms.org/Portals/19/assets/docs/References5garticle. pdf?ver=2017-03-10-112153-967.

34. Ramundo-Orlando A. "Effects of Millimeter Waves Radiation on Cell Membrane—A Brief Review." *Journal of Infrared, Millimeter, and Terahertz Waves.* Vol. 31, no. 12. (December 2010): 1400–11.

35. Kolomytseva MP, Gapeey AB, Sadovniko VB, Chemeris NK. "Suppression of Nonspecific Resistance of the Body under the Effect of Extremely High Frequency Electromagnetic Radiation of Low Intensity." *Biofizika (Biophysics).* Vol. 47, no. 1. (January–February 2002): 71–7.

36. Soghomonyan D, Trchounian K, Trchounian A. "Millimeter Waves or Extremely High Frequency Electromagnetic Fields in the Environment: What Are Their Effects on Bacteria?" *Applied Microbiology and Biotechnology.* Vol. 100, no. 11. (June 2016): 4761–4771. doi: 10.1007/s00253-016-7538-0.

37. Martin L. Pall, Ph.D. "5G: Great Risk for EU, U.S. and International Health! Compelling Evidence for Eight Distinct Types of Great Harm Caused by Electromagnetic Field (EMF) Exposures and the Mechanism That Causes Them." May 17, 2018. Page 81. https://peaceinspace.blogs.com/files/5g-emf-hazards--dr -martin-l.-pall--eu-emf2018-6-11us3.pdf.

38. Burrell L. "5G Radiation Dangers: 11 Reasons to Be Concerned." ElectricSense. Last modified April 24, 2019. https://www.electricsense.com/5g-radiation-dangers/.

39. Dr. Cindy Russell. "A 5G Wireless Future: Will It Give Us a Smart Nation or Contribute to an Unhealthy One?" *The Bulletin.* January–February 2017. https:// ecfsapi.fcc.gov/file/10308361407065/5%20G%20Wireless%20Future-SCCMA%20 Bulletin_FEb%202017_pdf.pdf.

40. References for "A 5G Wireless Future" by Dr. Cindy Russell (PDF). http:// www.sccma-mcms.org/Portals/19/assets/docs/References5garticle. pdf?ver=2017-03-10-112153-967.

41. Environmental Health Trust. "Letter to the FCC from Dr. Yael Stein MD in Opposition to 5G Spectrum Frontiers." July 9, 2016. https://ehtrust.org/letter-fcc -dr-yael-stein-md-opposition-5g-spectrum-frontiers/.

42. Grassroots Environmental Education. "5th Generation (5G) Wireless Communications Fact Sheet." Accessed April 14, 2019. https://www .telecompowergrab.org/uploads/3/8/5/9/38599771/5g_fact_sheet_v9.pdf.

43. Environmental Health Trust. "Letter to the FCC from Dr. Yael Stein MD in Opposition to 5G Spectrum Frontiers." July 9, 2016. https://ehtrust.org/letter-fcc -dr-yael-stein-md-opposition-5g-spectrum-frontiers/.

44. Shafirstein G, Moros EG. "Modelling Millimetre Wave Propagation and Absorption in a High Resolution Skin Model: the Effect of Sweat Glands." *Physics in Medicine & Biology.* Vol. 56, no. 5. (2011): 1329–39. doi: 10.1088/0031 -9155/56/5/007.

45. Environmental Health Trust. "Letter to the FCC from Dr. Yael Stein MD in Opposition to 5G Spectrum Frontiers." July 9, 2016. https://ehtrust.org/letter-fcc -dr-yael-stein-md-opposition-5g-spectrum-frontiers/.

46. Joint Non-Lethal Weapons Program. "Active Denial Technology Fact Sheet." U.S. Department of Defense. May 2016. https://jnlwp.defense.gov/Portals/50 /Documents/Press_Room/Fact_Sheets/ADT_Fact_Sheet_May_2016.pdf.

47. Environmental Health Trust. "Top Facts on 5G: What You Need to Know about 5G Wireless and 'Small' Cells." Accessed April 15, 2019. https://ehtrust.org/key -issues/cell-phoneswireless/5g-internet-everything/20-quick-facts-what-you -need-to-know-about-5g-wireless-and-small-cells/.

48. Nerkararyan AV, Shahinyan MA, Mikaelyan MS, Vardevanyan PO. "Effect of Millimeter Waves with Low Intensity on Peroxidase Total Activity and Isoenzyme Composition in Cells of Wheat Seedling Shoots." *International Journal of Scientific Research in Environmental Sciences.* Vol. 1, no. 9. (2013): 217– 223. doi: 10.12983/ijsres-2013-p217-223.

49. Sánchez-Bayo F, Wyckhuys CAG. "Worldwide Decline of the Entomofauna: A Review of Its Drivers." *Biological Conservation*. Vol. 232. (2019): 8–27. doi: 10.1016/j.biocon.2019.01.020.

50. Bond S, Wang K-K. "The Impact of Cell Phone Towers on House Prices in Residential Neighborhoods." *The Appraisal Journal*. Summer 2005. http://electromagnetichealth .org/wp-content/uploads/2014/06/TAJSummer05p256-277.pdf.

51. National Association of Realtors. "Cell Towers, Antennas Problematic for Buyers." *Realtor Magazine*. July 25, 2014. https://magazine.realtor/daily-news/2014/07/25 /cell-towers-antennas-problematic-for-buyers.

52. Ibid.

53. Office of Richard Blumenthal, United States Senator for Connecticut. "At Senate Commerce Hearing, Blumenthal Raises Concerns on 5G Wireless Technology's Potential Health Risks." February 7, 2019. https://www.blumenthal.senate.gov/ newsroom/press/release/at-senate-commerce-hearing-blumenthal-raises -concerns-on-5g-wireless-technologys-potential-health-risks.

54. "Scientists Warn of Potential Serious Health Effects of 5G." Environmental Health Trust. September 13, 2017. https://ehtrust.org/wp-content/uploads/Scientist-5G -appeal-2017.pdf.

55. "International Appeal: Stop 5G on Earth and in Space." June 7, 2019. https:// www.5gSpaceAppeal.org.

56. Maurizio Martucci. "'It Causes Damage to the Body!' Florence Brakes on 5G and Applies the Precautionary Principle. Motion in Defense of Health Approved (Almost) Unanimous." [Article in Italian.] Oasi Sana. April 5, 2019. https:// oasisana.com/2019/04/05/provoca-danni-al-corpo-firenze-frena-sul-5g-e-applica -il-principio-di-precauzione-approvata-con-voto-quasi-unanime-la-mozione-in -difesa-della-salute-notizia-esclusiva-oasi-sana/.

57. "Italian Court Orders Government To Launch Cell Phone Radiation Awareness Campaign." Environmental Health Trust. https://ehtrust.org/italian-court- orders-government-to-launch-cell-phone-radiation-awareness-campaign/.

58. Peter Winterman. "Chamber Wants Radiation Research First, Then 5G Network." [Article in Dutch.] *AD News*. April 4, 2019. https://www.ad.nl/tech/kamer-wil -eerst-stralingsonderzoek-dan-pas-5g-netwerk~ab567cd6/.

59. "Germans Petition Parliament to Stop 5G Auction on Health Grounds." Telecompaper. April 8, 2019. https://www.telecompaper.com/news/germans -petition-parliament-to-stop-5g-auction-on-health-grounds--1287962.

60. Anouch Seydtaghia. "5G: After the Vaud Moratorium, the Storm." [Article in French.] *Le Temps*. April 9, 2019. https://www.letemps.ch/suisse/5g-apres -moratoire-vaudois-tempete.

61. "Geneva Adopts Motion for a Moratorium on 5G." [Article in French.] *Le Temps*. April 11, 2019. www.letemps.ch/suisse/geneve-adopte-une-motion-un-moratoire-5g.

62. "A Municipality of Rome Votes against 5G: What Will the Giunta Do?" [Article in Italian.] *Terra Nuova*. March 28, 2019. http://www.terranuova.it/News/Attualita /Un-Municipio-di-Roma-vota-contro-il-5G-cosa-fara-la-Giunta.

63. Valery Kodachigov. "The Ministry of Defense Refused to Transmit to the Operators the Frequencies for 5G." [Article in Russian.] *Vedemosti*. March 28, 2019. https://www.vedomosti.ru/technology/articles/2019/03/28/797714 -minoboroni-otkazalos-peredavat-5g.

64. "Radiation Concerns Halt Brussels 5G Development, for Now." *The Brussels Times*. April 1, 2019. https://www.brusselstimes.com/brussels/55052/radiation -concerns-halt-brussels-5g-for-now/.

65. Bob Egelko. "Court Upholds SF's Right to Prevent Telecom Companies from Marring Scenic Views." *San Francisco Chronicle*. April 4, 2019. https://www. sfchronicle.com/bayarea/article/Court-upholds-SF-s-right-to-prevent -telecom-13742615.php.

66. "Exhibit 1: Small Cell 5G Health Study Resolution." Hallandale Beach, Florida. 2019. https://ehtrust.org/wp-content/uploads/Hallandale-Small-Cell-5G-Health -Study-Resolution.pdf.

67. "House Joint Resolution No. 13, Introduced by D. Dunn, A. Olsen." State of Montana. https://leg.mt.gov/bills/2019/billpdf/HJ0013. pdf?fbclid=IwAR1SPkpwFE99JZWKTMiVJfrw _IZ04LhvO6laVo7iQKZzGN67nfK7w9o88pE.

68. Keaton Thomas. "5G Wireless Technology Comes with Big Promises, but City of Portland Has Big Concerns." KATU News. March 12, 2019. https://katu.com /news/local/5g-wireless-technology-comes-with-big-promises-but-the-city-of -portland-has-big-concerns.

69. "Chapter 12.18 – Wireless Telecommunications Facilities in the Public Right-of-Way." City of Racho Palos Verdes Municipal Code. May 7, 2019. https://library .municode.com/ca/rancho_palos_verdes/codes/code_of _ordinances?nodeId=TIT12STSIPUPL_CH12.18WITEFAPURI-W.

70. New Hampshire HB522: Establishing a Commission to Study the Environmental and Health Effects of Evolving 5G Technology, adopted by both bodies in the 2019 legislative session. https://trackbill.com/bill/new-hampshire -house-bill-522-establishing-a-commission-to-study-the-environmental-and -health-effects-of-evolving-5g-technology/1630657/?fbclid=IwAR28psMtRFU7m BGMmA8SKxoS0AIkf8LzcQR7e7vO_MiifUzs0N4GfUNcLC4.

71. "Ordinance No. 819: An Urgency Ordinance of the Town Council of the Town of Fairfax Enacting Title 20 ('Telecommunications') of the Fairfax Municipal Code to Establish New Regulations for Wireless Telecommunications Facilities." Accessed April 5, 2019. https://storage.googleapis.com/proudcity/fairfaxca /uploads/2018/10/Ord-819-URGENCYsmall-cell.pdf.

72. "San Rafael City Council Agenda Report." December 17, 2018. https://ehtrust.org /wp-content/uploads/6.c-Small-Wireless-Facilities.pdf.

73. "Agenda Item Summary, City Council Meeting, November 5, 2018." City of Sonoma, California. https://sonomacity.civicweb.net/document/17797.

74. Adrian Rodriguez. "Ross Valley Officials Work to Tighten 5G Antenna Rules." *Marin Independent Journal*. October 27, 2018. https://www.marinij .com/2018/10/27/ross-valley-officials-work-to-tighten-5g-antenna-rules/.

75. Adrian Rodriguez. "California Town Looks for Alternatives to Small Cell Installations." *Marin Independent Journal.* October 5, 2018. https://www.govtech.com/network/California-Town-Looks-for-Alternatives-to-Small-Cell-Installations.html.

76. "Town of Burlington Policy, Applications for Small Cell Wireless Installations." Accepted by Board of Selectmen October 22, 2018. http://cms2.revize.com/revize/burlingtonma/Small.Cell.Wireless.Equiptment.Policy.Approved.10.22.2018.BURLINGTON.MA.pdf.

77. Rich Hosford. "Verizon Drops Small Cell Wireless Booster Application in Face of Fees." Burlington Cable Access Television. October 23, 2018. http://www.bcattv.org/bnews/top-stories/verizon-drops-small-cell-wireless-booster-application-in-face-of-fees/.

78. Glenn M. Parrish. "Cell Tower Ordinance Read for First Time at Council Meeting." *Booneville Democrat.* September 5, 2018. https://www.boonevilledemocrat.com/news/20180905/cell-tower-ordinance-read-for-first-time-at-council-meeting.

79. "Mill Valley Staff Report." September 6, 2018. http://cityofmillvalley.granicus.com/MetaViewer.php?view_id=2&clip_id=1290&meta_id=59943.

80. Petaluma Municipal Code, Ordinance 2674, passed November 19, 2018. https://www.codepublishing.com/CA/Petaluma/.

81. "Small Cell Towers Nixed in 7-Hour Monterey Planning Commission Meeting." *Cedar Street Times.* March 19, 2018. http://www.cedarstreettimes.com/18237-2/.

82. To see the code online go to https://qcode.us/codes/walnut/, click on "Title 6: Planning and Zoning," click on "Chapter 6.88: Antennas and Communication Facilities," click on "6.88.060: Design standards," see item "O."

83. Bob Fernandez. "Philly, Suburbs Brace for 'Attack of the Small Cells' Towers." *Philadelphia Inquirer.* June 1, 2017. https://www.philly.com/philly/business/comcast/philly-and-suburbs-brace-for-attack-of-the-small-cells-20170601.html?arc404=true.

84. William Kelly. "Official: Palm Beach Exempt from 5G Wireless Law." *Palm Beach Daily News.* May 3, 2017. https://www.palmbeachdailynews.com/news/20170503/official-palm-beach-exempt-from-5g-wireless-law.

85. "Part Eleven Zoning Ordinance." City of Mason, Ohio. Revised May 15, 2017. https://www.imaginemason.org/download/PDFs/building/MasonZoningCodev-05-15-2017.pdf.

86. "Town of Warren, Section 20 – Special Permit for Telecommunications Facilities and Towers." December 11, 2012. https://ehtrust.org/wp-content/uploads/Warren_Zoning_Telecom_Regs_-_December_11_2012-4.pdf.

87. C. Robert Gibson. "How a Mid-Sized Tennessee Town Took on Comcast, Revived Its Economy, and Did It With Socialism." Huffington Post. March 6, 2015 (updated May 6, 2015). http://www.huffingtonpost.com/carl-gibson/chattanooga-socialism_b_6812368.html.

88. Trevor Hughes. "Town Creates High-Speed Revolution, One Home at a Time." *USA Today.* November 19, 2014. https://www.usatoday.com/story/news/nation/2014/11/19/longmont-internet-service/19294335/.

89. Katherine Tweed. "Bell Labs Sets New Record for Internet over Copper." IEEE Spectrum. July 14, 2014. http://spectrum.ieee.org/tech-talk/telecom/internet /bell-labs-sets-new-record-for-internet-over-copper.

90. "New Method Examined to Bring Fiber Optics to Homes." *Durango Herald*. May 6, 2018. https://durangoherald.com/articles/221644.

Chapter 3: Cell Phones Are the Cigarettes of the 21st Century

1. Brandt AM. "Inventing Conflicts of Interest: A History of Tobacco Industry Tactics." *American Journal of Public Health*. Vol. 102, no. 1. (January 2012): 63–71. doi: 10.2105/AJPH.2011.300292.

2. Glantz SA, Slade J, Bero LA, Hanauer P, Barnes DE. *The Cigarette Papers*. 1998: University of California Press. Berkeley, California. Page 188.

3. Turner C and Spilich GJ. "Research into Smoking or Nicotine and Human Cognitive Performance: Does the Source of Funding Make a Difference?" *Addiction*. Vol. 92, no. 11. (1997): 1423–1426. https://pdfs.semanticscholar.org /d1ba/670b367bab2df3bd9ffcf5ae33d24c9688e3.pdf.

4. Ibid.

5. Brownell KC, Warner KE. "The Perils of History: Big Tobacco Played Dirty and Millions Died. How Similar is Big Food?" *Milbank Quarterly*. Vol. 87, no. 1. (2009): 259–294. doi: 10.1111/j.1468-0009.2009.00555.x.

6. Broder JM. "Cigarette Maker Concedes Smoking Can Cause Cancer." *New York Times*. March 21, 1997. https://www.nytimes.com/1997/03/21/us/cigarette -maker-concedes-smoking-can-cause-cancer.html.

7. Milberger S, Davis RM, Douglas CE, Beasley JK, Burns D, Houston T, Shopland D. "Tobacco Manufacturers' Defence against Plaintiffs' Claims of Cancer Causation: Throwing Mud at the Wall and Hoping Some of It Will Stick." *Tobacco Control*. Vol. 15, suppl. 4. (December 2006): iv17–iv26. doi: 10.1136/tc.2006.016956.

8. Andrew Dugan. "In U.S., Smoking Hits New Low at 16%." Gallup. July 24, 2018. https://news.gallup.com/poll/237908/smoking-rate-hits-new-low.aspx.

9. Centers for Disease Control and Prevention. "Smoking Leads to Disease and Disability and Harms Nearly Every Organ of the Body." Page last reviewed February 6, 2019. Accessed March 4, 2019. https://www.cdc.gov/tobacco/data _statistics/fact_sheets/fast_facts/index.htm.

10. Velicer, C, St Helen G, Glantz SA. "Tobacco Papers and Tobacco Industry Ties in Regulatory Toxicology and Pharmacology." *Journal of Public Health Policy*. Vol. 39, no. 1. (February 2018): 34-48. doi: 10.1057/s41271-017-0096-6.

11. Liu JJ, Bell CM, Matelski JJ, Detsky AS, Cram P. "Payments by US Pharmaceutical and Medical Device Manufacturers to US Medical Journal Editors: Retrospective Observational Study." *BMJ*. Vol. 359, no. j4619. (October 26, 2017). doi: 10.1136 /bmj.j4619.

12. Friedman L. "Financial Conflicts of Interest and Study Results in Environmental and Occupational Health Research." *Journal of Occupational and Environmental Medicine*. Vol. 58, no. 3. (March 2016): 238-47. doi: 10.1097/JOM.0000000000000671.

13. George Carlo. "The Latest Reassurance Ruse about Cell Phones and Cancer." Journal of the Australasian College of Nutritional and Environmental Medicine. Vol. 26, No. 1. (April, 2007).

14. "A Report on Non-Iodizing Radiation." Microwave News. Vol. 26, no. 4. (July, 2006) https://microwavenews.com/sites/default/files/docs/mwn.7-06.RR.pdf.

15. Huss A, Egger M, Hug K, Huwiler-Müntener K, Röösli M. "Source of Funding and Results of Studies of Health Effects of Mobile Phone Use: Systematic Review of Experimental Studies." Ciência & Saúde Coletiva. Vol. 13, no. 3 (2008). doi: 10.1590/S1413-81232008000300022.

16. Marino AA, Carruba S. "The Effects of Mobile-Phone Electromagnetic Fields on Brain Electrical Activity: A Critical Analysis of the Literature." Electromagnetic Biology and Medicine. Vol. 28, no. 3. (2009): 250–274. doi: 10.3109/15368370902918912.

17. Joel M. Moskowitz, "Government Must Inform Us of Cell Phone Risk." SFGate .com. July 25, 2013. http://www.sfgate.com/cgi-bin/article.cgi?f=/c/a/2010/04/27 /EDMB1D58TC.DTL#ixzz1qAghpiqI.

18. Panagopoulos DJ. "Comparing DNA Damage Induced by Mobile Telephony and Other Types of Man-Made Electromagnetic Fields." Mutation Research/Reviews in Mutation Research. Vol. 781. July–September 2019: 53–62. doi: 10.1016/j .mrrev.2019.03.003.

19. Daroit NB, Visioli F, Magnusson AS, Vieira GR, Rados PV. "Cell Phone Radiation Effects on Cytogenetic Abnormalities of Oral Mucosal Cells." Brazilian Oral Research. Vol. 29. (2015): 1–8. doi: 10.1590/1807-3107BOR-2015.vol29.0114.

20. Ibid.

21. D'Silva MH, Swer RT, Anbalagan J, Rajesh B. "Effect of Radiofrequency Radiation Emitted from 2G and 3G Cell Phone on Developing Liver of Chick Embryo - A Comparative Study." Journal of Clinical and Diagnostic Research for Doctors. Vol. 11, no. 7. (2017): 5–9. doi: 10.7860/JCDR/2017/26360.10275.

22. Panagopoulos D. "Mobile Telephony Radiation Effects on Insect Ovarian Cells. The Necessity for Real Exposures Bioactivity Assessment. The Key Role of Polarization, and the 'Ion Forced-Oscillation Mechanism.'" In Geddes CD (Ed.), Microwave Effects on DNA and Proteins. Springer, 2017.

23. Gevrek F, Aydin D, Ozsoy S, Aygun H, Bicer C. "Inhibition by Egb761 of the Effect of Cellphone Radiation on the Male Reproductive System." Bratislava Medical Journal. Vol. 118, no. 11. (2017): 676–683. doi: 10.4149/BLL_2017_128.

24. Çetkin M, Demirel C, Kızılkan N, Aksoy N, Erbağcı H. "Evaluation of the Mobile Phone Electromagnetic Radiation on Serum Iron Parameters in Rats." African Health Sciences. Vol. 17, no. 1. (2017): 186–189. doi: 10.4314/ahs.v17i1.23.

25. Shahin S, Singh SP, Chaturvedi CM. "Mobile Phone (1800 MHz) Radiation Impairs Female Reproduction in Mice, Mus Musculus, through Stress Induced Inhibition of Ovarian and Uterine Activity." Reproductive Toxicology. 73 (October 2017): 41–60. doi: 10.1016/j.reprotox.2017.08.001.

26. Zothansiama, Zosangzuali M, Lalramdinpuii M, Jagetia GC. "Impact of Radiofrequency Radiation on DNA Damage and Antioxidants in Peripheral Blood Lymphocytes of Humans Residing in the Vicinity of Mobile Phone Base

Stations." *Electromagnetic Biology and Medicine.* Vol. 36, no. 3. (2017): 295–305. doi: 10.1080/15368378.2017.1350584.

27. De Oliveira FM, Carmona AM, Ladeira C. "Is Mobile Phone Radiation Genotoxic? An Analysis of Micronucleus Frequency in Exfoliated Buccal Cells." *Mutation Research.* 822: (October 2017): 41–46. doi: 10.1016/j.mrgentox.2017.08.001.

28. Kalafatakis F, Bekiaridis-Moschou D, Gkioka E, Tsolaki M. "Mobile Phone Use for 5 Minutes Can Cause Significant Memory Impairment in Humans." *Hellenic Journal of Nuclear Medicine.* Vol. 20 supplement. (September 2017): 146–154.

29. Schauer I, Mohamad Al-Ali B. "Combined Effects of Varicocele and Cell Phones on Semen and Hormonal Parameters." *Wien Klin Wochenschrift.* Vol. 130, no. 9-10. (2018): 335–340. doi: 10.1007/s00508-017-1277-9.

30. Akdag M, Dasdag S, Canturk F, Akdag MZ. "Exposure to Non-Ionizing Electromagnetic Fields Emitted from Mobile Phones Induced DNA Damage in Human Ear Canal Hair Follicle Cells." *Electromagnetic Biology and Medicine.* Vol 37, no. 2. (2018): 66–75. doi: 10.1080/15368378.2018.1463246.

31. Fragopoulou AF, Polyzos A, Papadopoulou MD, Sansone A, Manta AK, Balafas E, Kostomitsopoulos N, Skouroliakou A, Chatgilialoglu C, Georgakilas A, Stravopodis DJ, Ferreri C, Thanos D, Margaritis LH. "Hippocampal Lipidome and Transcriptome Profile Alterations Triggered by Acute Exposure of Mice to GSM 1800 MHz Mobile Phone Radiation: An Exploratory Study." *Brain and Behavior.* Vol. 8, no. 6. (June 2018). doi: 10.1002/brb3.1001.

32. Ahmadi S, Alavi SS, Jadidi M, Ardjmand A. "Exposure to GSM 900-MHz Mobile Radiation Impaired Inhibitory Avoidance Memory Consolidation in Rat: Involvements of Opioidergic and Nitrergic Systems." *Brain Research.* Vol. 1701. (December 15, 2018): 36–45. doi: 10.1016/j.brainres.2018.07.016.

33. Shahbazi-Gahrouei D, Hashemi-Beni B, Moradi A, Aliakbari M, Shahbazi-Gahrouei S. "Exposure to Global System for Mobile Communication 900 MHz Cellular Phone Radiofrequency Alters Growth, Proliferation and Morphology of Michigan Cancer Foundation-7 Cells and Mesenchymal Stem Cells." *International Journal of Preventive Medicine.* Vol. 9. (June 19, 2018): 51. doi: 10.4103/ijpvm.IJPVM_75_17.

34. Bektas H, Bektas MS, Dasdag S. "Effects of Mobile Phone Exposure on Biochemical Parameters of Cord Blood: A Preliminary Study." *Electromagnetic Biology and Medicine.* Vol. 37, no. 4. (August 29, 2018): 184–191. doi: 10.1080/15368378.2018.1499033.

35. El-Maleky NF, Ebrahim RH. "Effects of Exposure to Electromagnetic Field from Mobile Phone on Serum Hepcidin and Iron Status in Male Albino Rats." *Electromagnetic Biology and Medicine.* Vol. 38, no. 1. (2019): 66–73. doi: 10.1080/15368378.2018.1531423.

36. Béres S, Németh Á, Ajtay Z, Kiss I, Németh B, Hejjel L. "Cellular Phone Irradiation of the Head Affects Heart Rate Variability Depending on Inspiration/Expiration Ratio." *In Vivo.* Vol. 32, no. 5. (2018): 1145–1153. doi: 10.21873/invivo.11357.

37. Shahabi S, Hassanzadeh Taji I, Hoseinnezhaddarzi M, Mousavi F, Shirchi S, Nazari A, Zarei H, Pourabdolhossein F. "Exposure to Cell Phone Radiofrequency Changes Corticotrophin Hormone Levels and Histology of the Brain and Adrenal Glands in Male Wistar Rat." *Iranian Journal of Basic Medical Sciences.* Vol. 21, no. 12. (December 2018): 1269–1274. doi: 10.22038 /ijbms.2018.29567.7133.

38. CTIA. "Overall Safety of Cell Phones." Cellphone Health Facts. Accessed February 12, 2019. https://www.wirelesshealthfacts.com/faq/.

39. Roberts C. "Do I Need to Worry about Radiation From WiFi and Bluetooth Devices?" *Consumer Reports*. March 1, 2018. https://www.consumerreports.org /radiation/do-i-need-to-worry-about-radiation-from-wifi-and-bluetooth-devices/.

40. National Toxicology Program. "Cell Phone Radio Frequency Radiation." Accessed February 14, 2019. https://ntp.niehs.nih.gov/results/areas/cellphones/index.html.

41. National Institute of Environmental Health Sciences. "NTP Releases Rodent Studies on Cell Phone Radiofrequency Radiation." Environmental Factor. June 2016. https://factor.niehs.nih.gov/2016/6/science-highlights/cellphones/index .htm.

42. Broad WJ. "Study of Cellphone Risks Finds 'Some Evidence' of Link to Cancer, at Least in Male Rats." *New York Times*. November 1, 2018. https://www.nytimes .com/2018/11/01/health/cellphone-radiation-cancer.html.

43. Knutson R. "Cellphone-Cancer Link Found in Government Study." *Wall Street Journal*. May 28, 2016. https://www.wsj.com/articles/cellphone-cancer-link -found-in-government-study-1464324146?mg=id-wsj.

44. "Telecommunications." Cornell Law School's Legal Information Institute. Accessed May 31, 2019. https://www.law.cornell.edu/uscode/text/47/332.

45. Norm Alster. *Captured Agency: How the Communications Commission Is Dominated by the Industry It Presumably Regulates*. Edmund J. Safra Institute for Ethics, Harvard University. Cambridge, Massachusetts. 2015.

46. Christopher Ketcham. "Warning: Your Cell Phone May Be Hazardous to Your Health." *GQ*. January 26 2010. https://www.gq.com/story/warning-cell-phone-radiation.

47. Daniel Lathro. "From Government Service to Private Practice: Writers of Telecom Law Move to K Street." Center for Public Integrity. October 28, 2004. http:// www.publicintegrity.org/2004/10/28/6597/government-service-private-practice.

48. Center for Responsive Politics. "AT&T, Inc: Summary." Open Secrets. Accessed March 4, 2019. https://www.opensecrets.org/lobby/clientsum .php?id=D000000076&year=2018.

49. Joel Moskowitz. "Cell Phones, Cell Towers, and Wireless Safety." https://www .youtube.com/watch?v=AgGRukb7qI4.

50. Lai H and Singh NP. "Acute Low-Intensity Microwave Exposure Increases DNA Single-Strand Breaks in Rat Brain Cells." *Bioelectromagnetics*. Vol. 16, no. 3. (1995): 207–210. doi: 10.1002/bem.2250160309.

51. "Motorola, Microwaves and DNA Breaks: 'War-Gaming' the Lai-Singh Experiments." *Microwave News*. Vol. 17, no. 1. January/February 1997: 13. https:// microwavenews.com/news/backissues/j-f97issue.pdf.

52. Frey AH, Feld SR, Frey B. "Neural Function and Behavior: Defining the Relationship." *Annals of the New York Academy of Sciences*. Vol. 247, no. 1. (February 1975): 433–439. https://nyaspubs.onlinelibrary.wiley.com/doi /abs/10.1111/j.1749-6632.1975.tb36019.x.

53. Christopher Ketcham. "Warning: Your Cell Phone May Be Hazardous to Your Health." *GQ*. January 25, 2010. https://www.gq.com/story/warning-cell-phone-radiation.

54. Paul Brodeur. *The Zapping of America: Microwaves, Their Deadly Risk and the Cover-Up.* Norton, 1977, p. 74.

55. Norm Alster. *Captured Agency: How the Federal Communications Commission Is Dominated by the Industries It Presumably Regulates.* Edmond J. Safra Center for Ethics, Harvard University. Cambridge, Massachusetts. 2015.

56. Alex Kotch of Sludge. "Revealed: How US Senators Invest in Firms They Are Supposed to Regulate." *The Guardian* and Sludge, an investigative news website focused on money in politics. September 19, 2019. https://amp.theguardian.com/us-news/2019/sep/19/us-senators-investments-conflict-of-interest?__twitter_impression=true.

57. Philip Shabecoff. "U.S. Sees Possible Cancer Tie to Electromagnetism." May 23, 1990. https://www.nytimes.com/1990/05/23/us/us-sees-possible-cancer-tie-to-electromagnetism.html.

58. "White House Report Argues EMFs Are Not a Public Health Issue." *Microwave News.* Vol. 12, no 6. (November/December 1992.) https://microwavenews.com/news/backissues/n-d92issue.pdf.

59. Portier CJ, Wolfe MS, editors. "Assessment of Health Effects from Exposure to Power-Line Frequency Electric and Magnetic Fields." National Institute of Environmental Health Sciences of the National Institutes of Health. 1998. http://niremf.ifac.cnr.it/docs/niehs98.pdf.

60. Yoram Wurmser. "Mobile Time Spent 2018: Will Smartphones Remain Ascendant?" June 18, 2018. https://www.emarketer.com/content/mobile-time-spent-2018.

61. Hardell L, Carlberg M, Mild KH. "Pooled Analysis of Case-Control Studies on Malignant Brain Tumours and the Use of Mobile and Cordless Phones Including Living and Deceased Subjects." *International Journal of Oncology.* Vol. 38, no 5. (2011): 1465–1474. doi: 10.3892/ijo.2011.947.

62. Danny Hakim. "At C.D.C., a Debate Behind Recommendations on Cellphone Risk." *New York Times.* January 1, 2016. https://www.nytimes.com/2016/01/02/technology/at-cdc-a-debate-behind-recommendations-on-cellphone-risk.html?_r=3.

63. "International Appeal: Scientists Call for Protection from Non-Ionizing Electromagnetic Field Exposure." EMFScientist.org. https://www.emfscientist.org/index.php/emf-scientist-appeal.

64. "ACS Responds to New Study Linking Cell Phone Radiation to Cancer." American Cancer Society. May 27, 2016. http://pressroom.cancer.org/NTP2016.

65. Proctor RN. "Tobacco and Health: Expert Witness Report Filed on Behalf of Plaintiffs in: 'The United States of America, Plaintiff, v. Philip Morris, Inc., et al., Defendants,' Civil Action No. 99-CV-02496 (GK)." May 10, 2002. http://www.columbia.edu/itc/hs/pubhealth/p9740/readings/tobacco-proctor.pdf.

66. Voosen P. "Hiroshima and Nagasaki Cast Long Shadows Over Radiation Science." *New York Times.* April 11, 2011. https://archive.nytimes.com/www.nytimes.com/gwire/2011/04/11/11greenwire-hiroshima-and-nagasaki-cast-long-shadows-over-99849.html?pagewanted=all.

67. Internal Brown & Williamson memo, August 21, 1969. https://www.industrydocumentslibrary.ucsf.edu/tobacco/docs/#id=qsdw0147.

Chapter 4: How EMFs Damage Your Body

1. Gultekin DH, Moeller L. "NMR Imaging of Cell Phone Radiation Absorption in Brain Tissue." *Proceedings of the National Academy of Sciences of the United States of America*. Vol. 110, no. 1. (January 2, 2013): 58–63. doi: 10.1073/pnas.1205598109.

2. Glaser, ZR, Ph.D. "Bibliography of Reported Biological Phenomena ('Effects') and Clinical Manifestations Attributed to Microwave and Radio-Frequency Radiation." Report No. 2, Revised. Naval Medical Research Institute. June 1971.

3. Goldsmith. JR. "Epidemiologic Evidence Relevant to Radar (Microwave) Effects." *Environmental Health Perspectives*. Vol. 105, suppl. 6. (1997): 1579–1587. doi: 10.1289/ehp.97105s61579.

4. Pall ML. "Wi-Fi Is an Important Threat to Human Health." *Environmental Research*. Vol. 164. (July 2018): 405–416. doi: 10.1016/j.envres.2018.01.035.

5. Pall ML. "How to Approach the Challenge of Minimizing Non-Thermal Health Effects of Microwave Radiation from Electrical Devices." *International Journal of Innovative Research in Engineering and Management*. Vol. 2, no. 5. (September 2015): 71–6.

6. Pall, ML. "Electromagnetic Fields Act via Activation of Voltage-Gated Calcium Channels to Produce Beneficial or Adverse Effects." *Journal of Cellular and Molecular Medicine*. Vol. 17, no. 8. (2013): 958–965. doi: 10.1111/jcmm.12088.

7. Piste P, Sayaji D, Avinash M. "Calcium and Its Role in Human Body." *International Journal of Research in Pharmaceutical and Biomedical Science*. Vol. 4. (2012): 2229–3701.

8. Demaurex N, Nunes P. "The Role of STIM and ORAI Proteins in Phagocytic Immune Cells." *American Journal of Physiology. Cell Physiology*. Vol. 310, no. 7. (April 2016): C496–C508. doi: 10.1152/ajpcell.00360.2015.

9. Walleczek J. "Electromagnetic Field Effects on Cells of the Immune System: The Role of Calcium Signaling." *FASEB Journal*. Vol. 6, no. 13. (1992): 3177–85. doi: 10.1096/fasebj.6.13.1397839.

10. Pall ML. "Wi-Fi Is an Important Threat to Human Health." *Environmental Research*. Vol. 164. (July 2018): 405–416. doi: 10.1016/j.envres.2018.01.035.

11. Pall ML. "Electromagnetic Fields Act via Activation of Voltage-Gated Calcium Channels to Produce Beneficial or Adverse Effects." *Journal of Cellular and Molecular Medicine*. Vol. 17, no. 8. (August 2013): 958–65. doi: 10.1111/jcmm.12088.

12. Vekaria HJ, et al. "Targeting Mitochondrial Dysfunction in CNS Injury Using Methylene Blue; Still a Magic Bullet?" *Neurochemical International*. Vol. 109. (October 2017): 117–125. doi: 10.1016/j.neuint.2017.04.004.

13. Pall ML. "Electromagnetic Fields Act Similarly in Plants as in Animals: Probable Activation of Calcium Channels via Their Voltage Sensor." *Current Chemical Biology*. Vol. 10, no. 1 (July 2016): 74–82. doi: 10.2174/2212796810666160419160433.

14. Santhosh Kumar S. "Colony Collapse Disorder (CCD) in Honey Bees Caused by EMF Radiation." *Bioinformation*. Vol. 14, no. 9. (December 21, 2018): 521–524. doi: 10.6026/97320630014521.

15. Dariusz Leszczy. "Henry Lai: Cautionary Words on 'Calcium Hypothesis' in the Science of EMF." *Between a Rock and a Hard Place* (blog). June 12, 2019. https://betweenrockandhardplace.wordpress.com/2019/06/12/henry-lai-cautionary-words-on-calcium-hypothesis-in-the-science-of-emf/.

16. Cheeseman KH, Slater TF. "An Introduction to Free Radical Biochemistry." *British Medical Bulletin*. Vol. 49, no. 3. (July 1993): 481–93. doi: 10.1093/oxfordjournals.bmb.a072625.

17. Sakihama Y, Maeda M, Hashimoto M, Tahara S, Hashidoko Y. "Beetroot Betalain Inhibits Peroxynitrite-Mediated Tyrosine Nitration and DNA Strand Damage." *Free Radical Research*. Vol. 46, no. 1. (2012): 93–9. doi: 10.3109/10715762.2011.641157.

18. Azizova OA, Panasenko OM, Vol'nova TV, Vladimirov YA. "Free Radical Lipid Oxidation Affects Cholesterol Transfer Between Lipoproteins and Erythrocytes." *Free Radical Biology & Medicine*. Vol. 7, no. 3. (1989): 251–7. doi: 10.1016/0891-5849(89)90132-9.

19. Lyras L, Perry RH, Perry EK, Ince PG, Jenner A, Jenner P, Halliwell B. "Oxidative Damage to Proteins, Lipids, and DNA in Cortical Brain Regions from Patients with Dementia with Lewy Bodies." *Journal of Neurochemistry*. Vol. 71, no. 1. (July 1998): 302–12. doi: 10.1046/j.1471-4159.1998.71010302.x.

20. Borys J, Maciejczyk M, Antonowicz B, Krętowski A, Sidun J, Domel E, Dąbrowski JR, Ładny JR, Morawska K, Zalewska A. "Glutathione Metabolism, Mitochondria Activity, and Nitrosative Stress in Patients Treated for Mandible Fractures." *Journal of Clinical Medicine*. Vol. 8, no. 1. (January 21, 2019): E127. doi: 10.3390/jcm8010127.

21. Tan DQ, Suda T. "Reactive Oxygen Species and Mitochondrial Homeostasis as Regulators of Stem Cell Fate and Function." *Antioxidants & Redox Signaling*. Vol. 29, no 2. (July 10, 2018): 149–168. doi: 10.1089/ars.2017.7273.

22. Cadet J, Douki T, Ravanat JL. "Oxidatively Generated Base Damage to Cellular DNA." *Free Radical Biology & Medicine*. Vol. 49, no. 1. (July 1, 2010): 9–21. doi: 10.1016/j.freeradbiomed.2010.03.025.

23. Pacher P, Beckman JS, Liaudet L. "Nitric Oxide and Peroxynitrite in Health and Disease." *Physiological Reviews*. Vol. 87, no. 1. (January 2007): 315–424. doi: 10.1152/physrev.00029.2006.

24. Reczek CR, Chandel NS. "ROS-Dependent Signal Transduction." *Current Opinion in Cell Biology*. Vol. 33. (April 2015): 8–13. doi: 10.1016/j.ceb.2014.09.010.

25. *Fat for Fuel*. Dr. Joseph Mercola. Hay House. Carlsbad, California. 2017.

26. Sohal RS, Weindruch R. "Oxidative Stress, Caloric Restriction, and Aging." *Science*. Vol. 273, no. 5271. (July 5, 1996): 59–63. doi: 10.1126/science.273.5271.59.

27. Salminena A, Kauppinenc A, Hiltunena M, Kaarnirantac K. "Krebs Cycle Intermediates Regulate DNA and Histone Methylation: Epigenetic Impact on the Aging Process." *Ageing Research Reviews*. Vol. 16. (July 2014): 45–65. doi: 10.1016/j.arr.2014.05.004.

28. Consales C, Merla C, Marino C, Benassi B. "Electromagnetic Fields, Oxidative Stress, and Neurodegeneration." *International Journal of Cell Biology*. Vol. 2012. (2012): 683897. doi: 10.1155/2012/683897.

29. Sawyer DT, Valentine J. "How Super Is Superoxide?" *Accounts of Chemical Research.* Vol. 14, no. 12. (December 1, 1981): 393–400.

30. Huie RE, Padmaja S. "The Reaction Rate of Nitric Oxide with Superoxide." *Free Radical Research Communications.* Vol. 18. (1993): 195–199.

31. Yetik-Anacak G, Catravas JD. "Nitric Oxide and the Endothelium: History and Impact on Cardiovascular Disease." *Vascular Pharmacology.* Vol. 45, no. 5. (November 2006): 268–276. doi: 10.1016/j.vph.2006.08.002.

32. Griffith TM, Edwards DH, Davies RL, Harrison TJ, Evans KT. "EDRF Co-ordinates the Behaviour of Vascular Resistance Vessels." *Nature.* Vol. 329. (1987): 442–445. https://www.nature.com/articles/329442a0.

33. Hibbs JB Jr. "Synthesis of Nitric Oxide from L-arginine: A Recently Discovered Pathway Induced by Cytokines with Antitumour and Antimicrobial Activities." *Research in Immunology.* Vol. 142, no. 7. (1991): 565–569. doi: 10.1016/0923 -2494(91)90103-P.

34. Förstermann U. "Nitric Oxide and Oxidative Stress in Vascular Disease." *Pflügers Archiv: European Journal of Physiology.* Vol. 459, no. 6. (May 2010): 923-39. doi: 10.1007/s00424-010-0808-2.

35. Ziche M, Morbidelli L. "Nitric Oxide and Angiogenesis." *Journal of Neuro-oncology.* Vol. 50, no. 1-2. (October-November 2000):13-48. doi: 10.1023/a:1006431309841.

36. Fode M, Jensen CFS, Østergren PB. "Sildenafil in Postprostatectomy Erectile Dysfunction (Perspective)." *International Journal of Impotence Research.* Vol. 31, no. 2. (March 2019): 61–64. doi: 10.1038/s41443-018-0102-y.

37. Pacher P, Szabo C. "Role of the Peroxynitrite-Poly(ADP-Ribose) Polymerase Pathway in Human Disease." *American Journal of Pathology.* Vol. 173, no. 1. (July 2008): 2–13. doi: 10.2353/ajpath.2008.080019.

38. Radi R. "Peroxynitrite, a Stealthy Biological Oxidant." *Journal of Biological Chemistry.* Vol. 288, no. 37. (September 13, 2013): 26464–26472. doi: 10.1074 /jbc.R113.472936.

39. Beckman JS, Beckman TW, Chen J, Marshall PA, Freeman BA. "Apparent Hydroxyl Radical Production by Peroxynitrite: Implications for Endothelial Injury from Nitric Oxide and Superoxide." *Proceedings of the National Academy of Sciences of the United States of America.* Vol. 87, no. 4. (February 1990): 1620–4. doi: 10.1073/pnas.87.4.1620.

40. Pacher P, Beckman JS, Liaudet L. "Nitric Oxide and Peroxynitrite in Health and Disease." *Physiological Reviews.* Vol. 87, no. 1. (January 2007); 315-424. doi: 10.1152/physrev.00029.2006.

41. Schwarz C, Kratochvil E, Pilger A, Kuster N, Adlkofer F, Rüdiger HW. "Radiofrequency Electromagnetic Fields (UMTS, 1,950 MHz) Induce Genotoxic Effects in Vitro in Human Fibroblasts but not in Lymphocytes." *International Archives of Occupational and Environmental Health.* Vol. 81, no. 6. (May 2008): 755–767. doi: 10.1007/s00420-008-0305-5.

42. Pall MP. "5G: Great Risk for EU, U.S. and International Health! Compelling Evidence for Eight Distinct Types of Great Harm Caused by Electromagnetic Field (EMF) Exposures and the Mechanism that Causes Them." EMF:data. May 17, 2018. https://www.emfdata.org/en/documentations/detail&id=243.

43. Lutz J, Adlkofer F. "Objections Against Current Limits for Microwave Radiation." Proceedings of the WFMN07, Chemnitz, Germany. (2007): 119–123. http://bemri.org/publications/icnirp/112-objections-against-the-current-limits-for-microwave-radiation.html.

44. Sivani S, Sudarsanam D. "Impacts of Radio-frequency Electromagnetic Field (RF-EMF) from Cell Phone Towers and Wireless Devices on Biosystem and Ecosystem – A Review." *Biology and Medicine*. Vol. 4, no. 4. (2012): 202–16. http://www.biolmedonline.com/Articles/Vol4_4_2012/Vol4_4_202-216_BM-8.pdf.

45. Cucurachi C, Tamis WL, Vijver MG, Peijnenburg WJ, Bolte JF, de Snoo GR. "A Review of the Ecological Effects of Radiofrequency Electromagnetic Fields (RF-EMF)." *Environment International*. Vol. 51. (2013): 116–40. doi: 10.1038/nature13290.

46. "Busy as a Bee: Pollinators Put Food on the Table." National Resources Defense Council. June, 2015. https://www.nrdc.org/sites/default/files/bee-deaths-FS.pdf.

47. Ellis J. "The Honey Bee Crisis." *Outlooks on Pest Management*. Vol. 23, no. 1. (February 2012): 34-40(6). doi: 10.1564/22feb10.

48. "Everything You Should Know About Colony Collapse Disorder and 'Disappearing' Bee Populations." ZME Science. April 3, 2019. https://geneticliteracyproject.org/2019/04/03/everything-you-should-know-about-colony-collapse-disorder-and-disappearing-bee-populations/.

49. Odemer R, Odemer F. "Effects of Radiofrequency Electromagnetic Radiation (RF-EMF) on Honey Bee Queen Development and Mating Success." *Science of the Total Environment*. Vol. 661. (April 15, 2019): 553-562. doi: 10.1016/j.scitotenv.2019.01.154.

50. Figueroa LL, Bergey EA. "Bumble Bees (Hymenoptera: Apidae) of Oklahoma: Past and Present Biodiversity." *Journal of the Kansas Entomological Society*. Vol. 88, no. 4. (October 1, 2015): 418-429. doi: 10.2317/0022-8567-88.4.418.

51. Favre D "Mobile Phone Induced Honeybee Worker Piping." *Apidologie*. Vol. 42. (2011): 270-9. https://link.springer.com/article/10.1007/s13592-011-0016-x.

52. Sharma VP and Kumar NK. "Changes in Honeybee Behaviour and Biology Under the Influence of Cellphone Radiations." *Current Science*. Vol. 98, no 10. (2010): 1376-8. https://www.researchgate.net/publication/225187745_Changes_in_honey_bee_behaviour_and_biology_under_the_influence_of_cell_phone_radiations.

53. Kimmel S, Kuhn J, Harst W, Stever H. "Electromagnetic Radiation: Influences on Honeybees (Apis mellifera)." *IIAS-InterSymp Conference*. 2007. https://www.researchgate.net/publication/228510851_Electromagnetic_Radiation_Influences_on_Honeybees_Apis_mellifera.

54. Harst W, Harst JK, Stever H. "Can Electromagnetic Exposure Cause a Change in Behaviour? Studying Possible Non-thermal Influences on Honey Bees – An Approach Within the Framework of Educational Informatics." *Acta Systemica-IIAS International Journal*. Vol 6, no. 1. (2006): 1-6. http://www.next-up.org/pdf/ICRW_Kuhn_Landau_study.pdf.

55. Margaritis LH, Manta AK, Kokkaliaris KD, Schiza D, Alimisis K, Barkas G, Georgiou E, Giannakopoulou O, Kollia I, Kontogianna G, Kourouzidou A, Myari A, Roumelioti F, Skouroliakou A, Sykioti V, Varda G, Xenos K, Ziomas K. "Drosophila Oogenesis as a Biomarker Responding to EMF Sources." *Electromagnetic Biology and Medicine*, vol. 33, no. 3, 2014, pp. 165-89. doi: 10.3109/15368378.2013.800102.

56. Sánchez-Bayo F, Wyckhuys KAG. "Worldwide Decline of the Entomofauna: A Review of its Drivers." *Biological Conservation*. Vol. 232. (2019): 8-27. doi: 10.1016/j.biocon.2019.01.020.

57. Damian Carrington. "Plummeting Insect Numbers 'Threaten Collapse of Nature." *The Guardian*. February 10, 2019. https://www.theguardian.com /environment/2019/feb/10/plummeting-insect-numbers-threaten-collapse-of -nature.

58. Pall M. "Electromagnetic Fields Act Similarly in Plants as in Animals: Probable Activation of Calcium Channels via Their Voltage Sensor." *Current Chemical Biology*. Vol. 10, no. 1. (2016). doi: 10.2174/2212796810666160419160433.

59. Soran, ML, Stan M, Niinemets Ü, Copolovici L. "Influence of Microwave Frequency Electromagnetic Radiation on Terpene Emission and Content in Aromatic Plants." *Journal of Plant Physiology*. Vol. 171, no. 15. (2014): 1436-43. doi: 0.1016/j.jplph.2014.06.013.

60. Beaubois E, Girard S, Lallechere S, Davies E, Paladian F, Bonnet P, Ledoigt G, Vian A. "Intercellular Communication in Plants: Evidence for Two Rapidly Transmitted Signals Generated in rRsponse to Electromagnetic Field Stimulation in Tomato." *Plant, Cell & Environment*. Vol. 30. (2007): 840-4. doi: 10.1111/j.1365-3040.2007.01669.x

61. Waldmann-Selsam C, Balmori-de la Puente A, Breunig H, Balmori A. "Radiofrequency Radiation Injures Trees Around Mobile Phone Base Stations." *Science of the Total Environment*. Vol. 572. (2016): 554-69. doi: 10.1016/j .scitotenv.2016.08.045.

62. Haggerty K. "Adverse Influence of Radio Frequency Background on Trembling Aspen Seedlings." *International Journal of Forestry Research*. Vol. 2010, no. 836278. (2010). doi: 10.1155/2010/836278.

63. Halgamuge MN. "Weak Radiofrequency Radiation Exposure from Mobile Phone Radiation on Plants." *Electromagnetic Biology and Medicine*. Vol. 36, no. 2. (2017): 213-235. doi: 10.1080/15368378.2016.1220389.

64. Grimaldi S, Pasquali R, Barbatano L, Lisi A, Santoro N, Serafino A, Pozzi D. "Exposure to a 50Hz Electromagnetic Field Induces Activation of the Epstein-Barr Virus Genome in Latently Infected Human Lyphoid Cells." *Journal of Environmental Pathology, Toxicology, and Oncology*. Vol. 16, no. 2-3. (1997): 205-7.

65. Dietrich Klinghardt. "Electromagnetic Fields: Their Effect on Your Biology and the Development of an Autistic Child." https://www.youtube.com/watch?v=qMAV -pZMlZs.

66. Voïchuk SI, Podgorskiï VS, Gromozova EN. "Effect of Radio-frequency Electromagnetic Radiation on Physiological Features of Saccharomyces Cerevisiae Strain UCM Y-517." *Microbiology Journal*. Vol. 66, no. 3. (May-June 2004): 51-57.

67. Hadjiloucas S, Chahal MS, Bowen JW. "Preliminary Results on the Non-thermal Effects of 200-350 GHz Radiation on the Growth Rate of S. cerevisiae cells in Microcolonies." *Physics in Medicine and Biology.* Vol. 47, no. 21. (November 7, 2002): 3831-9. doi: 10.1088/0031-9155/47/21/322.

68. Taheri M, Mortazavi SM, Moradi M, Mansouri S, Hatam GR, Nouri F. "Evaluation of the Effect of Radiofrequency Radiation Emitted From Wi-Fi Router and Mobile Phone Simulator on the Antibacterial Susceptibility of Pathogenic Bacteria *Listeria monocytogenes* and *Escherichia coli. Dose Response.*" Vol. 15, no. 1. (2017): 1559325816688527. doi: 10.1177/1559325816688527.

69. Hiscock HG, Mouritsen H, Manolopoulos DE, Hore PJ. "Disruption of Magnetic Compass Orientation in Migratory Birds by Radiofrequency Electromagnetic Fields." *Biophysical Journal.* Vol. 113, no. 7. (2017): 1475–1484. doi:10.1016/j.bpj.2017.07.031.

70. Malkemper EP, Eder SHK, Phillips JB, Winklhofer M, Hart V, Burda H. "Magnetoreception in the Wood Mouse (*Apodemus sylvaticus*): Influence of Weak Frequency-modulated Radio Frequency Fields." *Scientific Reports.* Vol. 4, no. 9917. (2015). https://www.nature.com/articles/srep09917.

71. Ernst DA, Lohmann, KJ."Effect of Magnetic Pulses on Caribbean Spiny Lobsters: Implications for Magnetoreception." *Journal of Experimental Biology.* Vol. 219, no. 12. (2016): 1827-32. 2016. doi: 10.1242/jeb.136036.

72. Balmori, A. "Mobile Phone Mast Effects on Common Frog (Rana temporaria) Tadpoles." *Electromagnetic Biology and Medicine.* Vol. 29, no. 1-2. (2010): 31-5. doi: 0.3109/15368371003685363.

73. Hillman D, Goeke CL, Moser R. "Electric and Magnetic Fields (EMF) Affect Milk Production and Behavior of Cows; Results Using Shielded Neutral Isolation Transformer." EE 12 International Conference on Production Diseases in Farm Animals, Michigan State University. Published by: Shocking News, 750 Berkshire Lane, East Lansing, Michigan. July 2004. http://www.electricalpollution.com /documents/Hillman/ShockingNewsv3-072004.pdf.

74. Nicholls B, Racey PA. "Bats Avoid Radar Installations: Could Electro-magnetic Fields Deter Bats from Colliding with Wind Turbines?" *PLOS One.* Vol. 3, no. e297. (2007). doi: 10.1371/journal.pone.0000297.

75. Morgan LL, Kesari S, Davis DL. "Why Children Absorb More Microwave Radiation Than Adults: The Consequences." *Journal of Microscopy and Ultrastructure.* Vol. 2, no 4. (December 2014): 197–204. doi: 10.1016/j.jmau.2014.06.005.

76. Ibid.

77. Bioelectric Shield. "The Risks of Cellphone Radiation for Children—and How to Protect Them." *Epoch Times.* February 27, 2017. https://www.theepochtimes .com/the-risks-of-cellphone-radiation-for-children-and-how-to-protect-them-2_2223846.html.

78. Melody Gutierrez, "State Kept Secret Guidelines on Safe Cell Phone Use." SFGate. March 3, 2017. https://www.sfgate.com/news/article/Judge-may-order-release-of -state-health-report-on-10973430.php.

79. Gandhi OP, Lazzi G, Furse CM. "Electromagnetic Absorption in the Human Head and Neck for Mobile Telephones at 835 and 1900 MHz." *IEEE Transactions on Microwave Theory and Techniques.* Vol. 44, no. 10. (1996): 1884–1897. doi: 10.1109/22.539947.

80. Gandhi OP, Morgan LL, Augusto de Salles A, Han Y, Herberman RB, Davis DL. "Exposure Limits: The Underestimation of Absorbed Cell Phone Radiation, Especially in Children." *Electromagnetic Biology and Medicine*. (2012): 1–18. doi: 10.3109/15368378.2011.622827.

81. International Agency for Research on Cancer. "Non-Ionizing Radiation, Part 2: Radiofrequency Electromagnetic Fields." Vol. 102. (2013): 44. https://monographs .iarc.fr/iarc-monographs-on-the-evaluation-of-carcinogenic-risks-to-humans-14/.

82. Divan HA, Kheifets L, Obel C, Olsen J. "Prenatal and Postnatal Exposure to Cell Phone Use and Behavioral Problems in Children." *Epidemiology*. Vol. 19, no. 4. (July 2008): 523–9. doi: 10.1097/EDE.0b013e318175dd47.

83. Ibid.

84. Divan HA, Kheifets L, Obel C, *Olsen J*. "Cell Phone Use and Behavioural Problems in Young Children." *Journal of Epidemiology and Community Health*. Vol. 66, no. 6. (June 2012): 524–529. doi: 10.1136/jech.2010.115402.

85. Li D, Ferber JR, Odouli R, Quesenberry, Jr CP. "A Prospective Study of In-Utero Exposure to Magnetic Fields and the Risk of Childhood Obesity." *Scientific Reports*. Vol. 2, no. 540. (2012). https://www.nature.com/articles/srep00540.

86. Li D, Chen H, Odouli R. "Maternal Exposure to Magnetic Fields During Pregnancy in Relation to the Risk of Asthma in Offspring." *Archives of Pediatric and Adolescent Medicine*. Vol. 165, no. 10. (October 2011): 945–950. doi: 10.1001/archpediatrics.2011.135.

87. Birks L, Guxens M, Papadopoulou E, Alexander J, Ballester F, Estarlich M, Gallastegi M, Ha M, Haugen M, Huss A, Kheifets L, Lim H, Olsen J, Santa-Marina L, Sudan M, Vermeulen R, Vrijkotte T, Cardis E, Vrijheid M. "Maternal Cell Phone Use During Pregnancy and Child Behavioral Problems in Five Birth Cohorts." *Environment International*. Vol. 104. (July 2017): 122–131. doi: 10.1016/j.envint.2017.03.024.

88. Li DK, Chen H, Ferber JR, Odouli R, Quesenberry C. "Exposure to Magnetic Field Non-Ionizing Radiation and the Risk of Miscarriage: A Prospective Cohort Study." *Scientific Reports*. Vol. 7, no 1. (December 13, 2017): 17541. doi: 10.1038 /s41598-017-16623-8.

89. Li DK, Chen H, Odouli R. "Maternal Exposure to Magnetic Fields During Pregnancy in Relation to the Risk of Asthma in Offspring." *Archives of Pediatrics and Adolescent Medicines*. Vol. 165, no. 10. (October 2011): 945–50. doi: 10.1001 /archpediatrics.2011.135.

90. Li DK, Ferber JR, Odouli R, Quesenberry CP Jr. "A Prospective Study of In-Utero Exposure to Magnetic Fields and the Risk of Childhood Obesity." *Scientific Reports*. Vol. 2. (July 27, 2012): 540. doi: 10.1038/srep00540.

91. Li DK. "Adverse Fetal and Childhood Health Effect of In-Utero Exposure to Magnetic Fields Non-ionizing Radiation." Division of Research, Kaiser Foundation Research Institute, Kaiser Permanente. Accessed August 15, 2019. https://www.healthandenvironment.org/docs/De-KunLiSlidesv3.2018-5-9.pdf.

92. Thomas S, Heinrich S, von Kries R, Radon K. "Exposure to Radio-Frequency Electromagnetic Fields and Behavioural Problems in Bavarian Children and Adolescents." *European Journal of Epidemiology*. Vol. 25, no. 2. (February 2010): 135–141. doi: 10.1007/s10654-009-9408-x.

93. Li DK. "Adverse Fetal and Childhood Health Effect of In-Utero Exposure to Magnetic Fields Non-ionizing Radiation." Division of Research, Kaiser Foundation Research Institute, Kaiser Permanente. Accessed August 15, 2019. https://www.healthandenvironment.org/docs/De-KunLiSlidesv3.2018-5-9.pdf.

94. Sage C, Burgio E. "Electromagnetic Fields, Pulsed Radiofrequency Radiation, and Epigenetics: How Wireless Technologies May Affect Childhood Development." *Child Development*. Vol. 89. (2018): 129–136. doi: 10.1111/cdev.12824.

95. Martin Pall. "The Autism Epidemic Is Caused by EMFs, Acting via Calcium Channels and Chemicals Acting via NMDA-Rs." AutismOne Media. June 10, 2015. https://www.youtube.com/watch?v=yydZZanRJ50.

96. Breitenkamp AF, Matthes J, Herzig S. "Voltage-Gated Calcium Channels and Autism Spectrum Disorders." *Current Molecular Pharmacology*. Vol. 8, no. 2. (2015): 123. doi: 10.2174/1874467208666150507105235.

97. Golomb, BA. "Diplomats' Mystery Illness and Pulsed Radiofrequency/Microwave Radiation." *Neural Computation*. (September 5, 2018): 1–104. doi: 10.1162 /neco_a_01133.

98. De Luca C, Chung Sheun Thai J, Raskovic D, Cesareo E, Caccamo D, Trukhanov A, Korkina L. "Metabolic and Genetic Screening of Electromagnetic Hypersensitive Subjects as a Feasible Tool for Diagnostics and Intervention." *Mediators of Inflammation*. Vol. 2014. (April 9, 2014). doi: 10.1155/2014/924184.

99. Lee SS, Kim HR, Kim MS, Park SH, Kim DW. "Influence of Smart Phone Wi-Fi Signals on Adipose-Derived Stem Cells." *Journal of Craniofacial Surgery*. Vol. 25, no. 5. (September 2014): 1902–1907. doi: 10.1097/SCS.0000000000000939.

100. Belyaev IY, Markovà E, Hillert L, Malmgren LO, Persson BR. "Microwaves from UMTS/GSM Mobile Phones Induce Long-Lasting Inhibition of 53BP1/gamma-H2AX DNA Repair Foci in Human Lymphocytes." *Bioelectromagnetics*. Vol. 30, no. 2. (February 2009): 129–141. doi: 10.1002/bem.20445.

101. Markovà E, Malmgren LO, Belyaev IY. "Microwaves from Mobile Phones Inhibit 53BP1 Focus Formation in Human Stem Cells More Strongly Than in Differentiated Cells: Possible Mechanistic Link to Cancer Risk." *Environmental Health Perspectives*. Vol. 118, no. 3. (March 1, 2010): 394–399. doi: 10.1289 /ehp.0900781.

102. Czyz J, Guan K, Zeng Q, Nikolova T, Meister A, Schönborn F, Schuderer J, Kuster N, Wobus AM. "High Frequency Electromagnetic Fields (GSM Signals) Affect Gene Expression Levels in Tumor Suppressor p53-Deficient Embryonic Stem Cells." *Bioelectromagnetics*. Vol. 25, no. 4. (May 2004): 296–307. doi: 10.1002/bem.10199.

103. Xu F, Bai Q, Zhou K, Ma L, Duan J, Zhuang F, Xie C, Li W, Zou P, Zhu C. "Age-Dependent Acute Interference with Stem and Progenitor Cell Proliferation in the Hippocampus after Exposure to 1800 MHz Electromagnetic Radiation." *Electromagnetic Biology and Medicine*. Vol. 36, no. 2. (2017): 213–35. doi: 10.1080/15368378.2016.

104. H. Bhargav, T.M. Srinivasan, S. Varambally, B.N. Gangadhar, P. Koka. "Effect of Mobile Phone-Induced Electromagnetic Field on Brain Hemodynamics and Human Stem Cell Functioning: Possible Mechanistic Link to Cancer Risk and Early Diagnostic Value of Electronphotonic Imaging." *Journal of Stem Cells*. Vol. 10, no. 4. (2015): 287–294. doi: jsc.2015.10.4.287.

105. Odaci E, Bas O, Kaplan S. "Effects of Prenatal Exposure to a 900 MHz Electromagnetic Field on the Dentate Gyrus of Rats: a Stereological and Histopathological Study." *Brain Research*. Vol. 1238 (October 31, 2008): 224–229. doi: 10.1016/j.brainres.2008.08.013.

106. Uchugonova A, Isemann A, Gorjup E, Tempea G, Bückle R, Watanabe W, König K. "Optical Knock Out of Stem Cells with Extremely Ultrashort Femtosecond Laser Pulses." *Journal of Biophotonics*. Vol. 1, no. 6. (2008): 463–469. doi: 10.1002/jbio.200810047.

107. Wang C, Wang X, Zhou H, Dong G, Guan X, Wang L, Xu X, Wang S, Chen P, Peng R, Hu X. "Effects of Microwave Exposure on BM-MSCs Isolated from C57BL/6 Mice." *PLoS One*. Vol. 10, no. 2. (2015): e0117550, doi: 10.1371/journal.pone.0117550.

108. Teven CM, Greives M, Natale RB, Su Y, Luo Q, He BC, Shenaq D, He TC, Reid RR. "Differentiation of Osteoprogenitor Cells Is Induced by High-Frequency Pulsed Electromagnetic Fields." *Journal of Craniofacial Surgery*. Vol. 23, no. 2. (March 2012): 586–593. doi: 10.1097/SCS.0b013e31824cd6de.

109. Xu F, Bai Q, Zhou K, Ma L, Duan J, Zhuang F, Xie C, Li W, Zou P, Zhu C. "Age-Dependent Acute Interference with Stem and Progenitor Cell Proliferation in the Hippocampus After Exposure to 1800 MHz Electromagnetic Radiation." *Electromagnetic Biology and Medicine*. Vol. 36, no. 2. (2017): 213–35. doi: 10.1080/15368378.2016.

110. Bhargav H, Srinivasan TM, Varambally S, Gangadhar BN, Koka P. "Effect of Mobile Phone-Induced Electromagnetic Field on Brain Hemodynamics and Human Stem Cell Functioning: Possible Mechanistic Link to Cancer Risk and Early Diagnostic Value of Electronphotonic Imaging." *Journal of Stem Cells*. Vol. 10, no. 4. (2015): 287–294. doi: jsc.2015.10.4.287.

111. Herbert MR, Sage C. "Autism and EMF? Plausibility of a Pathophysiological Link – Part I." *Pathophysiology*. Vol. 20, no. 3. (2013): 191–209. doi: 10.1016/j.pathophys.2013.08.001.

112. Mariea TJ, Carlo GL. "Wireless Radiation in the Etiology and Treatment of Autism: Clinical Observations and Mechanisms." *Journal of Australasian College of Nutrition and Environmental Medicine*. Vol. 26, no. 2. (2007): 3–7.

113. Thornton I. "Out of Time: A Possible Link Between Mirror Neurons, Autism and Electromagnetic Radiation." *Medical Hypotheses*. Vol. 67, no. 2. (2006): 378–382. doi: 10.1016/j.mehy.2006.01.032.

114. Currenti SA. "Understanding and Determining the Etiology of Autism." *Cellular Molecular Neurobiology*. Vol. 30, no. 2. (March 2010): 161–171. doi: 10.1007/s10571-009-9453-8.

115. Pino-Lopez M, Romero-Ayuso DM. "Parental Occupational Exposures and Autism Spectrum Disorder in Children." *Revista Española de Salud Pública*. Vol. 87. (2013): 73–85. doi: 10.4321/S1135-57272013000100008.

116. Kane RC. "A Possible Association Between Fetal/Neonatal Exposure to Radiofrequency Electromagnetic Radiation and the Increased Frequency of Autism Spectrum Disorders (ASD)." *Medical Hypotheses*. Vol. 62, no. 2. (2004): 195–197. doi: 10.1016/S0306-9877(03)00309-8.

117. Lathe R. "Electromagnetic Radiation and Autism." *E-Journal of Applied Psychology*. Vol. 5. (2009): 11–30. doi: 10.7790/ejap.v5i1.144.

118. Goldworthy A. "How Electromagnetically-induced Cell Leakage May Cause Autism." (2011). http://electromagnetichealth.org/wp-content/uploads/2011/05/Autism_2011_b.pdf.

119. Herbert MR, Sage C. "Autism and EMF? Plausibility of a Pathophysiological Link – Part I." *Pathophysiology.* Vol. 20, no. 3. (2013): 191–209. doi: 10.1016/j.pathophys.2013.08.001.

120. Herbert MR, Sage C. "Autism and EMF? Plausibility of a Pathophysiological Link-Part II." *Pathophysiology.* Vol. 20, no. 3. (June 2013): 211–234. doi: 10.1016/j.pathophys.2013.08.002.

121. Sullivan P. "Understanding Autism." 2013. https://www.youtube.com/watch?v=muMVAK19GTM.

122. "Data & Statistics on Autism Spectrum Disorder." Centers for Disease Control and Prevention. Accessed May 30, 2019. https://www.cdc.gov/ncbddd/autism/data.html.

123. Kogan MD, Vladutiu CJ, Schieve LA, Ghandour RM, Blumberg SJ, Zablotsky B, Perrin JM, Shattuck P, Kuhlthau KA, Harwood RL, Lu MC. "The Prevalence of Parent-Reported Autism Spectrum Disorder among US Children." *Pediatrics.* Vol. 142, no. 6. (December 2018): e20174161. doi: 10.1542/peds.2017-4161.

124. Katie Singer. "Calming Behavior in Children with Autism and ADHD." The Weston A. Price Foundation. August 22, 2016. https://www.westonaprice.org/health-topics/childrens-health/calming-behavior-children-autism-adhd/. Peter Sullivan. "Wireless and EMF Reduction for Autism." Clear Light Ventures. July 31, 2014. http://www.clearlightventures.com/blog/2014/07/emf-reduction-for-autism.html.

125. "Autism May Be Linked to Electromagnetic Radiation Levels In Mother's Bedroom During Pregnancy." Electromagnetichealth.org. Accessed May 30 2019. http://electromagnetichealth.org/media-stories/#Autism.

126. Adam Popescu. "Keep Your Head Up: How Smartphone Addiction Kills Manners and Moods." *New York Times.* January 25, 2018. https://www.nytimes.com/2018/01/25/smarter-living/bad-text-posture-neckpain-mood.html.

127. "The New Normal: Parents, Teens, and Devices around the World." Common Sense Media. Accessed May 30, 2019. https://www.commonsensemedia.org/research/The-New-Normal-Parents-Teens-and-Devices-Around-the-World.

128. Vernon L, Modecki KL, Barber BL. "Mobile Phones in the Bedroom: Trajectories of Sleep Habits and Subsequent Adolescent Psychosocial Development." *Child Development.* Vol. 89, no. 1. (January–February 2018): 66–77. doi: 10.1111/cdev.12836.

129. Twenge JM, Joiner TE, Rogers ML, and Martin GN. (2018). "Increases in Depressive Symptoms, Suicide-Related Outcomes, and Suicide Rates among U.S. Adolescents after 2010 and Links to Increased New Media Screen Time." *Clinical Psychological Science*, Vol. 6, no. 1. (2018): 3–17. doi: 10.1177/2167702617723376.

130. Hedegaard H, Curtin SC, Warner M. "Suicide Rates in the United States Continue to Increase." National Center of Health Statistics. NCHS Data Brief. No. 309. June 2018. https://www.cdc.gov/nchs/products/databriefs/db309.htm.

131. Anthony Cuthbertson. "iPhones Pose Suicide Risk to Teenagers, Apple Investors Warn." *Newsweek.* January 18, 2018. http://www.newsweek.com/iphones-pose-suicide-risk-teenagers-apple-investors-warn-773819.
    Lumb, David. "Kids Are Overusing iPhones, Warn Apple Investors." Engadget. January 8, 2018. https://www.engadget.com/2018/01/08/kids-are-overusing-iphones-warn-two-apple-investors/.

132. Juli Clover. "How to Use Screen Time in iOS 12." MacRumors. September 19, 2018. https://www.macrumors.com/how-to/how-to-use-screen-time-in-ios-12/.

133. Alissa J. Rubin and Elian Peltier. "France Bans Smartphones in Schools through 9th Grade. Will It Help Students?" *New York Times.* September 20, 2018. https://www.nytimes.com/2018/09/20/world/europe/france-smartphones-schools.html.

134. Mikko Ahonen, "Why Are Some Countries Removing Wi-Fi in Schools and Others Not?" Wireless Education. Accessed May 28, 2019. https://www.wirelesseducation.org/1073-2.

135. "Worldwide Precautionary Action." Parents for Safe Technology. Accessed May 28, 2019. http://www.parentsforsafetechnology.org/worldwide-countries-taking-action.html.

136. "Mobile Kids: The Parent, the Child and the Smartphone." Nielsen. February 28, 2017. https://www.nielsen.com/us/en/insights/news/2017/mobile-kids--the-parent-the-child-and-the-smartphone.html.
    "The Common Sense Census: Media Use by Kids Age Zero to Eight 2017." Common Sense Media. Accessed May 28, 2019. https://www.commonsensemedia.org/research/the-common-sense-census-media-use-by-kids-age-zero-to-eight-2017.

137. Jacqueline Howard. "When Kids Get Their First Cellphones around the World." CNN Health. December 11, 2017. https://www.cnn.com/2017/12/11/health/cell-phones-for-kids-parenting-without-borders-explainer-intl/.

138. "Quarter of Children Under Six Have a Smartphone, Study Finds." *The Independent.* April 8, 2018.

139. Monica Anderson and Jingjing Jiang. "Teens, Social Media & Technology 2018." Pew Research Center. May 31, 2018. https://www.pewinternet.org/2018/05/31/teens-social-media-technology-2018/.

Chapter 5: EMFs and Disease

1. Landgrebe M, Frick U, Hauser S, Hajak G, Langguth B. "Association of Tinnitus and Electromagnetic Hypersensitivity: Hints for a Shared Pathophysiology?" *PLoS One.* Vol. 4, no. 3. (2009): e5026. doi: 10.1371/journal.pone.0005026.

2. Mayo Clinic. "Tinnitus." Mayo Clinic. Accessed March 19, 2019. https://www.mayoclinic.org/diseases-conditions/tinnitus/symptoms-causes/syc-20350156.

3. Dobie RA. "A Review of Randomized Clinical Trials in Tinnitus." *Laryngoscope.* Vol. 109, no. 8. (August 1999): 1202–11. doi: 10.1097/00005537-199908000-00004.

4. Nittby H, Grafström G, Tian DP, Malmgren L, Brun A, Persson BR, Salford LG, Eberhardt J. "Cognitive Impairment in Rats after Long-Term Exposure to GSM-900 Mobile Phone Radiation." *Bioelectromagnetics.* Vol. 29, no. 3. (April 2008): 219–232. doi: 10.1002/bem.20386.

5. Krause CM, Pesonen M, Haarala BC, Hamalainen H. "Effects of Pulsed and Continuous Wave 902 MHz Mobile Phone Exposure on Brain Oscillatory Activity during Cognitive Processing." *Bioelectromagnetics*. Vol. 28, no. 4. (May 2007): 296–308. doi: 10.1002/bem.20300.

6. Papageorgiou CC, Nanou ED, Tsiafakis VG, Kapareliotis E, Kontoangelos KA, Capsalis CN, Rabavilas AD, Soldatos CR. "Acute Mobile Phone Effects on Pre-Attentive Operation." *Neuroscience Letters*. Vol. 397, no. 1–2. (April 2006): 99–103. doi: 10.1016/j.neulet.2005.12.001.

7. Maier R, Greter SE, Maier N. "Effects of Pulsed Electromagnetic Fields on Cognitive Processes - a Pilot Study on Pulsed Field Interference with Cognitive Regeneration." *Acta Neurologica Scandinavica*. Vol. 110, no. 1. (July 2004): 46–52. doi: 10.1111/j.1600-0404.2004.00260.x.

8. Hutter HP, Moshammer H, Wallner P, Cartellieri M, Denk-Linnert DM, Katzinger M, Ehrenberger K, Kundi M. "Tinnitus and Mobile Phone Use." Occupational *and Environmental Medicine*. Vol. 67, no. 12. (December 2010): 804–808. doi: 10.1136/oem.2009.048116.

9. Holgers K-M. "Tinnitus in 7-Year-Old Children." *European Journal of Pediatrics*. Vol. 162, no. 4. (April 2003): 276–78. doi: 10.1007/s00431-003-1183-1.

10. Holgers K-M and Juul J. "The Suffering of Tinnitus in Childhood and Adolescence." *International Journal of Audiology*. Vol. 45, no. 5. (May 2006): 267–72. doi: 10.1080/14992020500485668.

11. Bormusov E, Andle U, Sharon N, Schächter L, Lahav A, Dovrat A. "Non-Thermal Electromagnetic Radiation Damage to Lens Epithelium." *Open Ophthalmology Journal*. Vol. 2. (May 21, 2008): 102–106. doi: 10.2174/1874364100802010102.

12. Yu Y, Yao K. "Non-Thermal Cellular Effects of Low-Power Microwave Radiation on the Lens and Lens Epithelial Cells." *Journal of International Medical Research*. Vol. 38, no. 3. (June 2010): 729–736. doi: 10.1177/147323001003800301.

13. Parathath SR, Parathath S, Tsirka SE. "Nitric Oxide Mediates Neurodegeneration and Breakdown of the Blood-Brain Barrier in tPA-Dependent Excitotoxic Injury in Mice." *Journal of Cell Science*. Vol. 119. (January 15, 2006): 339–349. doi: 10.1242/jcs.02734.

14. Salford LG, Brun A, Sturesson K, Eberhardt JL, Persson BR. "Permeability of the Blood-Brain Barrier Induced by 915 MHz Electromagnetic Radiation, Continuous Wave and Modulated at 8, 16, 50, and 200 Hz." *Microscopy Research and Technique*. Vol. 27, no. 6. (April 15, 1994): 535–42. doi: 10.1002/jemt.1070270608.

15. Nittby H, Brun A, Eberhardt J, Malmgren L, Persson BR, Salford LG. "Increased Blood-Brain Barrier Permeability in Mammalian Brain 7 Days After Exposure to the Radiation from a GSM-900 Mobile Phone." *Pathophysiology*. Vol. 16, no. 2–3. (August 2009): 103–12. doi: 10.1016/j.pathophys.2009.01.001.

16. Tang J, Zhang Y, Yang L, Chen Q, Tan L, Zuo S, Feng H, Chen Z, Zhu G. "Exposure to 900 MHz Electromagnetic Fields Activates the mkp-1/ERK Pathway and Causes Blood-Brain Barrier Damage and Cognitive Impairment in Rats." *Brain Research*. Vol. 1601. (March 19, 2015): 92–101. doi: 10.1016/j.brainres.2015.01.019.

17. Salford LG, Nittby H, Persson BRR. "Effects of Electromagnetic Fields from Wireless Communication upon the Blood-Brain Barrier." Prepared for the

BioInitiative Working Group. September 2012. https://bioinitiative.org/wp -content/uploads/pdfs/sec10_2012_Effects_Electromagnetic_Fields_Wireless _Communication.pdf.

18. Bagheri Hosseinabadi M, Khanjani N, Ebrahimi MH, Haji B, Abdolahfard M. "The Effect of Chronic Exposure to Extremely Low-Frequency Electromagnetic Fields on Sleep Quality, Stress, Depression and Anxiety." *Electromagnetic Biology and Medicine*. Vol. 38, no. 1. (2019): 96–101. doi: 10.1080/15368378.2018.1545665.

19. Thomée S. "Mobile Phone Use and Mental Health. A Review of the Research That Takes a Psychological Perspective on Exposure." *International Journal of Environmental Research and Public Health*. Vol. 15, no. 12. (November 29, 2018): E2692. doi: 10.3390/ijerph15122692.

20. Ibrahim NK, Baharoon BS, Banjar WF, Jar AA, Ashor RM, Aman AA, Al-Ahmadi JR. "Mobile Phone Addiction and Its Relationship to Sleep Quality and Academic Achievement of Medical Students at King Abdulaziz University, Jeddah, Saudi Arabia." *Journal of Research in Health Science*. Vol. 18, no. 3. (August 4, 2018): e00420.

21. Zhang J, Sumich A, Wang G. "Acute Effects of Radiofrequency Electromagnetic Field Emitted by Mobile Phone on Brain Function." *Bioelectromagnetics*. Vol. 38, no. 5. (July 2017): 329–338. doi: 10.1002/bem.22052.

22. Matthew Walker. *Why We Sleep: Unlocking the Power of Sleep and Dreams*. Scribner's. New York City. 2018.

23. Griefahn B, Kunemund C, Blaszkewicz M, Lerchl A, Degen GH. "Effects of Electromagnetic Radiation (Bright Light, Extremely Low-Frequency Magnetic Fields, Infrared Radiation) on the Circadian Rhythm of Melatonin Synthesis, Rectal Temperature, and Heart Rate." *Industrial Health*. Vol. 40, no. 4. (October 2002): 320–7. doi: 10.2486/indhealth.40.320.
Reiter RJ. "Electromagnetic Fields and Melatonin Production." *Biomedicine & Pharmacotherapy*. Vol. 47, no. 10. (1993): 439–44.
Weydahl A, Sothern RB, Cornélissen G, Wetterberg L. "Geomagnetic Activity Influences the Melatonin Secretion at Latitude 70° N." *Biomedicine & Pharmacotherapy*. Vol. 55, Supplement 1. (November 11, 2000): s57–s62. doi: 10.1016/S0753-3322(01)90006-X.
Burch JB, Reif JS, Yost MG. "Geomagnetic Disturbances Are Associated with Reduced Nocturnal Excretion of a Melatonin Metabolite in Humans." *Neuroscience Letters*. Vol. 266, no. 3. (May 14, 1999): 209–12. doi: 10.1016/s0304 -3940(99)00308-0.
Reiter RJ. "Melatonin Suppression by Static and Extremely Low Frequency Electromagnetic Fields: Relationship to the Reported Increased Incidence of Cancer." *Review of Environmental Health*. Vol. 10, no. 3–4. (1994): 171–86.

24. Neil Cherry. "EMF/EMR Reduces Melatonin in Animals and People." September 2, 2002. https://hdl.handle.net/10182/3906.

25. Aynali G, Nazıroğlu M, Çelik Ö, Doğan M, Yarıktaş M, Yasan H. "Modulation of Wireless (2.45 GHz)-Induced Oxidative Toxicity in Laryngotracheal Mucosa of Rat by Melatonin." *European Archives of Oto-Rhino-Laryngology*. Vol. 270, no. 5. (May 2013): 1695–1700. doi: 10.1007/s00405-013-2425-0.

26. Mortazavi SM, Daiee E, Yazdi A, Khiabani K, Kavousi A, Vazirinejad R, Behnejad B, Ghasemi M, Mood MB. "Mercury Release from Dental Amalgam Restorations after Magnetic Resonance Imaging and Following Mobile Phone Use." *Pakistan Journal of Biological Sciences*. Vol. 11, no. 8. (April 15, 2008): 1142–6. doi:

10.3923/pjbs.2008.1142.1146.
Paknahad M, Mortazavi SM, Shahidi S, Mortazavi G, Haghani M. "Effect of Radiofrequency Radiation from Wi-Fi Devices on Mercury Release from Amalgam Restorations." *Journal of Environmental Health Science & Engineering.* Vol. 14, no. 12. (December 2016). doi: 10.1186/s40201-016-0253-z.

27. Mortazavi G, Mortazavi SAR, Mehdizadeh AR. "'Triple M' Effect: A Proposed Mechanism to Explain Increased Dental Amalgam Microleakage after Exposure to Radiofrequency Electromagnetic Radiation." *Journal of Biomedical Physics and Engineering.* Vol. 8, no. 1. (March 1, 2018): 141–146.

28. Hardell L, Carlberg M, Söderqvist F, Mild KH. "Case-Control Study of the Association between Malignant Brain Tumours Diagnosed between 2007 and 2009 and Mobile and Cordless Phone Use." *International Journal of Oncology.* Vol. 43, no. 6. (December 2013): 1833–45. doi: 10.3892/ijo.2013.2111.

29. Hardell L, Carlberg M, Söderqvist F, Mild KH. "Pooled Analysis of Case-Control Studies on Acoustic Neuroma Diagnosed 1997–2003 and 2007–2009 and Use of Mobile and Cordless Phones." *International Journal of Oncology.* Vol. 43, no. 4. (October 2013): 1036–44. doi: 10.3892/ijo.2013.2025.

30. Wang Y, Guo X. "Meta-Analysis of Association between Mobile Phone Use and Glioma Risk." *Journal of Cancer Research Therapies.* Vol. 12 supplement. (2016): C298–C300. doi: 10.4103/0973-1482.200759.

31. Carlberg M, Hardell L. "Evaluation of Mobile Phone and Cordless Phone Use and Glioma Risk Using the Bradford Hill Viewpoints from 1965 on Association or Causation." *BioMed Research International.* (2017): 9218486. doi: 10.1155/2017/9218486.

32. Hardell L. "Effects of Mobile Phones on Children's and Adolescents' Health: A Commentary." *Child Development.* Vol. 89, no. 1. (January 2018): 137–140. doi: 10.1111/cdev.12831.

33. Momoli F, Siemiatycki J, McBride ML, Parent ME, Richardson L, Bedard D, Platt R, Vrijheld M, Cardis E, Krewski D. "Probabilistic Multiple-Bias Modelling Applied to the Canadian Data From the INTERPHONE Study of Mobile Phone Use and Risk of Glioma, Meningioma, Acoustic Neuroma, and Parotid Gland Tumors." *American Journal of Epidemiology.* Vol. 186, no. 7. (2017): 885–893.

34. Hardell L, Carlberg M. "Use of Wireless Phones and Evidence for Increased Risk of Brain Tumors." Prepared for the BioInitiative Working Group. November 2017. https://bioinitiative.org/wp-content/uploads/2017/11/Hardell-2017-Sec11-Update-Use_of_Wireless_Phones.pdf.
Hardell L, Carlberg M, Kundi M. "Evidence for Brain Tumors and Acoustic Neuromas." Prepared for the BioInitiative Working Group. July 2007. https://bioinitiative.org/wp-content/uploads/pdfs/sec11_2007_Evidence_%20Effects_Brain_Tumors.pdf.
Hardell L, Carlberg M, Mild KH. "Use of Wireless Phones and Evidence for Increased Risk of Brain Tumors." Prepared for the BioInitiative Working Group. November 2012. https://bioinitiative.org/wp-content/uploads/pdfs/sec11_2012_Use_of_Wireless_Phones.pdf.
Kundi M. "Evidence for Brain Tumors (Epidemiological)." Prepared for the BioInitiative Working Group. September 2012. https://bioinitiative.org/wp-content/uploads/pdfs/sec11_2012_Evidence_%20Brain_Tumors.pdf.

35. Nadler DL and Zurbenko IG. "Estimating Cancer Latency Times Using a Weibull Model." *Advances in Epidemiology.* (2014): 746769. doi: 10.1155/2014/746769.

36. American Cancer Society. *Cancer Facts & Figures 2019*. Atlanta. 2019. https://www.cancer.org/content/dam/cancer-org/research/cancer-facts-and-statistics/annual-cancer-facts-and-figures/2019/cancer-facts-and-figures-2019.pdf.

37. James V. Grimaldi. "Verizon and AT&T Provided Cell Towers for McCain Ranch." *Washington Post*. October 16, 2008.

38. Morgan LL, Miller AB, Sasco A, Davis DL. "Mobile Phone Radiation Causes Brain Tumors and Should Be Classified as a Probable Human Carcinogen (2A) (Review)." *International Journal of Oncology*. Vol. 46, no. 5. (May 2015): 1865–1871. doi: 10.3892/ijo.2015.2908.
Bortkiewicz A, Gadzicka E, Szymczak W. "Mobile Phone Use and Risk for Intracranial Tumors and Salivary Gland Tumors – A Meta-Analysis." *International Journal of Occupational Medicine and Environmental Health*. Vol. 30, no. 1. (February 21, 2017): 27–43. doi: 10.13075/ijomeh.1896.00802.
Myung SK, Woong J, McDonnell D, Lee YJ, Kazinets G, Cheng C-T, Moskowitz JM. "Mobile Phone Use and Risk of Tumors: A Meta-Analysis." *Journal of Clinical Oncology*. Vol. 27, no. 33. (November 20, 2009): 5565–5572. doi: 10.1200/JCO.2008.21.6366.
Prasad M, Kathuria P, Nair P, Kumar A, Prasad K. "Mobile Phone Use and Risk of Brain Tumours: A Systematic Review of Association Between Study Quality, Source of Funding, and Research Outcomes." *Neurological Sciences*. Vol. 38, no. 5. (May 2017): 797. doi: 10.1007/s10072-017-2850-8.
Coureau G, Bouvier G, Lebailly P, Fabbro-Peray P, Gruber A, Leffondre K, Guillamo JS, Loiseau H, Mathoulin-Pélissier S, Salamon R, Baldi I. "Mobile Phone Use and Brain Tumours in the CERENAT Case-Control Study." *Occupational and Environmental Medicine*. Vol. 71, no. 7. (July 2014): 514–522. doi: 10.1136/oemed-2013-101754.

39. Michael Wyde. "NTP Toxicology and Carcinogenicity Studies of Cell Phone Radiofrequency Radiation." National Toxicology Program, National Institute of Environmental Health Sciences. June 8, 2016. https://ntp.niehs.nih.gov/ntp/research/areas/cellphone/slides_bioem_wyde.pdf.

40. Yang M, Guo W, Yang C, Tang J, Huang Q, Feng S, Jiang A, Xu X, Jiang G. "Mobile Phone Use and Glioma Risk: A Systematic Review and Meta-Analysis." *PLoS One*. Vol. 12, no. 5. (May 4, 2017): e0175136. doi: 10.1371/journal.pone.0175136.

41. Carlberg M, Hardell L. "Pooled Analysis of Swedish Case-Control Studies during 1997–2003 and 2007–2009 on Meningioma Risk Associated with the Use of Mobile and Cordless Phones." *Oncology Reports*. Vol. 33, no. 6. (June 2015): 3093–3098. doi: 10.3892/or.2015.3930.

42. Hardell L, Carlberg M. "Mobile Phones, Cordless Phones and the Risk for Brain Tumours." *International Journal of Oncology*. Vol. 35, no. 1. (July 2009): 5–17. doi: 10.3892/ijo_00000307.

43. Hardell L, Carlberg M, Hansson Mild K. "Use of Mobile Phones and Cordless Phones Is Associated with Increased Risk for Glioma and Acoustic Neuroma." *Pathophysiology*. Vol. 20, no. 2. (April 2013): 85–110. doi: 10.1016/j.pathophys.2012.11.001.

44. Hardell L, Carlberg M. "Mobile Phone and Cordless Phone Use and the Risk for Glioma – Analysis of Pooled Case-Control Studies in Sweden, 1997–2003 and 2007–2009." *Pathophysiology*. Vol. 22, no. 1. (March 2015): 1–13.

45. Philips A, Henshaw DL, Lamburn G, O'Carroll MJ. "Brain Tumours: Rise in Glioblastoma Multiforme Incidence in England 1995–2015 Suggests an Adverse

Environmental or Lifestyle Factor." *Journal of Environmental and Public Health*. Vol. 2018: 1–10. doi: 10.1155/2018/7910754.
"Incidence of Deadly Brain Tumours in England Doubled between 1995 and 2015." Powerwatch. September 7, 2018. https://www.powerwatch.org.uk /news/20180709-glioma-increase-paper.pdf.

46. Sage CL, "Evidence for Breast Cancer Promotion (Melatonin Studies in Cells and Animals)." Report for the BioInitiative Working Group. July 2007. https:// bioinitiative.org/wp-content/uploads/pdfs/sec14_2007_Evidence_For_Breast _Cancer_Promotion.pdf.

47. West JG, Kapoor NS, Liao SY, Chen JW, Bailey L, Nagourney RA. "Multifocal Breast Cancer in Young Women with Prolonged Contact between Their Breasts and Their Cellular Phones." *Case Reports in Medicine*. Vol. 2013. (2013): 354682. doi: 10.1155/2013/354682.

48. Balekouzou A, Yin P, Afewerky HK, Bekolo C, Pamatika CM, Nambei SW, Djeintote M, Doui Doumgba A, Mossoro-Kpinde CD, Shu C, Yin M, Fu Z, Qing T, Yan M, Zhang J, Chen S, Li H, Xu Z, Koffi B. "Behavioral Risk Factors of Breast Cancer in Bangui of Central African Republic: A Retrospective Case-Control Study." *PLoS One*. Vol. 12, no. 2. (February 8, 2017): e0171154. doi: 10.1371/journal.pone.0171154.

49. Çiğ B, Nazıroğlu M. "Investigation of the Effects of Distance from Sources on Apoptosis, Oxidative Stress and Cytosolic Calcium Accumulation via TRPV1 Channels Induced by Mobile Phones and Wi-Fi in Breast Cancer Cells." *Biochimica et Biophysica Acta (BBA)—Biomembranes*. Vol. 1848, no. 10, Part B. (October 2015): 2756–65. doi: 10.1016/j.bbamem.2015.02.013.

50. Esmekaya MA, Seyhan N, Kayhan H, Tuysuz MZ, Kurşun AC, Yağcı M. "Investigation of the Effects of 2.1 GHz Microwave Radiation on Mitochondrial Membrane Potential (ΔΨ m), Apoptotic Activity and Cell Viability in Human Breast Fibroblast Cells." *Cell Biochemistry and Biophysics*. Vol. 67, no. 3. (December 2013): 1371–8. doi: 10.1007/s12013-013-9669-6.

51. Coogan PF, Clapp RW, Newcomb PA, Wenzl TB, Bogdan G, Mittendorf R, Baron JA, Longnecker MP. "Occupational Exposure to 60-Hertz Magnetic Fields and Risk of Breast Cancer in Women." *Epidemiology*. Vol. 7, no. 5. (September 1, 1996): 459–464. doi: 10.1097/00001648-199609000-00001.
McElroy JA, Egan KM, Titus-Ernstoff L, Anderson HA, Trentham-Dietz A, Hampton JM, Newcomb PA. "Occupational Exposure to Electromagnetic Field and Breast Cancer Risk in a Large, Population-Based, Case-Control Study in the United States." *Journal of Occupational and Environmental Medicine*. Vol. 49, no. 3. (March 2007): 266–274. doi: 10.1097/JOM.0b013e318032259b.
Dosemeci M, Blair A. "Occupational Cancer Mortality Among Women Employed in the Telephone Industry." *Journal of Occupational Medicine*. Vol. 36, no. 11. (1994): 1204–1209. doi: 10.1097/00043764-199411000-00006.
Kliukiene J, Tynes T, Andersen A. "Follow-Up of Radio and Telegraph Operators with Exposure to Electromagnetic Fields and Risk of Breast Cancer." *European Journal of Cancer Prevention*. Vol. 12, no. 4. (2003): 301–307. doi: 10.1097/00008469-200308000-00010.

52. Zhang Y, Lai J, Ruan G, Chen C, Wang DW. "Meta-Analysis of Extremely Low Frequency Electromagnetic Fields and Cancer Risk: a Pooled Analysis of Epidemiologic Studies." *Environment International*. Vol. 88. (March 2016): 36–43. doi: 10.1016/j.envint.2015.12.012.

53. Wertheimer N, Leeper R. "Electrical Wiring Configurations and Childhood Cancer." *American Journal of Epidemiology.* Vol. 109, no 3. (March 1979): 273–284. doi: 10.1093/oxfordjournals.aje.a112681.

54. Savitz DA, Wachtel H, Barnes FA, John EM, Tvrdik JG. "Case-Control Study of Childhood Cancer and Exposure to 60-Hz Magnetic Fields." *American Journal of Epidemiology.* Vol. 128, no. 1. (July 1988): 21–38. doi: 10.1093/oxfordjournals.aje.a114943.

55. Kundi M. "Evidence for Childhood Cancers (Leukemia)." Prepared for the BioInitiative Working Group. September 2012. https://bioinitiative.org/wp-content/uploads/pdfs/sec12_2012_Evidence_%20Childhood_Cancers.pdf.

56. World Health Organization. "Extremely Low Frequency Fields." *Environmental Health Criteria No. 238.* (Updated August 4, 2016): 9. https://www.who.int/peh-emf/publications/elf_ehc/en/.

57. Yang Y, Jin X, Yan C, Tian Y, Tang J, Shen X. "Case-Only Study of Interactions between DNA Repair Genes (*hMLH1, APEX1, MGMT, XRCC1* and *XPD*) and Low-Frequency Electromagnetic Fields in Childhood Acute Leukemia." *Leukemia & Lymphoma.* Vol. 49, no. 12. (2008): 2344–2350. doi: 10.1080/10428190802441347.

58. "Faulty DNA Repair May Explain EMF Role in Childhood Leukemia." *Microwave News.* December 15, 2008. https://microwavenews.com/XRCC1.html.

59. Mejía-Aranguré JM, Bonilla M, Lorenzana R, Juárez-Ocaña S, de Reyes G, Pérez-Saldivar ML, González-Miranda G, Bernáledez-Ríos R, Ortiz-Fernández A, Ortega-Alvarez M, del Carmen Martínez-García M, Fajardo-Gutiérrez. "Incidence of Leukemias in Children from El Salvador and Mexico City between 1996 and 2000: Population-Based Data." *BMC Cancer.* Vol. 5. (2005): 33. doi: 10.1186/1471-2407-5-33.

60. Mejia-Arangure J, Fajardo-Gutierrez A, Perez-Saldivar M, Gorodezky C, Martinez-Avalos A, Romero-Guzman L, Campo-Martinez M, Flores-Lujano J, Salamanca-Gomez F, Velasquez-Perez L. "Magnetic Fields and Acute Leukemia in Children with Down Syndrome." *Epidemiology.* Vol. 18, no. 1. (January 2007): 158–161. doi: 10.1097/01.ede.0000248186.31452.be.

61. Centers for Disease Control and Prevention. "XRCC1 Allele and Genotyle Frequencies." Public Health Genomics. Accessed on March 7, 2019. https://www.cdc.gov/genomics/population/genvar/frequencies/XRCC1.htm#race.

62. Dixon RE, Cheng EP, Mercado JL, Santana LF. "L-Type Ca2+ Channel Function During Timothy Syndrome." *Trends in Cardiovascular Medicine.* Vol. 22, no. 3. (April 2012): 72–76. doi: 10.1016/j.tcm.2012.06.015.
Hsiao PY, Tien HC, Lo CP, Juang JM, Wang YH, Sung RJ. "Gene Mutations in Cardiac Arrhythmias: A Review of Recent Evidence in Ion Channelopathies." *Applications in Clinical Genetics.* Vol. 6. (January 18, 2013): 1–13. doi: 10.2147/TACG.S29676.
Tynes T, Hannevik M, Andersen A, Vistnes AI, Haldorsen T. "Incidence of Breast Cancer in Norwegian Female Radio and Telegraph Operators." *Cancer Causes & Control.* Vol. 7, no. 2. (March 1996): 197–204.
Kliukiene J., Tynes T., Andersen A. "Follow-Up of Radio and Telegraph Operators with Exposure to Electromagnetic Fields and Risk of Breast Cancer." *European*

Journal of Cancer Prevention. Vol. 12, no. 4. (August 2003): 301–7. doi: 10.1097/01 .cej.0000082602.47188.da.

63. Pall ML. "Microwave Electromagnetic Fields Act by Activating Voltage-Gated Calcium Channels: Why the Current International Safety Standards Do Not Predict Biological Hazard." *Journal of Cellular and Molecular Medicine.* Vol. 17, no. 8. (August 2013): 958–965. doi: 10.1111/jcmm.12088.

64. Braune S, Wrocklage C, Raczek J, Gailus T, Lücking CH. "Resting Blood Pressure Increase During Exposure to a Radio-Frequency Electromagnetic Field." *Research Letters.* Vol. 351, no. 9119. (June 20, 1998): 1857–1858. doi: 10.1016/s0140 -6736(98)24025-6.

65. John Schieszer. "Researcher: Turn off Cell Phones at BP Visits." *Renal & Urology News.* May 16, 2013. https://www.renalandurologynews.com/home/conference -highlights/american-society-of-hypertension/researcher-turn-off-cell-phones-at -bp-visits/.

66. Pedersen SA, Gaist D, Schmidt SAJ, Hömlich LR, Friis S, Pottegård A. "Hydrochlorothiazise Use and Risk of Nonmelanoma Skin Cancer: A Nationwide Case-Control Study from Denmark." *Journal of the American Academy of Dermatology.* Vol. 78, no. 4. (April 2018): 673–681. doi: 10.1016/j .jaad.2017.11.042.

67. "Facts & Statistics." Anxiety and Depression Association of America. Accessed March 7, 2019. https://adaa.org/about-adaa/press-room/facts-statistics.

68. Ruscio AM, Hallion LS, Lim CCW, Aguilar-Gaxiola S, Al-Hamzawi A, Alonso J, Andrade LH, Borges G, Bromet EJ, Bunting B, Caldas de Almeida JM, Demyttenaere K, Florescu S, de Girolamo G, Gureje O, Haro JM, He Y, Hinkov H, Hu C, de Jonge P, Karam EG, Lee S, Lepine JP, Levinson D, Mneimneh Z, Navarro-Mateu F, Posada-Villa J, Slade T, Stein DJ, Torres Y, Uda H, Wojtyniak B, Kessler RC, Chatterji S, Scott KM. "Cross-Sectional Comparison of the Epidemiology of DSM-5 Generalized Anxiety Disorder across the Globe." *JAMA Psychiatry.* Vol. 74, no. 5. (May 1, 2017): 465–475. doi: 10.1001 /jamapsychiatry.2017.0056.

69. "Majority of Americans Say They Are Anxious about Health; Millennials Are More Anxious than Baby Boomers." American Psychiatric Association. May 22, 2017. https://www.psychiatry.org/newsroom/news-releases/majority-of-americans -say-they-are-anxious-about-health-millennials-are-more-anxious-than-baby -boomers.

70. "Americans Say They Are More Anxious Than a Year Ago; Baby Boomers Report Greatest Increase in Anxiety." American Psychiatric Association. May 7, 2018. https://www.psychiatry.org/newsroom/news-releases/americans-say-they-are -more-anxious-than-a-year-ago-baby-boomers-report-greatest-increase-in- anxiety.

71. "Major Depression." National Institute of Mental Health. Updated February 2019. https://www.nimh.nih.gov/health/statistics/major-depression.shtml.

72. Söderqvist F, Carlberg M, Hardell L. "Use of Wireless Telephones and Self- Reported Health Symptoms: A Population-Based Study among Swedish Adolescents Aged 15–19 Years." *Environmental Health.* Vol. 7. (May 2008): 18. doi: 10.1186/1476-069X-7-18.

73. Hyman IE Jr, Sarb BA, Wise-Swanson BM. "Failure to See Money on a Tree: Inattentional Blindness for Objects That Guided Behavior." *Frontiers in Psychology.* Vol. 5. (April 23, 2014): 356. doi: 10.3389/fpsyg.2014.00356.

74. Ward AF, Duke K, Gneezy A, Bos MW. "Brain Drain: The Mere Presence of One's Own Smartphone Reduces Available Cognitive Capacity." *Journal of the Association for Consumer Research.* Vol. 2, no. 2. (April 2017).

75. Kolodynski AA, Kolodynska VV. "Motor and Psychological Functions of School Children Living in the Area of the Skrunda Radio Location Station in Latvia." *Science of the Total Environment.* Vol. 180, no. 1. (February 2, 1996): 87–93.

76. Pall ML. "Microwave Frequency Electromagnetic Fields (EMFs) Produce Widespread Neuropsychiatric Effects Including Depression." *Journal of Chemical Neuroanatomy.* Vol. 75, Part B. (September 2016): 43–51. doi: 10.1016/j .jchemneu.2015.08.001.

77. The research Pall based this statement on includes:
Berridge MJ. "Neuronal Calcium Signaling." *Neuron.* Vol. 21, no. 1. (July 1998): 13–26. doi: 10.1016/s0896-6273(00)80510-3.
Dunlap K, Luebke JL, Turner TJ. "Exocytic Ca Cannels in the Mammalian Central Nervous System." *Neuroscience.* Vol. 18, no 2. (February 1995): 89–98.
Wheeler DB, Randall A, Tsien RW. "Roles of N-type and Q-type Channels in Supporting Hippocampal Synaptic Transmission." *Science.* Vol. 264, no. 5155. (April 1, 1994): 107–111. https://science.sciencemag.org/content/264/5155/107.

78. Sundberg I, Ramklint M, Stridsberg M, Papadopoulos FC, Ekselius L, Cunningham JL. "Salivary Melatonin in Relation to Depressive Symptom Severity in Young Adults." *PLoS One.* Vol. 11, no. 4. (2016): e0152814. doi: 10.1371/journal. pone.0152814.

79. Oto R, Akdag Z, Dasdag S, Celik Y. "Evaluation of Psychologic Parameters in People Occupationally Exposed to Radiofrequencies and Microwaves." *Biotechnology & Biotechnology Equipment.* Vol. 8, no. 4. (1994): 71–74. doi: 10.1080/13102818.1994.10818812.

80. Thomée S, Härenstam A, Hagberg M. "Mobile Phone Use and Stress, Sleep Disturbances, and Symptoms of Depression Among Young Adults – a Prospective Cohort Study." *BMC Public Health.* Vol. 11. (January 31, 2011): 66. doi: 10.1186/1471-2458-11-66.

81. Glaser, ZR, Ph.D. "Bibliography of Reported Biological Phenomena ('Effects') and Clinical Manifestations Attributed to Microwave and Radio-Frequency Radiation." Report No. 2, Revised. Naval Medical Research Institute. June 1971.

82. Raines JK. "Electromagnetic Field Interactions with the Human Body: Observed Effects and Theories." National Aeronautics and Space Administration. Greenbelt, Maryland. April 9, 1981. https://ntrs.nasa.gov/search .jsp?R=19810017132.

83. Bolen SM. "Radiofrequency/Microwave Radiation Biological Effects and Safety Standards: A Review." U.S. Air Force Material Command, Griffiss Air Force Base. New York. 1994. https://apps.dtic.mil/dtic/tr/fulltext/u2/a282886.pdf.

84. Pall ML. "Microwave Frequency Electromagnetic Fields (EMFs) Produce Widespread Neuropsychiatric Effects Including Depression." *Journal of Chemical Neuroanatomy.* Vol. 75, Part B. (September 2016): 43–51. doi: 10.1016/j .jchemneu.2015.08.001.

85. Tolgskaya MS, Gordon ZV (Haigh B, Translator). *Pathological Effects of Radio Waves*. Consultants Bureau. New York/London. 1973.

86. Pall, M. "Microwave Frequency Electromagnetic Fields (EMFs) Produce Widespread Neuropsychiatric Effects Including Depression." *Journal of Chemical Neuroanatomy*. Vol. 75, part B. (September 2016): 43–51. doi: 10.1016/j .jchemneu.2015.08.001.

87. Sobel E, Davanipour Z, Sulkava R, Erkinjuntti T, Wikstrom J, Henderson VW, Buckwalter G, Bowman JD, Lee PJ. "Occupations with Exposure to Electromagnetic Fields: A Possible Risk Factor for Alzheimer's Disease." *American Journal of Epidemiology*. Vol. 142, no. 5. (September 1, 1995): 515–24. doi: 10.1093/oxfordjournals.aje.a117669.
Sobel E, Dunn M, Davanipour Z, Qian Z, Chui HC. "Elevated Risk of Alzheimer's Disease among Workers with Likely Electromagnetic Field Exposure." *Neurology*. Vol. 47, no. 6. (December 1996): 1477-81. doi: 10.1212/wnl.47.6.1477.
Savitz DA, Loomis DP, Tse CK. "Electrical Occupations and Neurodegenerative Disease: Analysis of U.S. Mortality Data." *Archives of Environmental Health*. Vol. 53, no. 1. (January–February 1998): 71–4. doi: 10.1080/00039899809605691.
Håkansson N, Gustavsson P, Johansen C, Floderus B. "Neurodegenerative Diseases in Welders and Other Workers Exposed to High Levels of Magnetic Fields." *Epidemiology*. Vol. 14, no. 4. (July 2003): 420–6; discussion 427–8.
Harmanci H, Emre M, Gurvit H, Bilgic B, Hanagasi H, Gurol E, Sahin H, Tinaz S. "Risk Factors for Alzheimer Disease: A Population-Based Case-Control Study in Istanbul, Turkey." *Alzheimer Disease & Associated Disorders*. Vol. 17, no. 3. (July–September 2003): 139–45.
Feychting M, Jonsson F, Pedersen NL, Ahlbom A. "Occupational Magnetic Field Exposure and Neurodegenerative Disease." *Epidemiology*. Vol. 14, no. 4. (July 2003): 413–9; discussion 427–8. doi: 10.1097/01.EDE.0000071409.23291.7b.
Röösli M, Lörtscher M, Egger M, Pfluger D, Schreier N, Lörtscher E, Locher P, Spoerri A, Minder C. "Mortality from Neurodegenerative Disease and Exposure to Extremely Low-Frequency Magnetic Fields: 31 Years of Observations on Swiss Railway Employees." *Neuroepidemiology*. Vol. 28, no. 4. (September 11, 2007): 197–206. doi: 10.1159/000108111.
Davanipour Z, Tseng CC, Lee PJ, Sobel E. "A Case-Control Study of Occupational Magnetic Field Exposure and Alzheimer's Disease: Results from the California Alzheimer's Disease Diagnosis and Treatment Centers." *BMC Neurology*. Vol. 7. (June 2007): 13. doi: 10.1186/1471-2377-7-13.
Park RM, Schulte PA, Bowman JD, Walker JT, Bondy SC, Yost MG, Touchstone JA, Dosemeci M. "Potential Occupational Risks for Neurodegenerative Diseases." *American Journal of Independent Medicine*. Vol. 48, no. 1. (July 2005): 63–77.

88. Huss A, Spoerri A, Egger M, Röösli M. "Residence Near Power Lines and Mortality from Neurodegenerative Diseases: Longitudinal Study of the Swiss Population." *American Journal of Epidemiology*. (November 5, 2008) [Epub ahead of print]. doi: 10.1093/aje/kwn297.

89. Salford LG, Brun AE, Eberhardt JL, Malmgren L, Persson BR. "Nerve Cell Damage in Mammalian Brain after Exposure to Microwaves from GSM Mobile Phones." *Environmental Health Perspectives*. Vol. 111, no. 7. (2003): 881–A408. doi: 10.1289/ehp.6039.

90. Jiang DP, Li J, Zhang J, Xu SL, Kuang F, Lang HY, Wang YF, An GZ, Li JH, Guo GZ. "Electromagnetic Pulse Exposure Induces Overexpression of Beta Amyloid Protein in Rats." *Archives of Medical Research*. Vol. 44, no. 3. (April 2013): 178–184. doi: 10.1016/j.arcmed.2013.03.005.

91. Soto-Gamez A, Quax WJ, Demaria M. "Regulation of Survival Networks in Senescent Cells: From Mechanisms to Interventions." *Journal of Molecular Biology.* Vol. 431, no. 15. (May 31, 2019): 2629-2643. doi: 10.1016/j. jmb.2019.05.036.

92. Pereira BI, Devine OP, Vukmanovic-Stejic M, Chambers ES, Subramanian P, Patel N, Virasami A, Sebire NJ, Kinsler V, Valdovinos A, LeSaux CJ, Passos JF, Antoniou A, Rustin MHA, Campisi J, Akbar AN. "Senescent Cells Evade Immune Clearance via HLA-E-Mediated NK and CD8+ T Cell Inhibition." *Nature Communications.* Vol. 10, no. 1. (2019): 2387. doi: 10.1038/s41467-019-10335-5.

93. Bevington M. "The Prevalence of People with Restricted Access to Work in Man-Made Electromagnetic Environments." *Journal of Environment and Health Science.* Vol. 5. (January 18, 2019.) doi: 10.15436/2378-6841.19.2402.

94. Irigaray P, Caccamo D, Belpomme D. "Oxidative Stress in Electrohypersensitivity SelfReporting Patients: Results of a Prospective in Vivo Investigation with Comprehensive Molecular Analysis." *International Journal of Molecular Medicine.* Vol. 42, no. 4. (October 2018): 1885–1898. doi: 10.3892/ijmm.2018.3774.

95. EHS & MCS Research and Treatment European Group. "Hypothesis of Common Patho-Physiological Mechanisms Accounting for the Co-Occurrence of EHS and MCS." Accessed April 4, 2019. http://www.ehs-mcs.org/en/patho-physiological -mechanisms_178.html.

96. De Luca C, Chung Sheun Thai J, Raskovic D, Cesareo E, Caccamo D, Trukhanov A, Korkina L. "Metabolic and Genetic Screening of Electromagnetic Hypersensitive Subjects as a Feasible Tool for Diagnostics and Intervention." *Mediators of Inflammation.* Vol. 2014, no. 2. (April 9, 2014). doi: 10.1155/2014/924184.

97. Golomb, BA. "Diplomats' Mystery Illness and Pulsed Radiofrequency/Microwave Radiation." *Neural Computation.* (September 5, 2018): 1–104. doi: 10.1162 /neco_a_01133.

98. Omura Y, Losco M, Omura AK, Yamamoto S, Ishikawa H, Takeshige C, Shimotsuura Y, Muteki T. "Chronic or Intractable Medical Problems Associated with Prolonged Exposure to Unsuspected Harmful Environmental Electric, Magnetic or Electro-Magnetic Fields Radiating in the Bedroom or Workplace and Their Exacerbation by Intake of Harmful Light and Heavy Metals from Common Sources." *Acupuncture & Electro-Therapeutics Research.* Vol. 16, no. 3–4. (1991): 143–77.

99. Landgrebe M, Frick U, Hauser S, Hajak G, Langguth B. "Association of Tinnitus and Electromagnetic Hypersensitivity: Hints for a Shared Pathophysiology?" *PLoS One.* Vol. 4, no. 3. (March 27, 2009): e5026. doi: 10.1371/journal .pone.0005026.

100. Administrative Appeals Tribunal of Australia. "McDonald and Comcare." Last updated February 28, 2013. http://www7.austlii.edu.au/cgi-bin/viewdoc/au /cases/cth/aat/2013/105.html.

101. "Gadget 'Allergy': French Woman Wins Disability Grant." BBC News. August 27, 2015. https://www.bbc.com/news/technology-34075146.

102. Scott O'Connell. "Judge Rules in Favor of Southboro School in Wifi Sickness Case." *Worcester Telegram & Gazette.* https://www.telegram.com/news/20180611 /judge-rules-in-favor-of-southboro-school-in-wifi-sickness-case.

103. Mascarenhas MN, Flaxman SR, Boerma T, Vanderpoel S, Stevens GA. "National,

Regional, and Global Trends in Infertility Prevalence since 1990: A Systematic Analysis of 277 Health Surveys." *PLoS Medicine*. Vol. 9, no. 12. (December 2012): e1001356. doi: 10.1371/journal.pmed.1001356.

104. Brugh VM, Lipshultz LI. "Male Factor Infertility: Evaluation and Management." *Medical Clinics of North America*. Vol. 88. no. 2. (March 2004): 367–85. doi: 10.1016/S0025-7125(03)00150-0.
Hirsh A. "Male Subfertility." *BMJ*. Vol. 327. (2003): 669. doi: 10.1136 /bmj.327.7416.669.

105. Philips A, Philips J. "The Adverse Effects of Electromagnetic Fields on Reproduction." EMFFields.org. (2013). http://www.powerwatch.org.uk/library /downloads/emf-reproduction-2014-03.pdf.

106. Wertheimer N, Leeper E. "Possible Effects of Electric Blankets and Heated Waterbeds on Fetal Development." *Bioelectromagnetics*. Vol. 7, no. 1. (1986): 13–22. doi: 10.1002/bem.2250070103.

107. Mascarenhas MN, Flaxman SR, Boerma T, Vanderpoel S, Stevens GA. "National, Regional, and Global Trends in Infertility Prevalence Since 1990: A Systematic Analysis of 277 Health Surveys." *PLoS Medicine*. Vol 9, no. 12. (December 2012): e1001356. doi: 10.1371/journal.pmed.1001356.

108. Carlsen E, Giwercman A, Keiding N, Skakkebæk NE. "Evidence for Decreasing Quality of Semen During Past 50 years." *BMJ*. Vol. 305, no. 6854. (September 12, 1992): 609–613. doi: 10.1136/bmj.305.6854.609.

109. Gorpinchenko I, Nikitin O, Banyra O, Shulyak A. "The Influence of Direct Mobile Phone Radiation on Sperm Quality." *Central European Journal of Urology*. Vol. 67, no. 1. (2014): 65–71. doi: 10.5173/ceju.2014.01.art14.

110. Agarwal A, Deepinder F, Sharma RK, Ranga G, Li J. "Effect of Cell Phone Usage on Semen Analysis in Men Attending Infertility Clinic: An Observational Study." *Fertility and Sterility*. Vol. 89. (2008): 124–128. doi: 10.1016/j .fertnstert.2007.01.166.

111. Agarwal A, Desai NR, Makker K, Varghese A, Mouradi R, Sabanegh E, Sharma R. "Effects of Radiofrequency Electromagnetic Waves (RF-EMW) from Cellular Phones on Human Ejaculated Semen: An in Vitro Pilot Study." *Fertility and Sterility*. Vol. 92, no. 4. (October 2009): 1318–1325. doi: 10.1016/j .fertnstert.2008.08.022.

112. Li DK, Yan B, Li Z, Gao E, Miiao M, Gong D, Weng X, Ferber JR, Yuan W. "Exposure to Magnetic Fields and the Risk of Poor Sperm Quality." *Reproductive Toxicology*. Vol. 29, no. 1. (January 2010): 86–92. doi: 10.1016/j .reprotox.2009.09.004.

113. Kesari KK, Agarwal A, Henkel R. "Radiations and Male Fertility." *Reproductive Biology and Endocrinology*. Vol. 16, no. 1. (December 9, 2018): 118. doi: 10.1186 /s12958-018-0431-1.

114. Adams JA, Galloway TS, Mondal D, Esteves SC, Mathews M. "Effect of Mobile Telephones on Sperm Quality: A Systematic Review and Meta-Analysis." *Environment International*. Vol. 70. (September 2014): 106-112. doi: 10.1016/j .envint.2014.04.015.
La Vignera S, Condorelli RA, Vicari E, D'Agata R, Calogero AE. "Effects of the

Exposure to Mobile Phones on Male Reproduction: A Review of the Literature."
Journal of Andrology. Vol. 33, no. 3. (May–June 2012): 350–6. doi: 10.2164
/jandrol.111.014373.
Desai NR, Kesari KK, Agarwal A. "Pathophysiology of Cell Phone Radiation:
Oxidative Stress and Carcinogenesis with Focus on Male Reproductive System."
Reproductive Biology and Endocrinology. Vol. 7. (October 22, 2009): 114. doi:
10.1186/1477-7827-7-114.
Dama MS, Bhat MN. "Mobile Phones Affect Multiple Sperm Quality Traits: A
Meta-Analysis." *F1000 Research.* Vol. 2. (February 12, 2013): 40. doi: 10.12688
/f1000research.2-40.v1.
Liu K, Li Y, Zhang G, Liu J, Cao J, Ao L, Zhang S. "Association between Mobile
Phone Use and Semen Quality: A Systemic Review and Meta-Analysis."
Andrology. Vol. 2. (2014): 491–501. doi: 10.1111/j.2047-2927.2014.00205.x.
Houston B, Nixon B, King B, De Iuliis G, Aitken R. "The Effects of
Radiofrequency Electromagnetic Radiation on Sperm Function." *Reproduction.*
Vol. 152, no. 6. (2016): R263-R276. doi: 10.1530/REP-16-0126.
La Vignera S, Condorelli RA, Vicari E, D'Agata R, Calogero AE. "Effects of the
Exposure to Mobile Phones on Male Reproduction: A Review of the Literature."
Journal of Andrology. Vol. 33, no. 3. (May–June 2012): 350–6. doi: 10.2164
/jandrol.111.014373.

115. Santini SJ, Cordone V, Falone S, Mijit M, Tatone C, Amicarelli F, Di Emidio G.
"Role of Mitochondria in the Oxidative Stress Induced by Electromagnetic Fields:
Focus on Reproductive Systems." *Oxidative Medicine and Cellular Longevity.* Vol.
2018, no. 3. (November 2018): article ID 5076271. doi: 10.1155/2018/5076271.

116. Kesari KK, Behari J. "Evidence for Mobile Phone Radiation Exposure
Effects on Reproductive Pattern of Male Rats: Role of ROS." *Electromagnetic
Biology and Medicine.* Vol. 31, no. 3. (September 2012): 213–22. doi:
10.3109/15368378.2012.700292.

117. Meena R, Kumari K, Kumar J, Rajamani P, Verma HN, Kesari KK. "Therapeutic
Approaches of Melatonin in Microwave Radiations-Induced Oxidative Stress-
Mediated Toxicity on Male Fertility Pattern of Wistar Rats." *Electromagnetic
Biology and Medicine.* Vol. 33, no. 2. (June 2014): 81–91.

118. Simon Khalaf and Lali Kesiraju. "U.S. Consumers Time-Spent on Mobile Crosses
5 Hours a Day." *Flurry Analytics Blog.* March 2, 2017. https://www.flurry.com
/blog/post/157921590345/us-consumers-time-spent-on-mobile-crosses-5.

119. Xu YQ, Li BH, Cheng HM. "High-Frequency Electromagnetic Field Exposure on
Reproductive and Endocrine Functions of Female Workers." [Article in Chinese.]
*Zhonghua Lao Dong Wei Sheng Zhi Ye Bing Za Zhi (Chinese Journal of Industrial
Hygiene and Occupational Diseases).* Vol. 26, no. 6. (2008): 332–5.

120. Wojsiat J, Korczyński J, Borowiecka M, Żbikowska HM. "The Role of Oxidative
Stress in Female Infertility and in Vitro Fertilization." [Article in Polish.] *Postepy
Higieny i Medycyny Doswiadczalnej.* Vol. 71. (May 9, 2017): 359–366.

121. Gul A, Çelebi H, Uğraş S. "The Effects of Microwave Emitted by Cellular Phones
on Ovarian Follicles in Rats." *Archives of Gynecology and Obstetrics.* Vol. 280.
(November 2009): 729–33. doi: 10.1007/s00404-009-0972-9.

122. Augner C, Hacker GW. "Are People Living Next to Mobile Phone Base Stations More
Strained? Relationship of Health Concerns, Self-Estimated Distance to Base Station,
and Psychological Parameters." *Indian Journal of Occupational and Environmental
Medicine.* Vol. 13, no. 3. (2009): 141–5. doi: 10.4103/0019-5278.58918.

Augner C, Hacker GW, Oberfeld G, Florian M, Hitzl W, Hutter J, Pauser G. "Effects of Exposure to GSM Mobile Phone Base Station Signals on Salivary Cortisol, Alpha-Amylase, and Immunoglobulin A." *Biomedical and Environmental Sciences.* Vol. 23, no. 3. (June 2010): 199–207. doi: 10.1016/S0895-3988(10)60053-0.

123. Mary Brophy Marcus. "Stress May Diminish a Woman's Fertility, Study Suggests." HealthDay. March 24, 2014.
Lynch CD, Sundaram R, Maisog JM, Sweeney AM, Buck Louis GM. "Preconception Stress Increases the Risk of Infertility: Results from a Couple-Based Prospective Cohort Study—the LIFE Study." *Human Reproductive.* Vol. 29, no. 5. (May 2014): 1067–75. doi: 10.1093/humrep/deu032.

124. Li D-K, Chen H, Ferber JR, Odouli R, Quesenberry C. "Exposure to Magnetic Field Non-Ionizing Radiation and the Risk of Miscarriage: A Prospective Cohort Study." *Scientific Reports.* Vol. 7, no. 1. (2017): 17541. doi: 10.1038/s41598-017 -16623-8.

125. Li D-K, Odouli R, Wi S, Janevic T, Golditch I, Bracken TD, Senior R, Rankin R, Iriye R. "A Population-Based Prospective Cohort Study of Personal Exposure to Magnetic Fields During Pregnancy and the Risk of Miscarriage." *Epidemiology.* Vol. 13, no. 1. (January 2002): 9–20.

Lee GM, Neutra RR, Hristova L, Yost M, Hiatt RA. "A Nested Case-Control Study of Residential and Personal Magnetic Field Measures and Miscarriages." *Epidemiology.* Vol. 13, no. 1. (January 2002): 21–31.

126. Chen H, Qu Z, Liu W. "Effects of Simulated Mobile Phone Electromagnetic Radiation on Fertilization and Embryo Development." *Fetal and Pediatric Pathology.* Vol. 36, no. 2. (April 2017): 123–9. doi: 10.1080/15513815.2016.1261974.

Chapter 6: How Do You Repair EMF-Related Damage?

1. Hopp AK, Grüter P, Hottiger MO. "Regulation of Glucose Metabolism by NAD+ and ADP-Ribosylation." *Cells.* Vol. 8, no. 8. (August 2019): 890. doi: 10.3390 /cells8080890.

2. Virág L, Szabo C. "The Therapeutic Potential of Poly(ADP-ribose) Polymerase Inhibitors." *Pharmacological Reviews.* Vol. 54, no. 3. (September 2002): 375–429.

3. Shall S, de Murcia G. "Poly(ADP-ribose) Polymerase-1: What Have We Learned from the Deficient Mouse Model?" *Mutation Research.* Vol. 460, no. 1. (June 30, 2000): 1–15.

4. Alemasova EE, Lavrik OI. "Poly(ADP-ribosyl)ation by PARP1: Reaction Mechanism and Regulatory Proteins." *Nucleic Acids Research.* Vol. 47, no. 8. (February 25, 2019): 3811–3827. doi: 10.1093/nar/gkz120.

5. Schraufstatter IU, Hinshaw DB, Hyslop PA, Spragg RG, Cochrane CG. "Oxidant Injury of Cells. DNA Strand-Breaks Activate Polyadenosine Diphosphate-Ribose Polymerase and Lead to Depletion of Nicotinamide Adenine Dinucleotide." *Journal of Clinical Investigation.* Vol. 77, no. 4. (April 1, 1986): 1312–1320. doi: 10.1172/JCI112436.

6. Bai P. "PARP-1 Inhibition Increases Mitochondrial Metabolism through SIRT1 Activation." *Cell Metabolism.* Vol. 13, no. 4. (April 6, 2011): 461–46.

7. Pirinen E, Cantó C, Jo YS, Morato L, Zhang H, Menzies KJ, Williams EG,

Mouchiroud L, Moullan N, Hagberg C, Li W, Timmers S, Imhof R, Verbeek J, Pujol A, van Loon B, Viscomi C, Zeviani M, Schrauwen P, Sauve AA, Schoonjans K, Auwerx J. ""Pharmacological Inhibition of Poly(ADP-Ribose) Polymerases Improves Fitness and Mitochondrial Function in Skeletal Muscle." *Cell Metabolism*. Vol. 19, no. 6. (June 3, 2014): 1034–41. doi: 10.1016/j .cmet.2014.04.002.

8. Massudi H, Grant R, Braidy N, Guest J, Farnsworth B, Guillemin GJ. "Age-Associated Changes in Oxidative Stress and NAD+ Metabolism in Human Tissue." *PLoS One*. Vol. 7, no. 7. (2012): e42357.

9. Braidy N, Guillemin GJ, Mansour H, Chan-Ling T, Poljak A, Grant R. "Age Related Changes in NAD+ Metabolism, Oxidative Stress, and Sirt1 Activity in Wistar Rats." *PLoS One*. Vol. 6, no. 4. (April 26, 2011): e19194.

10. Makvandi M, Sellmyer MA, Mach RH. "Inflammation and DNA Damage: Probing Pathways to Cancer and Neurodegeneration." *Drug Discovery Today: Technologies*. Vol. 25. (November 2017): 37–43. doi: 10.1016/j.ddtec.2017.11.001.

11. Berger, F. "The New Life of a Centenarian: Signalling Functions of NAD(P)." *Trends in Biochemical Sciences*. Vol. 29, no. 3. (2004): 111–118. doi: 10.1016/j .tibs.2004.01.007.

12. Warburg O, Pyridine CW. "Pyridine, the Hydrogen Transfusing Component of Fermentative Enzymes." *Helvetica Chimica Acta*. Vol. 19. (1936): 79–88.

13. Sinclair DA, Guarente L. "Unlocking the Secrets of Longevity Genes." *Scientific American*. Vol. 294, no. 3. (March 2006): 48–51, 54–7.

14. Romani M. "Niacin: An Old Lipid Drug in a New NAD+ Dress." *Journal of Lipid Research*. Vol. 60, no. 4. (April 2019): 741–746. doi: 10.1194/jlr.S092007.

15. Braidy N, Berg J, Clement J, Khorshidi F, Poliak A, Javasena T, Grant R, Sachdev P. "Role of NAD+ and Related Precursors as Therapeutic Targets for Age-Related Degenerative Diseases: Rationale, Biochemistry, Pharmacokinetics, and Outcomes." *Antioxidants & Redox Signal*. Vol. 30, no. 2. (January 10, 2019): 251–294. doi: 10.1089/ars.2017.7269.

16. Ansari HR, Raghava GP. "Identification of NAD Interacting Residues in Proteins." *BMC Bioinformatics*. Vol. 11. (March 30, 2010): 160.

17. Placzek S, Schomburg I, Chang A, Jeske L, Ulbrich M, Tillack J, Schomburg D. "BRENDA in 2017: New Perspectives and New Tools in BRENDA." *Nucleic Acids Research*. Vol. 45. (January 4, 2017): D380–D388.

18. Conze D, Brenner C, Kruger CL. "Safety and Metabolism of Long-Term Administration of NIAGEN (Nicotinamide Riboside Chloride) in a Randomized, Double-Blind, Placebo-Controlled Clinical Trial of Healthy Overweight Adults." *Scientific Reports*. Vol. 9, no. 1. (July 5, 2019): 9772. doi: 10.1038/s41598-019 -46120-z.

19. Canto C, Menzies KJ, and Auwerx J. "NAD(+) Metabolism and the Control of Energy Homeostasis: A Balancing Act Between Mitochondria and the Nucleus." *Cellular Metabolism*. Vol. 22. (2015): 31–53.

20. Won SJ, Choi BY, Yoo BH, Sohn M, Ying W, Swanson R, Suh SW. "Prevention of Traumatic Brain Injury Induced Neuron Death by Intranasal Delivery of NAD+." *Journal of Neurotrauma*. Vol. 29, no. 7. (May 1, 2012): 1401–1409.

21. Zhang M, Ying W. "NAD Deficiency Is a Common Central Pathological Factor of a Number of Diseases and Aging: Mechanisms and Therapeutic Implications." *Antioxidants & Redox Signaling.* (February 7, 2018.)

22. Hosseini L, Vafaee MS, Mahmoudi J, Badalzadeh R. "Nicotinamide Adenine Dinucleotide Emerges as a Therapeutic Target in Aging and Ischemic Conditions." *Biogerontology.* (March 5, 2019). doi: 10.1007/s10522-019-09805.

23. Csiszar A, Tarantini S, Yabluchanskiy A, Balasubramanian P, Kiss T, Farkas E, Baur JA, Ungvari ZI. "Role of Endothelial NAD+ Deficiency in Age-Related Vascular Dysfunction." *American Journal of Physiology-Heart and Circulatory Physiology.* (2019). doi: 10.1152/ajpheart.00039.2019.

24. Poulos LH, Poulos TL. "Structure-Function Studies on Nitric Oxide Synthases." *Journal of Inorganic Biochemistry.* Vol. 99, no. 1. (January 2005): 293–305.

25. Bradshaw P. "Cytoplasmic and Mitochondrial NADPH-Coupled Redox Systems in the Regulation of Aging." *Nutrients.* Vol. 11, no. 3. (February 27, 2019): 504. doi: 10.3390/nu11030504.

26. Placzek S, Schomburg I, Chang A, Jeske L, Ulbrich M, Tillack J, Schomburg D. "BRENDA in 2017: New Perspectives and New Tools in BRENDA." *Nucleic Acids Research.* Vol. 45. (January 4, 2017): D380–D388.

27. Curtis W, Kemper ML, Miller AL, Pawlosky R, King MT, Veech RL. "Mitigation of Damage from Reactive Oxygen Species and Ionizing Radiation by Ketone Body Esters." In *Ketogenic Diet and Metabolic Therapies: Expanded Roles in Health and Disease.* (Masino SA, ed.). Oxford University Press, Oxford. 2017. Pages 254–270.

28. Harman D. "Free Radical Theory of Aging: An Update: Increasing the Functional Life Span." *Annals of the New York Academy of Sciences.* Vol. 1067. (May 2006): 10–21.

29. LaBaron TW, Laher I, Kura B, Slezak J. "Hydrogen Gas: From Clinical Medicine to an Emerging Ergogenic Molecule for Sports Athletes." *Canadian Journal of Physiology and Pharmacology.* (April 10, 2019.) doi: 10.1139/cjpp-2019-0067.

30. Selman C, McLaren JS, Meyer C, Duncan JS, Redman P, Collins AR, Duthie GG, Speakman JR. "Life-Long Vitamin C Supplementation in Combination with Cold Exposure Does Not Affect Oxidative Damage or Lifespan in Mice, but Decreases Expression of Antioxidant Protection Genes." *Mechanisms of Ageing and Development.* Vol. 127, no. 12. (December 2006): 897–904.

31. Ernst IM, Pallauf K, Bendall JK, Paulsen L, Nikolai S, Huebbe P, Roeder T, Rimbach G. "Vitamin E Supplementation and Lifespan in Model Organisms." *Ageing Research Reviews.* Vol. 12, no. 1. (January 2013): 365–375. doi: 10.1016/j.arr.2012.10.002.

32. Bradshaw P. "Cytoplasmic and Mitochondrial NADPH-Coupled Redox Systems in the Regulation of Aging." *Nutrients.* Vol. 11, no. 3. (February 27, 2019): 504. doi: 10.3390/nu11030504.

33. Zhu XH, Lu M, Lee BY, Ugurbil K, Chen W. "In Vivo NAD Assay Reveals the Intracellular NAD Contents and Redox State in Healthy Human Brain and Their Age Dependences." *Proceedings of the National Academy of Sciences of the United States of America.* Vol. 112, no. 9. (March 3, 2015): 2876–2881.

34. Pollak N, Dolle C, Ziegler M. "The Power to Reduce: Pyridine Nucleotides—Small Molecules with a Multitude of Functions." *Biochemistry Journal.* Vol. 402. (March 1, 2007): 205–218. doi: 10.1042/BJ20061638.

35. Panday A, Sahoo MK, Osorio D, Batra S. "NADPH Oxidases: An Overview from Structure to Innate Immunity-Associated Pathologies." *Cellular & Molecular Immunology*. Vol. 12, no. 1. (January 12, 2015): 5–23. doi: 10.1038/cmi.2014.89.

36. Brandes RP, Kreuzer J. "Vascular NADPH Oxidases: Molecular Mechanisms of Activation." *Cardiovascular Research*. Vol. 65, no. 1. (January 1, 2005): 16–27.

37. Bradshaw P. "Cytoplasmic and Mitochondrial NADPH-Coupled Redox Systems in the Regulation of Aging." *Nutrients*. Vol. 11, no. 3. (February 27, 2019): 504. doi: 10.3390/nu11030504.

38. Pacher P, Beckman JS, Liaudet L. "Nitric Oxide and Peroxynitrite in Health and Disease." *Physiological Reviews*. Vol. 87, no. 1. (January 2007): 315–424.

39. Slezák J, Kura B, Frimmel K, Zálešák M, Ravingerová T, Viczenczová C, Okruhlicová L', Tribulová N. "Preventive and Therapeutic Application of Molecular Hydrogen in Situations with Excessive Production of Free Radicals." *Physiological Research*. Vol. 65, no. 1. (September 19, 2016): S11-S28.

40. Ohta S. "Molecular Hydrogen as a Novel Antioxidant: Overview of the Advantages of Hydrogen for Medical Applications." *Methods in Enzymology*. Vol. 555. (2015): 289–317. doi: 10.1016/bs.mie.2014.11.038.

41. Zhai X, Chen X, Ohta S, and Sun X. "Review and Prospect of the Biomedical Effects of Hydrogen." *Medical Gas Research*. Vol. 4, no 1. (2014): 19. doi: 10.1186/s13618-014-0019-6.

42. Gao Q, Song H, Wang XT, Liang Y, Xi YJ, Gao Y, Guo QJ, LeBaron T, Luo YX, Li SC, Yin X, Shi HS, Ma YX. "Molecular Hydrogen Increases Resilience to Stress in Mice." *Scientific Reports*. Vol. 7, no. 1. (2017): 9625. doi: 10.1038/s41598-017-10362-6.

43. Sato Y, Kajiyama S, Amano A, Kondo Y, Sasaki T, Handa S, Takahashi R, Fukui M, Hasegawa G, Nakamura N, Fujinawa H, Mori T, Ohta M, Obayashi H. Maruyama N, Ishigami A. "Hydrogen-Rich Pure Water Prevents Superoxide Formation in Brain Slices of Vitamin C-Depleted SMP30/GNL Knockout Mice." *Biochemical and Biophysical Research and Communications*. Vol. 375, no. 3. (October 24, 2008): 346–350. doi: 10.1016/j.bbrc.2008.08.020.

44. LeBaron TW, Laher I, Kura B, Slezak J. "Hydrogen Gas: From Clinical Medicine to an Emerging Ergogenic Molecule for Sports Athletes." *Canadian Journal of Physiology and Pharmacology*. Vol. 97, no. 9. (September 2019): 797–807. doi: 10.1139/cjpp-2019-0067.

45. Kang KM, Kang YN, Choi IB, Gu Y, Kawamura T, Toyoda Y, Nakao A. "Effects of Drinking Hydrogen-Rich Water on the Quality of Life of Patients Treated with Radiotherapy for Liver Tumors." *Medical Gas Research*. 2011 Jun 7; 1 (1): 11. doi: 10.1186/2045-9912-1-11.

46. Yang Q, Ji G, Pan R, Zhao Y, Yan P. "Protective Effect of Hydrogen-Rich Water on Liver Function of Colorectal Cancer Patients Treated with mFOLFOX6 Chemotherapy." *Molecular and Clinical Oncology*. Vol. 7, no. 5. (November 2017): 891–896. doi: 10.3892/mco.2017.1409.

47. Batra V, Kislay B. "Mitigation of Gamma-Radiation Induced Abasic Sites in Genomic DNA by Dietary Nicotinamide Supplementation: Metabolic Up-Regulation of NAD+ Biosynthesis." *Mutation Research/Fundamental and Molecular Mechanisms of Mutagenesis*. Vol. 749, no. 1–2. (2013): 28–38.

Braidy N, Guillemin GJ, Mansour H, Chan-Ling T, Poljak A, Grant R. "Age Related Changes in NAD+ Metabolism Oxidative Stress and Sirt1 Activity in Wistar Rats." *PLoS One*. Vol. 6, no. 4. (April 26, 2011): e19194.

48. Sheng C, Chen H, Wang B, Liu T, Hong Y, Shao J, He X, Ma Y, Nie H, Liu N, Xia W, Ying W. "NAD+ Administration Significantly Attenuates Synchrotron Radiation X-Ray-Induced DNA Damage and Structural Alterations of Rodent Testes." *International Journal of Physiology, Pathophysiology and Pharmacology.* Vol. 4, no. 1. (2012): 1–9.

49. Ma Y, Nie H, Sheng C, Chen H, Wang B, Liu T, Shao J, He X, Zhang T, Zheng C, Xia W, and Ying W. "Roles of Oxidative Stress in Synchrotron Radiation X-Ray-Induced Testicular Damage of Rodents." *International Journal of Physiology Pathophysiology and Pharmacology*. Vol. 4, no. 2. (2012): 108–114.

50. Fessel JP, Oldham W. "Pyridine Dinucleotides from Molecules to Man." *Antioxidants & Redox Signaling*. Vol. 28, no. 3. (January 20, 2018): 180–212.

51. Rajman L, Chwalek K, Sinclair DA. "Therapeutic Potential of NAD-Boosting Molecules: The in Vivo Evidence." *Cellular Metabolism*. Vol. 27, no. 3. (March 6, 2018): 529–547.

52. Erdelyi K, Bakondi E, Gergely P, Szabó C, Virág L. "Pathophysiologic Role of Oxidative Stress-Induced Poly(ADP-ribose) Polymerase-1 Activation: Focus on Cell Death and Transcriptional Regulation." *Cellular and Molecular Life Sciences*. Vol. 62, no. 7–8. (April 2005): 751–759.

53. Clement J, Wong M, Poljak A, Sachdev P, Braidy N. "The Plasma NAD+ Metabolome Is Dysregulated in 'Normal' Aging. *Rejuvenation Research*. Vol. 22, no. 2. (April 2019): 121–130. doi: 10.1089/rej.2018.2077.

54. Laliotis GP, BizelisI, Rogdakis R. "Comparative Approach of the de novo Fatty Acid Synthesis (Lipogenesis) between Ruminant and Non Ruminant Mammalian Species: From Biochemical Level to the Main Regulatory Lipogenic Genes." *Current Genomics*. Vol. 11, no. 3. (May 2010): 168–183. doi: 10.2174/138920210791110960.

55. Fang EF, Lautrup S, Hou Y, Demarest TG, Croteau DL, Mattson MP, Bohr VA. "NAD(+) in Aging: Molecular Mechanisms and Translational Implications." *Trends in Molecular Medicine*. Vol. 23, no. 10. (October 2017): 899–916. doi: 10.1016/j.molmed.2017.08.001.

56. Katsyuba E, Auwerx J. "Modulating NAD(+) Metabolism, from Bench to Bedside." *EMBO Journal*. Vol. 36, no. 18. (September 15, 2017): 2670–2683. doi: 10.15252 /embj.201797135.

57. Rajman L, Chwalek K, Sinclair DA. "Therapeutic Potential of NAD-Boosting Molecules: The in vivo Evidence." *Cellular Metabolism*. Vol. 27, no. 3. (March 6, 2018): 529–547.

58. Yoshino J, Baur JA, Ima SI. "NAD(+) Intermediates: The Biology and Therapeutic Potential of NMN and NR." *Cellular Metabolism*. Vol. 27, no. 3. (March 6, 2018): 513–528.

59. Grant RS, Kapoor V. "Murine Glial Cells Regenerate NAD, After Peroxide-Induced Depletion, Using Either Nicotinic Acid, Nicotinamide, or Quinolinic Acid as Substrates." *Journal of Neurochemistry*. Vol. 70, no. 4. (April 1998): 1759–1763.

60. Elvehjem CA, Madden RJ, Strong FM, Woolley DW. "The Isolation and Identification of the Anti-Black Tongue Factor." *Nutrition Reviews*. Vol. 32, no. 2. (February 1974): 48–50.

61. Mannar V, Hurrell R., editors. *Food Fortification in a Globalized World*. London: Academic Press/Elsevier, 2017.

62. Kirkland JB. "Niacin Status and Treatment-Related Leukemogenesis." *Molecular Cancer Therapeutics*. Vol. 8, no. 4. (April 2009): 725–732.

63. Kirkland JB. "Niacin Status Impacts Chromatin Structure." *Journal of Nutrition*. Vol. 139, no. 12. (December 2009): 2397–2401.

64. Kirkland JB. "Niacin Status and Genomic Instability in Bone Marrow Cells; Mechanisms Favoring the Progression of Leukemogenesis." *Subcellular Biochemistry*. Vol. 56. (2012): 21–3.

65. Kirkland JB. "Niacin Requirements for Genomic Stability." *Mutation Research*. Vol. 733, no. 1–2. (May 1, 2012): 14–20.

66. Menon RM, Gonzalez MA, Adams MH, Tolbert DS, Leu JH, Cefali EA. "Effect of the Rate of Niacin Administration on the Plasma and Urine Pharmacokinetics of Niacin and Its Metabolites." *Journal of Clinical Pharmacology*. Vol. 47, no. 6. (June 2007): 681–68.

67. Peled T. "Nicotinamide, a SIRT1 Inhibitor, Inhibits Differentiation and Facilitates Expansion of Hematopoietic Progenitor Cells with Enhanced Bone Marrow Homing and Engraftment." *Experimental Hematology*. Vol. 40, no. 4. (April 2012): 342–55.

68. Gaikwad A, Long DJ 2nd, Stringer JL, Jaiswal AK. "In Vivo Role of NAD(P) H:Quinone Oxidoreductase 1 (NQO1) in the Regulation of Intracellular Redox State and Accumulation of Abdominal Adipose Tissue." *Journal of Biological Chemistry*. Vol. 276, no. 25. (June 22, 2001); 22559–64.

69. Yaku K, Okabe K, Nakagawa T. "NAD Metabolism: Implications in Aging and Longevity." *Ageing Research Reviews*. Vol. 47. (November 2018): 11–7. doi: 10.1016/j.arr.2018.05.006.

70. Müller F. "Flavin Radicals: Chemistry and Biochemistry." *Free Radical Biology and Medicine*. Vol. 3, no. 3. (1987): 215–30.

71. Garber K. "Biochemistry: A Radical Treatment." *Nature*. Vol. 489. (2012) S4–6.

72. Mathew ST, Bergström P, Hammarsten O. "Repeated Nrf2 Stimulation Using Sulforaphane Protects Fibroblasts from Ionizing Radiation." *Toxicology and Applied Pharmacology*. Vol. 276, no. 3. (May 2014): 188–194.

73. Reisman SA, Lee CY, Meyer CJ, Proksch JW, Sonis ST, Ward KW. "Topical Application of the Synthetic Triterpenoid RTA 408 Protects Mice from Radiation-Induced Dermatitis." *Radiation Research*. Vol. 181, no. 5. (May 2014): 512–520.

74. Iranshahy M, Iranshahi M, Abtahi SR, Karimi G. "The Role of Nuclear Factor Erythroid 2-Related Factor 2 in Hepatoprotective Activity of Natural Products: A Review." *Food and Chemical Toxicology*. Vol. 120. (October 2018): 261–276. doi: 10.1016/j.fct.2018.07.024.

75. O'Connell MA, Hayes JD. "The Keap1/Nrf2 Pathway in Health and Disease: From the Bench to the Clinic." *Biochemical Society Transactions*. Vol. 43. (2015):

687–689.

76. Marik PE, Khangoora V, Rivera R, Hooper MH, Catravas J. "Hydrocortisone, Vitamin C, and Thiamine for the Treatment of Severe Sepsis and Septic Shock: A Retrospective Before-After Study." *Chest.* Vol. 151, no. 6. (June 2017): 1229–1238. doi: 10.1016/j.chest.2016.11.036.

77. Hershey TB, Kahn JM. "State Sepsis Mandates—A New Era for Regulation of Hospital Quality." *New England Journal of Medicine.* Vol. 376, no. 24. (June 15, 2017): 2311–2313. doi: 10.1056/NEJMp1611928.

78. Shin TG, Kim YJ, Ryoo SM, Hwang SY, Jo IJ, Chung SP, Choi SH, Suh GJ, Kim WY. "Early Vitamin C and Thiamine Administration to Patients with Septic Shock in Emergency Departments: Propensity Score-Based Analysis of a Before-and-After Cohort Study." *Journal of Clinical Medicine.* Vol. 8, no. 1. (January 16, 2019): E102. doi: 10.3390/jcm8010102.

79. Balakrishnan M, Gandhi H, Shah K, Pandya H, Patel R, Keshwani S, Yadav N. "Hydrocortisone, Vitamin C and Thiamine for the Treatment of Sepsis and Septic Shock Following Cardiac Surgery." *Indian Journal of Anaesthesia.* Vol. 62, no. 12. (December 2018): 934-939. doi: 10.4103/ija.IJA_361_18.

80. Marik PE. "Hydrocortisone, Ascorbic Acid and Thiamine (HAT Therapy) for the Treatment of Sepsis. Focus on Ascorbic Acid." *Nutrients.* Vol. 10, no. 11. (November 14, 2018): E1762. doi: 10.3390/nu10111762.

81. Moskowitz A, Andersen LW, Huang DT, Berg KM, Grossestreuer AV, Marik PE, Sherwin RL, Hou PC, Becker LB, Cocchi MN, Doshi P, Gong J, Sen A, Donnino MW. "Ascorbic Acid, Corticosteroids, and Thiamine in Sepsis: A Review of the Biologic Rationale and the Present State of Clinical Evaluation." *Critical Care.* Vol. 22, no. 1. (October 29, 2018): 283. doi: 10.1186/s13054-018-2217-4.

82. Surh YJ, Kundu JK, Na HK. "Nrf2 as a Master Redox Switch in Turning on the Cellular Signaling Involved in the Induction of Cytoprotective Genes by Some Chemopreventive Phytochemicals." *Planta Medica.* Vol. 74, no. 13. (October 2008): 1526–39.

83. Nakagawa F, Morino K, Ugi S, Ishikado A, Kondo K, Sato D, Konno S, Nemoto K, Kusunoki C, Sekine O, Sunagawa A, Kawamura M, Inoue N, Nishio Y, Maegawa H. "4-Hydroxy Hexenal Derived from Dietary n-3 Polyunsaturated Fatty Acids Induces Anti-Oxidative Enzyme Heme Oxygenase-1 in Multiple Organs." *Biochemical and Biophysical Research Communications.* Vol. 443, no. 3. (2014): 991–996.

84. Kumar H, Kim IS, More SV, Kim BW, Choi DK. "Natural Product-Derived Pharmacological Modulators of Nrf2/ARE Pathway for Chronic Diseases." *Natural Products Reports.* Vol. 31, no. 1. (January 2014): 109–139.

85. Lewis KN, Mele J, Hayes JD, Buffenstein R. "Nrf2, a Guardian of Healthspan and Gatekeeper of Species Longevity." *Integrative and Comparative Biology.* Vol. 50, no. 5. (November 2010): 829–843.

86. Kapeta S, Chondrogianni N, Gonos ES. "Nuclear Erythroid Factor 2-Mediated Proteasome Activation Delays Senescence in Human Fibroblasts." *Journal of Biological Chemistry.* Vol. 285, no. 11. (March 12, 2010): 8171–8184.

87. Jódar L, Mercken EM, Ariza J, Younts C, González-Reyes JA, Alcaín FJ, Burón I, de Cabo R, Villalba JM. "Genetic Deletion of Nrf2 Promotes Immortalization and

Decreases Life Span of Murine Embryonic Fibroblasts." *Journals of Gerontology. Series A: Biological Sciences and Medical Sciences*. Vol. 66A, no. 3. (March 2011): 247–256.

88. Takahashi A, Ohtani N, Yamakoshi K, Iida S, Tahara H, Nakayama K, Nakayama KI, Ide T, Saya H, Hara E. "Mitogenic Signalling and the p16INK4a-Rb Pathway Cooperate to Enforce Irreversible Cellular Senescence." *Nature Cell Biology*. Vol. 8, no. 11. (2006): 1291–1297.

89. Gounder SS, Kannan S, Devadoss D, Miller CJ, Whitehead KJ, Odelberg SJ. Firpo MA, Paine R 3rd, Hoidal JR, Abel ED, Rajasekaran NS. "Impaired Transcriptional Activity of Nrf2 in Age-Related Myocardial Oxidative Stress Is Reversible by Moderate Exercise Training." *PLoS One*. Vol. 7, no. 9. (2012): e45697.

90. Pall ML, Levine S. "Nrf2, a Master Regulator of Detoxification and also Antioxidant, Anti-Inflammatory and Other Cytoprotective Mechanisms, Is Raised by Health Promoting Factors." *Sheng Li Xue Bao (Acta Physiologica Sinica)*. Vol. 67, no. 1. (February 25, 2015): 1–18.

91. Pearson KJ, Lewis KN, Price NL, Chang JW, Perez E, Cascajo MV, Tamashiro KL, Poosala S, Csiszar A, Ungvari Z, Kensler TW, Yamamoto M, Egan JM, Longo DL, Ingram DK, Navas P, de Cabo R. "Nrf2 Mediates Cancer Protection but Not Prolongevity Induced by Caloric Restriction." Proceedings of the National Academy of Sciences of the United States of America. Vol. 105, no. 7. (2008): 2325–2330.

92. Bishop NA, Guarente L. "Two Neurons Mediate Diet-Restriction-Induced Longevity in C. Elegans." *Nature*. Vol. 447, no. 7144. (2007): 545–549.

93. Sykiotis GP, Habeos IG, Samuelson AV, Bohmann D. "The Role of the Antioxidant and Longevity-Promoting Nrf2 Pathway in Metabolic Regulation." *Current Opinions in Clinical Nutrition and Metabolic Care*. Vol. 14, no. 1. (January 2011): 41–48.

94. Martín-Montalvo A, Villalba JM, Navas P, de Cabo R. "NRF2, Cancer and Calorie Restriction." *Oncogene*. Vol. 30, no. 5. (February 3, 2011): 505–520.

95. Ungvari Z, Parrado-Fernandez C, Csiszar A, de Cabo R. "Mechanisms Underlying Caloric Restriction and Lifespan Regulation: Implications for Vascular Aging." *Circulation Research*. Vol. 102, no. 5. (March 14, 2008): 519–528.

96. Lei P, Tian S, Teng C, Huang L, Liu X, Wang J, Zhang Y, Li B, Shan Y. "Sulforaphane Improves Lipid Metabolism by Enhancing Mitochondrial Function and Biogenesis in Vivo and In Vitro." *Molecular Nutrition & Food Research*. Vol. 63, no. 4. (February 2019): e1800795. doi: 10.1002 /mnfr.201800795.

97. Huang DD, et al "Nrf2 Deficiency Exacerbates Frailty and Sarcopenia by Impairing Skeletal Muscle Mitochondrial Biogenesis and Dynamics in an Age-Dependent Manner." *Experimental Gerontology*. Vol. 119. (January 25, 2019): 617–3. doi: 10.1016/j.exger.2019.01.022.

98. Piechota-Polanczyk A, Kopacz A, Kloska D, Zgrapan B, Neumayer C, Grochot-Przeczek A, Huk I, Brostjan C, Dulak J, Jozkowicz A."Simvastatin Treatment Upregulates HO-1 in Patients with Abdominal Aortic Aneurysm but Independently of Nrf2." *Oxidative Medicine and Cellular Longevity*. Vol. 2018, no. 28. (March 2018.) doi: 10.1155/2018/2028936.

99. Smith RE, Tran K, Smith CC, McDonald M, Shejwalkar P, Hara K"The Role of the

Nrf2/ARE Antioxidant System in Preventing Cardiovascular Diseases." *Oxidative Medicine and Cellular Longevity.* Vol. 4, no. 4. (December 2016): 34.

100. Jang HJ, Hong EM, Kim M, Kim JH, Jang J, Park SW, Byun HW, Koh DH, Choi MH, Kae SH, Lee J. "Simvastatin Induces Heme Oxygenase-1 via NF-E2-Related Factor 2 (Nrf2) Activation through ERK and PI3K/Akt Pathway in Colon Cancer." *Oncotarget.* Vol. 7, no. 29. (July 19, 2016): 46219-46229. doi: 10.18632/oncotarget.10078.

101. Leonardo CC, Doré S. "Dietary Flavonoids Are Neuroprotective through Nrf2-Coordinated Induction of Endogenous Cytoprotective Proteins." *Nutritional Neuroscience.* Vol. 14, no. 5. (September 2011): 226–236. doi: 10.1179/1476830511Y.0000000013.

102. Kumar H, Kim IS, More SV, Kim BW, Choi DK. "Natural Product-Derived Pharmacological Modulators of Nrf2/ARE Pathway for Chronic Disease." *Natural Products Reports.* Vol. 31, no. 1. (January 2014): 109–139.

103. Baird L, Dinkova-Kostova AT. "The Cytoprotective Role of the Keap1-Nrf2 Pathway." *Archives of Toxicology.* Vol. 85, no. 4. (April 2011): 241–272.

104. Gao B, Doan A, Hybertson BM. "The Clinical Potential of Nrf2 Signaling in Degenerative and Immunological Disorders." *Journal of Clinical Pharmacology.* Vol. 6. (2014): 19–34.

105. Sandberg M, Patil J, D'Angelo B, Weber SG, Mallard C. "NRF2-Regulation in Brain Health and Disease: Implication of Cerebral Inflammation." *Neuropharmacology.* Vol. 79. (2014): 298–306. doi: 10.1016/j .neuropharm.2013.11.004.

106. Seo HA, Lee IK. "The Role of Nrf2: Adipocyte Differentiation, Obesity, and Insulin Resistance." *Oxidative Medicine and Cellular Longevity.* Vol. 2013. (2013): 184598.

107. Pedruzzi LM, Stockler-Pinto MB, Leite M Jr., Mafra D. "Nrf2-keap1 System Versus NF-κB: The Good and the Evil in Chronic Kidney Disease?" *Biochimie.* Vol. 94, no. 12. (December 2012): 2461–2466. doi: 10.1016/j.biochi.2012.07.015.

108. Smolarek AK, So JY, Thomas PE, Lee HJ, Paul S, Dombrowski A, Wang CX, Saw CL, Khor TO, Kong AN, Reuhl K, Lee MJ, Yang CS, SUh N. "Dietary Tocopherols Inhibit Cell Proliferation, Regulate Expression of ERα, PPARγ, and Nrf2, and Decrease Serum Inflammatory Markers During the Development of Mammary Hyperplasia." *Molecular Carcinogenesis.* Vol. 52. (2013): 514–525. doi: 10.1002 /mc.21886.

109. Chen L, Yang R, Qiao W, Zhang W, Chen J, Mao L, Goltzman D, Miao D. "1,25-Dihydroxyvitamin D Exerts an Antiaging Role by Activation of Nrf2-Antioxidant Signaling and Inactivation of p16/p53-Senescence Signaling." *Aging Cell.* Vol. 18. (March 24, 2019): e 12951. doi: 10.1111/acel.12951.

110. Chen H, Xie K, Han H, Li Y, Liu L, Yang T, Yu Y. "Molecular Hydrogen Protects Mice Against Polymicrobial Sepsis by Ameliorating Endothelial Dysfunction via an Nrf2/HO-1 Signaling Pathway." *International Immunopharmacology.* Vol. 28, no. 1. (September 2015): 643–54.

111. Yu J, Zhang W, Zhang R, Jiang G, Tang H, Ruan X, Ren P, Lu B. "Molecular Hydrogen Attenuates Hypoxia/Reoxygenation Injury of Intrahepatic Cholangiocytes by Activating Nrf2 Expression." *Toxicology Letters.* Vol. 238, no.

3. (November 4, 2015): 11–9. doi: 10.1016/j.toxlet.2015.08.010.

112. Kawamura T, Wakabayashi N, Shigemura N, Huang CS, Masutani K, Tanaka Y, Noda K, Peng X, Takahashi T, Billiar TR, Okumura M, Toyoda Y, Kensler TW, Nakao A. "Hydrogen Gas Reduces Hyperoxic Lung Injury via the Nrf2 Pathway in Vivo." *American Journal of Physiology-Lung Cellular and Molecular Physiology.* Vol. 304, no. 10. (May 15, 2013): L646–L656. doi: 10.1152/ajplung.00164.2012.

113. Huang C, Wu J, Chen D, Jin J, Wu Y, Chen Z. "Effects of Sulforaphane in the Central Nervous System." *European Journal of Pharmacology.* Vol. 853. (June 15, 2019): 153–168. doi: 10.1016/j.ejphar.2019.03.010.

114. Singh S, Dubey V, Meena A, Siddiqui L, Maruya AK, Luqman S. "Rutin Restricts Hydrogen Peroxide-Induced Alterations by Up-Regulating the Redox-System: An in Vitro, in Vivo and in Silico Study." *European Journal of Pharmacology.* Vol. 835. (July 31, 2018): 115–125. doi: 10.1016/j.ejphar.2018.07.055.

115. Tian R. "Rutin Ameliorates Diabetic Neuropathy by Lowering Plasma Glucose and Decreasing Oxidative Stress via Nrf2 Signaling Pathway in Rats." *European Journal of Pharmacology.* Vol. 771. (January 15, 2016): 84–92. doi: 10.1016/j.ejphar.2015.12.021.

116. Chaiprasongsuk A, Onkoksoong T, Pluemsamran T, Limsaengurai S, Panich U. "Photoprotection by Dietary Phenolics against Melanogenesis through Nrf2-Dependent Antioxidant Responses." *Redox Biology.* Vol. 8. (August 2016): 79–90. doi: 10.1016/j.redox.2015.12.006.

117. Lee YJ, Lee DM, Lee SH. "Nrf2 Expression and Apoptosis in Quercetin-Treated Malignant Mesothelioma Cells" *Molecules and Cells.* Vol. 38, no. 5. (May 31, 2015): 416–425. doi: 10.14348/molcells.2015.2268.

118. Sun GY, Chen Z, Jasmer KJ, Chuang DY, Gu Z, Hannink M, Simonyi A. "Quercetin Attenuates Inflammatory Responses in BV-2 Microglial Cells: Role of MAPKs on the Nrf2 Pathway and Induction of Heme Oxygenase-1." *PLoS One.* Vol. 10, no. 10. (October 27, 2015): e0141509. doi: 10.1371/journal.pone.0141509.

119. Jin Y, Huang ZL, Li L, Yang Y, Wang CH, Wang ZT, Ji LL. "Quercetin Attenuates Toosendanin-Induced Hepatotoxicity through Inducing the Nrf2/GCL/GSH Antioxidant Signaling Pathway." *Acta Pharmacologica Sinica.* Vol. 40, no. 1. (January 2019): 75–85. doi: 10.1038/s41401-018-0024-8.

120. Miltonprabu S, Tomczyk M, Skalicka-Wózniak K, Rastrelli L, Daglia M, Nabavi SF, Alavian SM, Nabavi SM. "Hepatoprotective Effect of Quercetin: From Chemistry to Medicine." *Food and Chemical Toxicology.* Vol. 108, Part B. (October 2017): 365–374. doi: 10.1016/j.fct.2016.08.034.

121. Iranshahy M, Iranshsahi M, Abtahi SR, Karimi G. "The Role of Nuclear Factor Erythroid 2-Related Factor 2 in Hepatoprotective Activity of Natural Products: A Review." *Food and Chemical Toxicology.* Vol. 120. (October 2018): 261–276. doi: 10.1016/j.fct.2018.07.024.

122. Lu C, Zhang F, Xu W, Wu X, Lian N, Jin H, Chen Q, Chen L, Shao J, Wu L, Lu Y, Zheng S. "Curcumin Attenuates Ethanol-Induced Hepatic Steatosis through Modulating Nrf2/FXR Signaling in Hepatocytes." *IUBMB Life.* Vol. 67, no. 8. (August 2015 Aug): 645–58. doi: 10.1002/iub.1409.

123. Chen B, Zhang Y, Wang Y, Rao J, Jiang X, Xu Z. "Curcumin Inhibits Proliferation of Breast Cancer Cells through Nrf2-Mediated Down-Regulation of Fen1 Expression." *Journal of Steroid Biochemistry and Molecular Biology.* Vol. 143.

(September 2014): 11–8. doi: 10.1016/j.jsbmb.2014.01.009.

124. Zhang H, Zheng W, Feng X, Yang F, Qin H, Wu S, Hou DX, Chen J. "Nrf2–ARE Signaling Acts as Master Pathway for the Cellular Antioxidant Activity of Fisetin." *Molecules.* Vol. 24, no. 4. (2018): 708. doi: 10.3390/molecules24040708.

125. Elshaer M, Chen Y, Wang XJ, Tang X. "Resveratrol: An Overview of Its Anti-Cancer Mechanisms." *Life Sciences.* Vol. 207. (August 15, 2018): 340–349. doi: 10.1016/j.lfs.2018.06.028.

126. Cheng L, Jin Z, Zhao R, Ren K, Deng C, Yu S. "Resveratrol Attenuates Inflammation and Oxidative Stress Induced by Myocardial Ischemia-Reperfusion Injury: Role of Nrf2/ARE Pathway." *International Journal of Clinical and Experimental Medicine.* Vol. 8, no. 7. (2015): 10420–10428.

127. Singh B, Shoulson R, Chatterjee A, Ronghe A, Bhat NK, Dim DC, Bhat HK. "Resveratrol Inhibits Estrogen-Induced Breast Carcinogenesis through Induction of NRF2-Mediated Protective Pathways." *Carcinogenesis.* 2014 Aug; 35 (8): 1872–1880. doi: 10.1093/carcin/bgu120.

128. Kanzaki H, Shinohara F, Itohiya-Kasuya K, Ishikawa M, Nakamura Y. "Nrf2 Activation Attenuates Both Orthodontic Tooth Movement and Relapse." *Journal of Dental Research.* Vol. 94, no. 6. (June 2015): 787–94. doi: 10.1177/0022034515577814.
Kanlaya R, Khamchun S, Kapincharanon C, Thongboonkerd V. "Protective Epigallocatechin-3-Gallate (EGCG) via Nrf2 Pathway against Oxalate-Induced Epithelial Mesenchymal Transition (EMT) of Renal Tubular Cells." *Scientific Reports.* Vol. 6. (2016): 30233. doi: 10.1038/srep30233.

129. Wang D, Wang Y, Wan X, Yang CS, Zhang J. "Green Tea Polyphenol (-)-Epigallocatechin-3-Gallate Triggered Hepatotoxicity in Mice: Responses of Major Antioxidant Enzymes and the Nrf2 Rescue Pathway." *Toxicology and Applied Pharmacology.* Vol. 283, no. 1. (February 15, 2015): 65–74. doi: 10.1016/j.taap.2014.12.018.

130. Ibid.

131. Massini L, Rico D, Martin-Diana A, Barry-Ryan C. "Valorisation of Apple Peels." *European Journal of Food Research & Review.* Vol. 3, no. 1. (2013): 1–15. doi: 10.21427/D7R32T.

132. Shoji T, Akazome Y, Kanda T, Ikeda M. "The Toxicology and Safety of Apple Polyphenol Extract." *Food and Chemical Toxicology.* Vol. 42, no. 6. (2004): 959–967.

133. Li Y, Guo C, Yang J, Wei J, Xu J, Cheng S. "Evaluation of Antioxidant Properties of Pomegranate Peel Extract in Comparison with Pomegranate Pulp Extract." *Food Chemistry.* Vol. 96, no. 2. (2006): 254–260. doi: 10.1016/j.foodchem.2005.02.033.

134. Zhai X. Zhu C, Zhang Y, Sun J, Alim A, Yang X. "Chemical Characteristics, Antioxidant Capacities and Hepatoprotection of Polysaccharides from Pomegranate Peel." *Carbohydrate Polymers.* Vol. 202. (December 15, 2018): 461–469. doi: 10.1016/j.carbpol.2018.09.013.

135. Imperatori F, Barlozzari G, Scardigli A, Romani A, Macri G, Polinori N, Bernin R, Santi L. "Leishmanicidal Activity of Green Tea Leaves and Pomegranate Peel Extracts on *L. infantum*." *Natural Products Research.* (June 4, 2018): 1–7. doi:

10.1080/14786419.2018.1481841.

136. Ho CY, Cheng YT, Chau CF, Yen GC. "Effect of Diallyl Sulfide on in Vitro and in Vivo Nrf2-Mediated Pulmonic Antioxidant Enzyme Expression via Activation ERK/p38 Signaling Pathway." *Journal of Agricultural and Food Chemistry*. Vol. 60. (2012): 100–107. doi: 10.1021/jf203800d.

137. Colín-González AL, Santana RA, Silva-Islas CA, Chánez-Cárdenas ME, Santamaría A, Maldonado PD. "The Antioxidant Mechanisms Underlying the Aged Garlic Extract and S-Allylcysteine-Induced Protection." *Oxidative Medicine and Cellular Longevity*. Vol. 2012, no. 3. (May 2012): 907162. doi: 10.1155/2012/907162.

138. Hsieh TC, Elangovan S, Wu JM. "Differential Suppression of Proliferation in MCF-7 and MDA-MB-231 Breast Cancer Cells Exposed to Alpha-, Gamma- and Delta-Tocotrienols Is Accompanied by Altered Expression of Oxidative Stress Modulatory Enzymes." *Anticancer Research*. Vol. 30. (2010): 4169–4176.

139. Sontag TJ, Parker RS. "Influence of Major Structural Features of Tocopherols and Tocotrienols on Their Omega-Oxidation by Tocopherol-Omega-Hydroxylase." *Journal of Lipid Research*. Vol. 48, no. 5. (May 2007): 1090–1098.

140. Esatbeyoglu T, Rodriguez-Werner M, Schlösser A, Winterhalter P, Rimbach G. "Fractionation, Enzyme Inhibitory and Cellular Antioxidant Activity of Bioactives from Purple Sweet Potato (Ipomoea Batatas)." *Food Chemistry*. Vol. 221. (April 15, 2017): 447–456. doi: 10.1016/j.foodchem.2016.10.077.

141. Hwang YP, Choi JH, Choi JM, Chung YC, Jeong HG. "Protective Mechanisms of Anthocyanins from Purple Sweet Potato Against Tert-Butyl Hydroperoxide-Induced Hepatotoxicity." *Food and Chemical Toxicology*. Vol. 49, no. 9. (September 2011): 2081–9. doi: 10.1016/j.fct.2011.05.021.

142. Hwang YP, Choi JH, Yun HJ, Han EH, Kim HG, Kim JY, Park BH, Khanal T, Choi JM, Chung YC, Jeong HG. "Anthocyanins from Purple Sweet Potato Attenuate Dimethylnitrosamine-Induced Liver Injury in Rats by Inducing Nrf2-Mediated Antioxidant Enzymes and Reducing COX-2 and iNOS Expression." *Food and Chemical Toxicology*. Vol. 49, no. 1. (January, 2011): 93–9. doi: 10.1016/j.fct.2010.10.002.

143. Wu Q, Wang HD, Zhang X, Yu Q, Li W, Zhou ML, Wang XL."Astaxanthin Activates Nuclear Factor Erythroid-Related Factor 2 and the Antioxidant Responsive Element (Nrf2-ARE) Pathway in the Brain after Subarachnoid Hemorrhage in Rats and Attenuates Early Brain Injury." *Marine Drugs*. Vol. 12, no. 12. (December 2014): 6125–6141. doi: 10.3390/md12126125.

144. Saw CL, Yang AY, Guo Y, Kong AN. "Astaxanthin and Omega-3 Fatty Acids Individually and in Combination Protect Against Oxidative Stress via the Nrf2-ARE Pathway." *Food and Chemical Toxicology*. Vol. 62. (December 2013): 869–75. doi: 10.1016/j.fct.2013.10.023.

145. Feng Y, Chu A, Luo Q, Wu M, Shi X, Chen Y. "The Protective Effect of Astaxanthin on Cognitive Function via Inhibition of Oxidative Stress and Inflammation in the Brains of Chronic T2DM Rats." *Frontiers in Pharmacology*. Vol. 9. (July 2018): 748. doi: 10.3389/fphar.2018.00748.

146. Saito H. "Toxico-Pharmacological Perspective of the Nrf2- Keap1 Defense System against Oxidative Stress in Kidney Diseases." *Biochemical Pharmacology*. Vol. 85,

no. 7. (April 2013): 865–872. doi: 10.1016/j.bcp.2013.01.006.

147. Pedruzzi LM, Stockler-Pinto MB, Leite M Jr, Mafra D. "Nrf2-keap1 System Versus NF-κB: The Good and the Evil in Chronic Kidney Disease?" *Biochimie.* Vol. 94, no. 12. (December 2012): 2461–2466. doi: 10.1016/j.biochi.2012.07.015.

148. Loboda A, Rojczyk-Golebiewska E, Bednarczyk-Cwynar B, Lucjusz Z, Jozkowicz A, Dulak J. "Targeting nrf2-Mediated Gene Transcription by Triterpenoids and Their Derivatives." *Biomolecules & Therapeutics (Seoul).* Vol. 20. (2012): 499–505. doi: 10.4062/biomolther.2012.20.6.499.

149. Vomhof-Dekrey EE, Picklo MJ Sr. "The Nrf2-Antioxidant Response Element Pathway: A Target for Regulating Energy Metabolism." *Journal of Nutritional Biochemistry.* Vol. 23, no. 10. (October 2012): 1201–1206. doi: 10.1016/j.jnutbio.2012.03.005.

150. Liby KT, Sporn MB. "Synthetic Oleanane Triterpenoids: Multifunctional Drugs with a Broad Range of Applications for Prevention and Treatment of Chronic Disease." *Pharmacological Reviews.* Vol. 64, no. 4. (October 2012): 972–1003. doi: 10.1124/pr.111.004846.

151. Jiang XY, Zhu XS, Xu HY, Zhao ZX, Li SY, Li SZ, Cai JH, Cao JM. "Diallyl Trisulfide Suppresses Tumor Growth through the Attenuation of Nrf2/Akt and Activation of p38/JNK and Potentiates Cisplatin Efficacy in Gastric Cancer Treatment." *Acta Pharmacologica Sinica.* Vol. 38, no. 7. (July 2017): 1048-1058. doi: 10.1038/aps.2016.176.

152. Yang CM, Huang SM, Liu CL, Hu ML. "Apo-8'-Lycopenal Induces Expression of HO-1 and NQO-1 via the ERK/p38- Nrf2-ARE Pathway in Human HepG2 Cells." *Journal of Agricultural and Food Chemistry.* Vol. 60, no. 6. (February 2012): 1576–1585. doi: 10.1021/jf204451n.

153. Linnewiel K, Ernst H, Caris-Veyrat C, Ben-Dor A, Kampf A, Salman H, Danilenko M, Levy J, Sharoni Y. "Structure Activity Relationship of Carotenoid Derivatives in Activation of the Electrophile/Antioxidant Response Element Transcription System." *Free Radical Biology & Medicine.* Vol. 47, no. 5. (September 2009): 659–667.

154. Zhang M, Wang S, Mao L, Leak RK, Shi Y, Zhang W, Hu X, Sun B, Cao G, Gao Y, Xu Y, Chen J, Zhang F. "Omega-3 Fatty Acids Protect the Brain against Ischemic Injury by Activating Nrf2 and Upregulating Heme Oxygenase 1." *Journal of Neuroscience.* Vol. 34. (2014): 1903–1915. doi: 10.1016/j .freeradbiomed.2009.06.008.

155. Nakagawa F, Morino K, Ugi S, Ishikado A, Kondo K, Sato D, Konno S, Nemoto K, Kusunoki C, Sekine O, Sunagawa A, Kawamura M, Inoue N, Nishio Y, Maegawa H. "4-Hydroxy Hexenal Derived from Dietary n-3 Polyunsaturated Fatty Acids Induces Anti-Oxidative Enzyme Heme Oxygenase-1 in Multiple Organs." *Biochemistry and Biophysical Research Communications.* Vol. 43. (2014): 991–996. doi: 10.1016/j.bbrc.2013.12.085.

156. Maher J, Yamamoto M. "The Rise of Antioxidant Signaling—The Evolution and Hormetic Actions of Nrf2." *Toxicology in Applied Pharmacology.* Vol. 244, no. 1. (April 2010): 4–15.

157. Ahmadi Z, Ashrafizadeh M. "Melatonin as a Potential Modulator of Nrf2." *Fundamental & Clinical Pharmacology.* (July 8, 2019). doi: 10.1111/fcp.12498.

158. Uwitonze AM, Razzaque MS. "Role of Magnesium in Vitamin D Activation and Function." *Journal of the American Osteopathic Association.* Vol. 118, no. 3.

(March 1, 2018): 181–189. doi: 10.7556/jaoa.2018.037.

159. Houston M. "The Role of Magnesium in Hypertension and Cardiovascular Disease." *Journal of Clinical Hypertension (Greenwich)*. Vol. 13, no. 11. (November 2011): 843–7. doi: 10.1111/j.1751-7176.2011.00538.x.

160. Bertinato J. "Magnesium Deficiency: Prevalence, Assessment, and Physiological Effects." *Handbook of Famine, Starvation, and Nutrient Deprivation*. December 2016. doi: 10.1007/978-3-319-40007-5_6-1.

161. Liu G, Weinger JG, Lu ZL, Xue F, Sadeghpour S. "Efficacy and Safety of MMFS-01, a Synapse Density Enhancer, for Treating Cognitive Impairment in Older Adults: A Randomized, Double-Blind, Placebo-Controlled Trial." *Journal of Alzheimer's Disease*. Vol. 49, no. 4. (2016): 971–90.

Chapter 7: How to Reduce Your EMF Exposure

1. Wall S, Wang ZM, Kendig T, Dobraca D, Lipsett M. "Real-World Cell Phone Radiofrequency Electromagnetic Field Exposures." *Environmental Research*. Vol. 171. (April 2019): 581–592. doi: 10.1016/j.envres.2018.09.015.

2. Havas M, Illiatovitch M, Proctor C. "Teacher Student Response to the Removal of Dirty Electricity." Presented at 3rd International Workshop on the Biological Effects of EMFS, October 4–8, 2004. Kos, Greece. http://electricalpollution.com/documents/WWcolour.pdf.

3. Wilkins A, Veitch J, Lehman B. "LED Lighting Flicker and Potential Health Concerns: IEEE Standard PAR1789 Update." Institute of Electrical and Electronics Engineers. September 1, 2010. Doi: 10.1109/ECCE.2010.5618050.https://ece.northeastern.edu/groups/power/lehman/Publications/Pub2010/2010_9_Wilkins.pdf

4. David Goldman. "Your Samsung TV Is Eavesdropping on Your Private Conversations." CNN Business. February 10, 2015. https://money.cnn.com/2015/02/09/technology/security/samsung-smart-tv-privacy/index.html.

5. Matt Day, Giles Turner, and Natalia Drozdiak. "Amazon Workers Are Listening to What You Tell Alexa." Bloomberg. April 10, 2019. https://www.bloomberg.com/news/articles/2019-04-10/is-anyone-listening-to-you-on-alexa-a-global-team-reviews-audio.

6. Samuel Burke. "Google Admits Its New Smart Speaker Was Eavesdropping on Users." CNN Business. October 12, 2017. https://money.cnn.com/2017/10/11/technology/google-home-mini-security-flaw/index.html.

7. Davies N, Griffin DW. "Effect of Metal-Framed Spectacles on Microwave Radiation Hazards to the Eyes of Humans." *Medical and Biological Engineering and Computing*. Vol. 27, no. 22. (March 1989): 191–97.

8. "How Safe Is a Wireless Baby Monitor?" CBS Local 2, posted by EMFAnalysis on November 22, 2014. https://www.youtube.com/watch?v=1WONwXP5lvM.

9. "EMF Radiation Blocked! Smart Meter EMF Radiation Protection." Smart Meter Guard. January 24, 2013. https://www.youtube.com/watch?v=cmS5pVEZHzg.

Chapter 8: The Path from Here

1. Mark Hertsgaard and Mark Dowie. "How Big Wireless Made Us Think That Cell Phones Are Safe: A Special Investigation." *The Nation.* March 29, 2018. https://www.thenation.com/article/how-big-wireless-made-us-think-that-cell-phones-are-safe-a-special-investigation/.

2. Sarah Ryle. "Insurers Balk at Risk from Phones." *The Guardian.* April 10, 1999. https://www.theguardian.com/uk/1999/apr/11/sarahryle.theobserver.

3. "Lloyd's Emerging Risks Team Report." November 2010, version 2.0. http://s3.amazonaws.com/eakes-production/file_attachments/25/lloyds_of_london_emf_final_november_2010.pdf. (From https://www.joneakes.com/jons-fixit-database/2235-lloyds-of-london-bails-out-of-the-cell-phone-health-debate.)

4. MedSurance A&M Policy Document. U.S. Version 3.2 CFC Underwriting (backed by Lloyd's of London). http://www.eperils.com/pol/cfc-a&mcmb-v32.pdf.

5. Available from the company's website, at https://investor.crowncastle.com/financial-information/annual-reports.

6. Timothy Schoechle, Ph.D. "Re-Inventing Wires: The Future of Landlines and Networks." The National Institute for Science, Law, and Public Policy. 2008. http://electromagnetichealth.org/wp-content/uploads/2018/02/ReInventing-Wires-1-25-18.pdf.

Appendix A: Damaging Effects of Excessive Peroxynitrite

1. Pacher P, Beckman JS, Liaudet L. "Nitric Oxide and Peroxynitrite in Health and Disease." *Physiological Reviews.* Vol. 87, no. 1. (January 2007): 315-424. doi: 10.1152/physrev.00029.2006.

2. Arteel GE, Briviba K, Sies H. "Protection Against Peroxynitrite." *FEBS Letters.* Vol. 445, no. 2-3. (1999): 226–230. doi: 10.1016/s0014-5793(99)00073-3.

3. Salvemini D, Doyle TM, Cuzzocrea S. "Superoxide, Peroxynitrite and Oxidative/Nitrative Stress in Inflammation." *Biochemical Society Transactions.* Vol. 34, part 5. (November 2006): 965-70. doi: 10.1042/BST0340965.

4. Bartesaghi S, Radi R. "Fundamentals on the Biochemistry of Peroxynitrite and Protein Tyrosine Nitration." *Redox Biology.* Vol. 14. (April 2018): 618–625. doi: 10.1016/j.redox.2017.09.009.

5. Choudhari S, Chaudhary M, Badge S, Gadbail AR, Joshi V. "Nitric Oxide and Cancer: A Review." *World Journal of Surgical Oncology.* Vol. 11. (May 30, 2013): 118. doi: 10.1186/1477-7819-11-118.

6. Singh IN, Sullivan PG, Hall ED. "Peroxynitrite-Mediated Oxidative Damage to Brain Mitochondria: Protective Effects of Peroxynitrite Scavengers." *Journal of Neuroscience Research.* Vol. 85, no. 10. (August 1, 2007): 2216-2223. doi: 10.1002/jnr.21360.

7. Cai Z, Yan LJ. "Protein Oxidative Modifications: Beneficial Roles in Disease and Health." *Journal of Biochemical and Pharmacological Research.* Vol. 1, no. 1. (March 2013): 15-26.

8. Nita M, Grzybowski A. "The Role of the Reactive Oxygen Species and Oxidative Stress in the Pathomechanism of the Age-Related Ocular Diseases and Other Pathologies of the Anterior and Posterior Eye Segments in Adults." *Oxidative Medicine and Cellular Longevity.* Vol. 2016. (2016): 3164734. doi: 10.1155/2016/3164734.

9. MacMillan-Crow LA, Thompson JA. "Tyrosine Modifications and Inactivation of Active Site Manganese Superoxide Dismutase Mutant (Y34F) by Peroxynitrite." *Archives of Biochemistry and Biophysics.* Vol. 366, no. 1. (June 1, 1999): 82-88. doi: 10.1006/abbi.1999.1202.

10. Van der Veen RC, Roberts LJ. "Contrasting Roles for Nitric Oxide and Peroxynitrite in the Peroxidation of Myelin Lipids." *Journal of Neuroimmunology.* Vol. 95, no. 1-2. (March 1, 1999): 1-7. doi: 10.1016/s0165-5728(98)00239-2.

11. Schmidt P, Youhnovski N, Daiber A, Balan A, Arsic M, Bachschmid M, Przybylski M, Ullrich V. "Specific Nitration at Tyrosine 430 Revealed by High Resolution Mass Spectrometry as Basis for Redox Regulation of Bovine Prostacyclin Synthase." *Journal of Biological Chemistry.* Vol. 278, no. 15. (April 11, 2003): 12813-12819. doi: 10.1074/jbc.M208080200.

12. Bartesaghi S, Radi R. "Fundamentals on the Biochemistry of Peroxynitrite and Protein Tyrosine Nitration." *Redox Biology.* Vol. 14. (April 2018): 618–625. doi: 10.1016/j.redox.2017.09.009.

13. Lee DY, Wauquier F, Eid AA, Roman LJ, Ghosh-Choudhury G, Khazim K, Block K, Gorin Y. "NADPH Oxidase Mediates Peroxynitrite-Dependent Uncoupling of Endothelial Nitric-Oxide Synthase and Fibronectin Expression in Response to Angiotensin II: Role of Mitochondrial Reactive Oxygen Species." *Journal of Biological Chemistry.* Vol. 288, no. 40 (October 4, 2013): 28668-28686. doi: 10.1074/jbc.M113.470971.

14. Gochman E, Mahajna J, Reznick AZ. "NF-κB Activation by Peroxynitrite through IκBα-Dependent Phosphorylation versus Nitration in Colon Cancer Cells." *Anticancer Research.* Vol. 31, no. 5. (May 2011): 1607-1617.

15. Kuzkaya N, Weissmann N, Harrison DG, Dikalov S. "Interactions of Peroxynitrite with Uric Acid in the Presence of Ascorbate and Thiols: Implications for Uncoupling Endothelial Nitric Oxide Synthase." *Biochemical Pharmacology.* Vol. 70, no. 3. (August 1, 2005): 343-354. doi: 10.1016/j.bcp.2005.05.009.

16. Pall ML. "The NO/ONOO-Cycle as the Central Cause of Heart Failure." *International Journal of Molecular Sciences.* Vol. 14, no. 11. (November 2013): 22274–22330. doi: 10.3390/ijms141122274.

17. Case AJ. "On the Origin of Superoxide Dismutase: An Evolutionary Perspective of Superoxide-Mediated Redox Signaling." *Antioxidants (Basel).* Vol. 6, no. 4 (October 30, 2017): 82. doi: 10.3390/antiox6040082.

INDEX

ACKNOWLEDGMENTS

It took me three years to compile the information for and write this book and there were many people who helped to improve my ability to translate much of this complex and technical information so it would serve as a practical guide for you.

Would first like to express my appreciation to my sister Janet, who has worked with me since I first started my medical practice in 1985. She now serves as chief editor for my website, mercola.com, and has greatly helped with the editing of this book, for which I am grateful.

Kate Hanley is a professional writer and helped to convert my initial drafts into more compelling reader-friendly text that will make it more usable for you.

I also asked many of the leading experts on various aspects of EMF science to review the portions of this manuscript that relate to their areas of expertise. I am thankful for all of their thoughtful comments, additions, and recommendations:

- Brian Hoyer is an expert in EMF remediation who has personally helped me remediate my home and remove stealth EMF sources. He added valuable perspectives in Chapter 7 on how to remediate your home. He is in the process of training others so they can provide similar service. His website is https://shielded-healing.com/.

- Martha Herbert, M.D., Ph.D., is an assistant professor of neurology at Harvard Medical School, a pediatric neurologist and neuroscientist at the Massachusetts General Hospital in Boston, and an affiliate of the Harvard-MIT-MGH Martinos Center for Biomedical Imaging, where she is director of the TRANSCEND Research Program (Treatment Research and Neuroscience Evaluation of Neurodevelopmental Disorders).

- Stephanie Seneff, Ph.D., is a senior research scientist at the Computer Science and Artificial Intelligence Laboratory of the Massachusetts Institute of Technology. She has published groundbreaking research on the molecular mechanisms of how glyphosate damages humans.

- Sharon Goldberg, M.D., is a board-certified internal medicine practitioner and a voluntary associate professor at the University of New Mexico School of Medicine.

- Magda Haavas, Ph.D., is an associate professor at Trent University. Since the 1990s, Dr. Havas's research has investigated the biological effects of electromagnetic pollution including radio frequency radiation, electromagnetic fields, dirty electricity, and ground current. She works with diabetics as well as with individuals who have multiple sclerosis, tinnitus, chronic fatigue, fibromyalgia and those who are electrically hypersensitive. She also conducts research on sick-building syndrome as it relates to power quality in schools.

- James Clement is one of the leading clinical researchers on life extension and NAD+. He ran the Supercentenarian Research Study (www.supercentenarianstudy.com) and is founder of the 501(c)(3) non-profit scientific research organization Betterhumans (www.betterhumans.org).

- Peter Sullivan is the founder and CEO of Clear Light Ventures, Inc., a prominent funder of environmental health research. He is based in Silicon Valley and has had many personal and family experiences with recovering from EMF exposures.

- Nicolas Pineault is a health journalist who has published more than 1,500 online articles through a daily newsletter called Nick & Gen's Healthy Life. In 2017, he authored *The Non-Tinfoil Guide to EMFs*—an unconventional book that combines common sense and humor to tackle the very serious topic of electromagnetic pollution and its effects on human health.

- Oram Miller is a leader in the field of building biology. He remediates many homes and is an active teacher to those seeking to learn this field. He provided valuable insights on the remediation strategies in Chapter 7, as he is in the trenches every day helping people sort through their EMF challenges.

- Alasdair Phillips is an electrical engineer who has been instrumental in organizing international conferences on the causes of childhood cancer. He is one of the leading experts on the biological effects of EMFs in the UK. His websites are emfields-solutions.com and power-watch.org.uk.

- Lloyd Burrell is an EMF author and founder of the site https://www.electricsense.com, which has helped thousands sort through the confusing topic of EMF pollution and provided powerful practical resources, and also contributed to the meter options in the resource section.

- Arthur Firstenberg is a passionate advocate of EMF safety. He has written two books, *Microwaving Our Planet: The Environmental Impact of the Wireless Revolution* and *The Invisible Rainbow*.

- Alex Tarnava is a brilliant researcher whose work has allowed the practical application of molecular hydrogen as a tool to improve health.

ABOUT THE AUTHOR

Dr. Joseph Mercola is a physician and *New York Times* best-selling author. He was voted the Ultimate Wellness Game Changer by the *Huffington Post* and has been featured in several national media outlets, including *Time* magazine, the *Los Angeles Times*, CNN, Fox News, ABC News, *TODAY*, and *The Dr. Oz Show*. He founded hjs website: mercola.com in 1997 well before Google, Amazon and Facebook, and it has been the most visited natural health site on the web for the last 15 years.

Website: mercola.com

Hay House Titles of Related Interest

YOU CAN HEAL YOUR LIFE, the movie,
starring Louise Hay & Friends
(available as a 1-DVD program, an expanded 2-DVD set,
and an online streaming video)
Learn more at www.hayhouse.com/louise-movie

THE SHIFT, the movie, starring Dr. Wayne W. Dyer
(available as a 1-DVD program, an expanded 2-DVD set,
and an online streaming video)
Learn more at www.hayhouse.com/the-shift-movie

***

KETOFAST: Rejuvenate Your Health with a Step-by-Step Guide
to Timing Your Ketogenic Meals, by Dr. Joseph Mercola

SUPERFUEL: Ketogenic Keys to Unlock the Secrets of Good Fats, Bad Fats,
and Great Health, by Dr. James DiNicolantonio and Dr. Joseph Mercola

FAT FOR FUEL: A Revolutionary Diet to Combat Cancer, Boost Brain Power,
and Increase Your Energy, by Dr. Joseph Mercola

All of the above are available at your local bookstore,
or may be ordered by contacting Hay House (see next page).

We hope you enjoyed this Hay House book. If you'd like to receive our online catalog featuring additional information on Hay House books and products, or if you'd like to find out more about the Hay Foundation, please contact:

Hay House, Inc., P.O. Box 5100, Carlsbad, CA 92018-5100
(760) 431-7695 or (800) 654-5126
(760) 431-6948 (fax) or (800) 650-5115 (fax)
www.hayhouse.com® • www.hayfoundation.org

———

Published in Australia by: Hay House Australia Pty. Ltd.,
18/36 Ralph St., Alexandria NSW 2015
Phone: 612-9669-4299 • *Fax:* 612-9669-4144
www.hayhouse.com.au

Published in the United Kingdom by: Hay House UK, Ltd.,
The Sixth Floor, Watson House, 54 Baker Street, London W1U 7BU
Phone: +44 (0)20 3927 7290 • *Fax:* +44 (0)20 3927 7291
www.hayhouse.co.uk

Published in India by: Hay House Publishers India,
Muskaan Complex, Plot No. 3, B-2, Vasant Kunj, New Delhi 110 070
Phone: 91-11-4176-1620 • *Fax:* 91-11-4176-1630
www.hayhouse.co.in

———

Access New Knowledge.
Anytime. Anywhere.

Learn and evolve at your own pace
with the world's leading experts.

www.hayhouseU.com

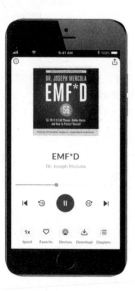

Free e-newsletters
from Hay House, the Ultimate
Resource for Inspiration

Be the first to know about Hay House's free downloads, special offers, giveaways, contests, and more!

 Get exclusive excerpts from our latest releases and videos from *Hay House Present Moments*.

 Our *Digital Products Newsletter* is the perfect way to stay up-to-date on our latest discounted eBooks, featured mobile apps, and Live Online and On Demand events.

 Learn with real benefits! *HayHouseU.com* is your source for the most innovative online courses from the world's leading personal growth experts. Be the first to know about new online courses and to receive exclusive discounts.

 Enjoy uplifting personal stories, how-to articles, and healing advice, along with videos and empowering quotes, within *Heal Your Life*.

Sign Up Now!

Get inspired, educate yourself, get a complimentary gift, and share the wisdom!

Visit www.hayhouse.com/newsletters to sign up today!